MW01621199

Prentice Hall Advanced Reference Series 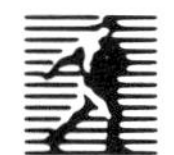

Physical and Life Sciences

PRENTICE HALL
Biophysics and Bioengineering Series

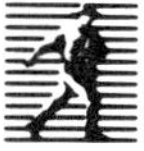

Abraham Noordergraaf, Series Editor

AGNEW AND MCCREERY, EDS. *Neural Prostheses: Fundamental Studies*
ALPEN *Radiation Biophysics*
DAWSON *Engineering Design of the Cardiovascular System of Mammals*
GANDHI, ED. *Biological Effects and Medical Applications of Electromagnetic Energy*
LLEBOT AND JOU *Introduction to the Thermodynamics of Biological Processes*
RIDEOUT *Mathematical and Computer Modeling of Physiological Systems*

FORTHCOMING BOOKS IN THIS SERIES (*tentative titles*)

COLEMAN *Integrative Human Physiology: A Quantitative View of Homeostasis*
FOX *Fundamentals of Medical Imaging*
GRODZINSKY *Fields, Forces, and Flows in Biological Tissues and Membranes*
HUANG *Principles of Biomedical Image Processing*
MAYROVITZ *Analysis of Microcirculation*
SCHERER *Respiratory Fluid Mechanics*
VAIDHYANATHAN *Regulation and Control in Biological Systems*
WAAG *Theory and Measurement of Ultrasound Scattering in Biological Media*

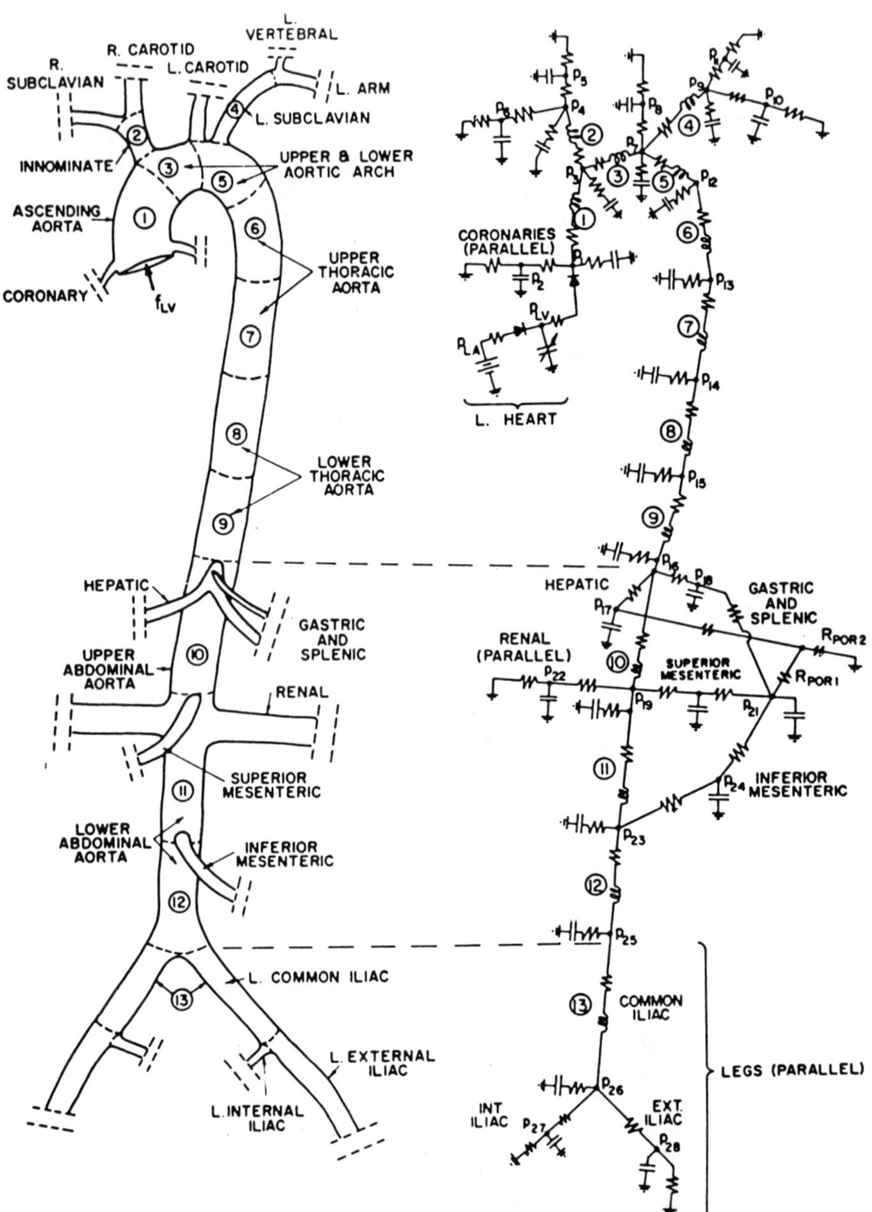

The human arterial system, shown on the left above may be discretized into thirteen major and thirteen minor segments for modeling, as shown in convenient circuit form on the right. The thirty-nine first-order differential equations describing this model may be solved by computer methods to find good approximations to pressure, flow and volume waveforms. (From Snyder-68 in references in Chap. 4, with permission).

Mathematical and Computer Modeling of Physiological Systems

Vincent C. Rideout

Electrical and Computer
Engineering Department
Department of Anesthesiology

University of Wisconsin-Madison

PRENTICE HALL
Englewood Cliffs, New Jersey 07632

Library of Congress Cataloging-in-Publication Data

Rideout, Vincent C.
Mathematical and computer modeling of physiological systems / Vincent C. Rideout.
p. cm.
Includes bibliographical references and index.
ISBN 0-13-563354-0
1. Physiology—Computer simulation. 2. Physiology—Mathematical models. I. Title.
QP33.6.D38R53 1991
612'.001'13—dc20 90-40755
CIP

Editorial/production supervision
and interior design: Laura A. Huber
Cover design: Wanda Lubelska Design
Manufacturing buyers: Kelly Behr/Susan Brunke
Acquisitions Editor: Mike Hays

Prentice Hall Advanced Reference Series
Prentice Hall Biophysics and Bioengineering Series

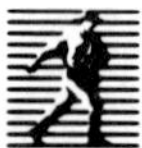

The publisher offers discounts on this book when ordered in bulk quantities. For more information, write:

Special Sales/College Marketing
College Technical and Reference Division
Prentice Hall
Englewood Cliffs, New Jersey 07632

Printed in the United States of America
10 9 8 7 6 5 4 3 2 1

ISBN 0-13-563354-0

Prentice-Hall International (UK) Limited, *London*
Prentice-Hall of Australia Pty. Limited, *Sydney*
Prentice-Hall Canada Inc., *Toronto*
Prentice-Hall Hispanoamericana, S.A., *Mexico*
Prentice-Hall of India Private Limited, *New Delhi*
Prentice-Hall of Japan, Inc., *Tokyo*
Simon & Schuster Asia Pte. Ltd., *Singapore*
Editora Prentice-Hall do Brasil, Ltda., *Rio de Janeiro*

Dedicated to the memory of my son
Vincent Leo Rideout

Contents

Preface

This book was written to assist students and researchers needing an introduction to physiological modeling using the powerful personal computers and convenient software now available at reasonable cost. The author has used an IBM/AT with Fortran software and ACSL, a differential equation–solving program that translates system equations into Fortran for solution. Other computers of the same or better speed and memory may be used, with ACSL or related software, as discussed in Appendix A. Students in the author's classes in modeling have used ACSL (and thus Fortran) working from terminals attached to a large mainframe computer; other students have used workstations.

A primary objective of this book is to provide the reader with a guide to mathematical modeling techniques and computer simulation methods for systems such as the respiratory, the cardiovascular, and the human thermal control systems. Of particular interest to the author is the combination of models for fluid pressure-flow systems with models for transport of substances carried into, through, and/or out of the body; such combined models are called *multiple models* in this book.

One might think that large multiple models representing the interconnection and action of dozens of differential equations would be too complex for many users, particularly students. This book attempts to show that the computer hardware and software now available, together with the modular principles of multiple modeling, make possible the simulation of more complete systems even for students who are new to computer modeling. The emphasis here on physically based modeling (as opposed to black box modeling), together with multiple modeling, leads to less approximation due to omission of subsystems and easier adjustment of the model detail to suit the needs of a given project. To save the users of this book time and effort in typing up code, many of the simulation programs discussed are provided on a disk available separately; these programs may be used for practice, but also will lead, it is hoped, to the development of new programs by modifying, combining, simplifying, or expanding the models as needed.

Acknowledgments

For the models in this book, as well as the modeling methods and the computer methods used here, the author owes much to many workers in this field. They include Jan Beneken, Gene Blackstone, Bram Noordergraaf, Fred Grodins, Jim Bassingthwaighte, Arthur Guyton, Ty Smith and Kiichi Sagawa, to name but a few. Here at Wisconsin, Frank Sasse and Ben Rusy in Anesthesiology, Jim Will in Veterinary Science, Dan Geisler in Neurophysiology and Ed Kendrick in Physiology have been most helpful over the years. My graduate students were a great source of help and inspiration: among the many who worked with me were my doctoral students, —Don Dick, Maurice Snyder, Dan Rukavina, Jim Sims, Yasu Fukui, John Gianunzio, Pao-Ping Chang, John Slate, George Szils, and Robert Tham. Helga Fack provided most of the artwork, and Al Moucha assisted in some changes and additions. Of great assistance in the final efforts of completing the manuscript were Liz Krug, working on problems of English expression, Jon Pfeffer and Jesse Olson, checking programs and designing student exercises, and Joe Gauthier, of Mitchell and Gauthier Associates, providing assistance in the more difficult aspects of ACSL programming.

Vincent C. Rideout
Madison, Wisconsin

1 Introduction to Biomodeling

1.0 SCOPE AND PURPOSE

This book is about the *mathematical modeling* of physiological systems and the *computer simulation* of these models; such modeling may be referred to as medical modeling or biomodeling. The word *system* means an interconnected set of elements that function in some coordinated fashion. Thus the human heart, with its muscles, nerves, and blood, may be regarded as a system; however, the heart is merely a subsystem of the entire circulatory system, which in turn is a subsystem of the entire body, which also contains many other subsystems such as the respiratory and renal systems.

The mathematical modeling of a physiological system results in a description in terms of equations, usually differential equations, chosen to describe the dynamic aspects of the system. Computers and numerical analysis software suitable for the simulation of such sets of differential equations are usually essential for the study of any but the simplest of models.

Although physiological modeling is now much more readily accepted than in recent decades when computers first began to make the easy simulation of models possible, such activities are still regarded with a certain suspicion because models often have severe limitations despite their complexities and costs. However, Rosenblueth and Wiener (Rosenblueth-45) most clearly expressed the importance of modeling when they pointed out that "partial models, imperfect as they may be, are the only means developed by science for understanding the universe." A number of introductory articles have appeared that deal with the philosophy and the rudiments of biomedical modeling (Apter-70, Groth-84, Bekey-77 and Bassingthwaighte-85); these and some of the several papers dealing with the history of modeling (referred to in the next section) may be of interest.

The mathematics and physiological knowledge needed to model many of the important biosystems have been available for some time, but the computers required were, until rather recently, quite large and expensive, and the specialized software needed was not generally available. Now powerful desktop computers and workstations with high level languages (see Section 2.4) make it relatively cheap and easy to simulate systems without simplifying them unrealistically.

Biomodeling has three principal uses:

1. *Research,* where it assists in verification of hypotheses and helps determine what tests will reveal more about the system being studied.
2. *Teaching and training,* as in medical school use of Dickinson's models, such as MacMan (Dickinson-73), MacPuf (Dickinson-72a) and MacPee (Dickinson-72b).
3. *Clinical applications,* where models may relate to diagnosis or aid in the determination of drug regimens. Another kind of clinical application is in the design of prostheses, such as artificial limbs, hearing aids, or automated insulin infusion systems (Hinds-83, Schils-83).

We will be concerned with all three uses, and it is quite possible for a given model to serve any or all of them. However, the design goals of a model are important, and attempts will be made to point out how models may be modified to suit the needs of a given study without omitting essential parts or adding more complexity than can be conveniently handled.

The modeling considered in this book relates particularly to the cardiovascular, respiratory, and endocrine systems, to the kinetics and dynamics of natural and pharmaceutical substances in the bloodstream and tissues, and to temperature regulation and heat transfer in the body. Certain aspects of the central nervous system are important to the effective modeling of these systems, particularly the feedback control or autonomic regulation systems of the body (Harmon-68). However, neural modeling cannot be treated in detail here, nor can some of the important mathematically oriented approaches to the detailed modeling required in problems such as the uptake of oxygen in tissue (Reneau-67).

When modeling physiological systems, we are concerned with various kinds of transport, as follows:

1. *Momentum transport.* In the wave equations describing blood flow, we are concerned with momentum, blood viscosity, and the elasticity of the vessel walls in determining pressures and flows of the system (see Chapter 4).
2. *Mass transport.* Blood carries many important substances, such as oxygen, carbon dioxide, and pharmaceutical substances. The diffusion of these substances into or out of tissue is often essential in a model.
3. *Energy transport.* The blood in our veins, as well as the air we breathe, carries heat energy; this heat may diffuse through tissues, though in a way different than the mass diffusion referred to above. Also, energy transformation, as well as transport, occurs in muscle tissue.
4. *Information transport.* Information is carried throughout the body by nerve fibers, much as messages are transmitted in a communication system. Hormones also carry information, moving mostly with the aid of the bloodstream (Slent-72).

A model requiring consideration of three of these kinds of transport (momentum, mass, and information) might be used to study computer control of the administration of halothane anesthesia (Lampard-73). Figure 1.0.1 shows such a model in block form (Fukui-81a, 81b, Schils-87). With adequate detail in the various blocks, this model might be set up on a computer to study the interaction of computer control of anesthesia with blood pressure control in the body (Tham-88). Furthermore, if body temperature were of importance, still another submodel might be added for heat flow and temperature regulation (see Chapter 7).

This model does not show the details that are required in each block, but it does illustrate the *modular* aspects of a typical model of rather advanced form and shows a few of the signal interconnections required. The difficulty of setting up and using such a model is greatly reduced by the modular form adopted here, giving what will be termed a *multiple model* (discussed in detail in Chapter 6). The simplification results because the individual blocks can be set up separately for study and test before combining them into the complete model (actually the model is never complete; here it might be desirable to add a carbon dioxide transport submodel, for example). Mass transport models are introduced in Chapter 3, models of blood pressure and flow in Chapter 4, and respiratory models of both kinds in Chapter 5, together with a first example of a simulation using multiple modeling.

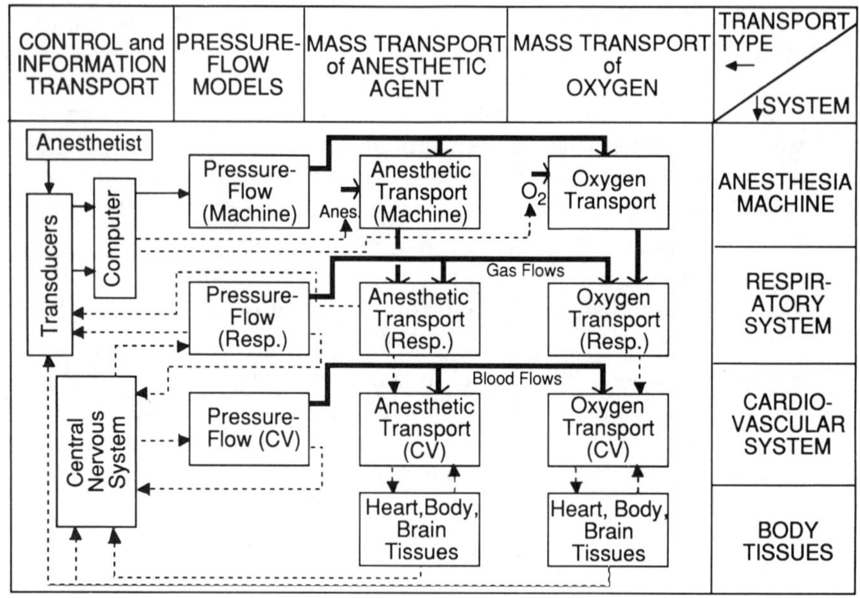

Figure 1.0.1. Block diagram of a model of computer-controlled halothane anesthesia. In this model a control-system computer accepts halothane end-tidal level and oxygen partial pressure signals from transducers. These inputs and a set-point input provided by the anesthetist are used to activate the controls of the anesthesia machine according to some chosen computer algorithm, and this in turn causes desired levels of halothane and oxygen to be maintained. The model also has interconnected blocks (eleven in all) for pressure-flow dynamics and for halothane and oxygen transport in the anesthesia machine, the respiratory system, the cardiovascular system, and the body tissues.

Large multiple models of this kind require that a number of algebraic and differential equations be written for each block and (still more difficult) that reasonably correct numerical values be determined for use in these equations. The determination and checking of the equations and their associated numerical values may require animal experimentation and human clinical data, unless adequate information is available in the literature. In fact, the work of building a model is itself a most important learning experience. In typical research uses of the model, experiments will be run that correspond to problems too difficult or tedious to solve by hand calculation. It is interesting that such studies often indicate that the model may be greatly simplified, something that may be important in redesigns of the anesthesia controller. Thus an example much like the one in Figure 1.0.1 (discussed in some detail in Chapter 6) may bear upon all three of the uses of biomodeling: teaching, research, and clinical applications.

1.1 HISTORY OF PHYSIOLOGICAL SYSTEM MODELING

Modeling may be said to go as far back as medical research, and today's modelers will find it instructive to study medical history. Certainly Harvey was modeling in 1628 when he showed that blood flows around the body in a complete loop (Harvey-41), and Starling was modeling when he described the principle we refer to as Starling's law (that the more the ventricles are filled, the more strongly the blood is pumped out by them). But Harvey's observations were structural, and Starling's law is qualitative. We are concerned with the *quantitative* modeling of dynamic physiological systems; such modeling requires the use of differential equations, and their simulation using a computer requires numerical estimates of parameters and of initial values of variables.

Because modeling of physiological systems has been so widely used (though not always recognized as such), a historical review in any detail would resemble the history of the development of physiology. If we limit our concerns to mathematical modeling, it will be found that such applications have been concerned with physiology on the one hand and with the computing tools available on the other. Thus early use of mathematics often resulted in handy formulas such as the Moens-Korteweg expression for arterial wave velocity and the Poiseuille expression for resistance to laminar flow in cylindrical vessels (see Chapter 4); often, however, the observed physiological relationships could only be expressed graphically.

The description of such aspects of system dynamics as fluid flow or body motion requires that sets of differential equations be written, and these equations usually contain nonlinearities such that closed-form mathematical solutions cannot be obtained. Thus, as pointed out, computers and numerical analysis are essential in modeling, and the history of biological modeling is closely related to the development of such tools (Sargent-82, Beltrami-87).

The first computers to be available and useful to physiology modelers were the analog computers, or differential analyzers, which have been described in many engineering textbooks (Hausner-71). These computers evolved from awkward mechanical machines toward the end of World War II, first appearing in vacuum tube form and later with transistors. The basic element in these electronic machines, the operational amplifier, could be used to add, subtract, and (most importantly) to integrate time-varying electrical signals. With some difficulty, certain nonlinear operations could be performed, and these machines began to be widely used in the study and design of such complex systems as the control of aircraft by autopilot.

It was soon recognized that these computers could also be used to run simulations of any physiological system that could be adequately described in mathematical form. Early studies often related to the cardiovascular or respiratory system and to the feedback control loops associated with such systems (Warner-62, Grodins-59), and one cardiovascular model (McLeod-66) became important as a simulation benchmark. In Britain there appeared some early anesthesia models (Mapleson-73) that were to have many descendants, and what we might call the Dutch school of cardiovascular modeling appeared with the work of Beneken and others, all using analog computers (Beneken-65, Noordergraaf-63, Jager-65).

As better analog machines appeared, with some logical abilities, they were often combined with a digital computer to give what was called a *hybrid computer.* Such simulation machines, combining the speed of the parallel analog computer with the logic and memory capabilities of the serial digital computer, could simulate very large system models at speeds that are still hard to match with the modern supercomputers. Detailed and sophisticated cardiovascular system models began to appear (Dick-68, Skalak-72, Snyder-72), while Fukui showed (Fukui-71) that it was possible to have a pulsatile cardiovascular-respiratory multiple model that would run at 60 times real time, making runs of several hours of real time in as many minutes of computer time. Reviews and collections of some of these efforts have been provided (Beneken-72, Rideout-76, Milhorn-74, and Coleman-77).

The hybrid machines were (and are) costly, and programming and setup were awkward. The digital machines steadily improved in speed and memory size, and their convenience in programming, program storage, and handling of logic resulted in their being used more and more, particularly as specialized simulation languages became available. Languages such as ACSL (Advanced Continuous Simulation Language), which sort equations and translate them into Fortran before compiling and running, offer great convenience and power and are now widely used (see Appendix A). Therefore, the use of all-digital simulation increased during the 1970s, particularly among those investigators concerned with the respiratory system. Dynamic models of respiratory mechanics appeared (Yamamoto-75, Jackson-73) together with models of respiratory control (Grodins-59, 78), and in some cases, respiratory control was combined with cardiovascular control in large models (Fukui-71).

Neural modeling and endocrine system modeling have also been vigorously pursued, despite the complexities of these systems (Harmon-68, Garfinkel-80). The movements of pharmaceutical substances within the body (pharmacokinetics) is commonly studied using computer models (Himmelstein-79). Sensing systems, particularly the eye and the ear, have received much model-aided study. The perceived need to automate the administration of drugs, as well as such natural substances as insulin, led to modeling studies of the feedback systems used to control infusion pumps, and of the interaction of these systems with the control systems of the body. Prosthetic devices such as aortic balloon pumps and myoelectric limbs also required modeling studies (see Chapter 8).

In this brief review of medical modeling history, many references have been made to recent advances in computer design. Nevertheless, the size and complexity of models are often limited by the speed and cost of the computers available rather than by the needs of the problem and the abilities of the user. We have noted that even the largest and most costly supercomputers cannot always match the speed of the parallel analog machines in hybrid combination with a digital computer. However, more and more powerful personal computers and workstations as well as parallel simulation computers (Almasi-89) are beginning to appear and may soon be expected to provide the means for speedier solutions at reasonable cost.

1.2 ANIMAL MODELS AND CLINICAL OBSERVATIONS

The systems of the human body are much like those of other animals, particularly other mammals. Physiologists have taken advantage of these similarities to study many aspects of physiological systems in animals; these studies, combined with data on humans obtained by clinical observation, have been most important in the development of our store of physiological knowledge.

Researchers using animals because of their resemblance to humans use the term *animal model,* whereas engineers would use the more descriptive *animal analog*. Note that the mathematical or computer model begins as a simplified representation of a real system with all unwanted subsystems removed, whereas the analogous (animal) system may include subsystems that are not of immediate interest or importance. Also note that animals may differ markedly from humans in some aspects; thus, for example, the spleen in dogs is much more important as a place for storage, or sequestering of blood, than in humans. Nevertheless, resemblances in the amazingly complex physiological systems in different mammalian species are more important than differences (see Section 2.7), and animal studies can provide researchers with information that they could never get solely from clinical observations.

Mathematical and computer modeling in research is therefore an adjunct to animal studies and clinical observations. A typical application in simulation studies is to set up what is known to exist and thought to be important in the way of subsystems in a model and then to "exercise" this model to verify that the entire system is correctly represented and can be used for some limited predictions. Such studies can in turn indicate necessary animal and clinical studies. It is important to note that the biological variability that is so important in real physiological systems does not appear in computer models unless purposely included.

The role of computer models compared with animal models is, or should be, of somewhat more importance in classroom demonstrations as in research; suggestions for their use in teaching have appeared (Randall-87, Dickinson-73). Somewhat more ambitious plans for computer models to be used as trainers for medical students have been described (Dickinson-72a,-72b,73). Application of such model-based training methods seems to be of most interest to anesthesiologists, and has long been pursued by N. Ty Smith, and more recently by Schwid (Schwid-86, -87).

1.3 OTHER KINDS OF MODELING

Physical models can be built using mechanical parts and flowing liquids, and have been useful in teaching and for certain aspects of research (Philip-89). Such models, though, are often difficult to build and use. Moreover, they are not easily adaptable to cases of interest unless computers and electromechanical devices are incorporated. Thus the knowledge required to construct physical models of physiological systems may lead back to the mathematical-computer kind of models discussed in this book.

In addition to the continuous system modeling that we are concerned with in this book, there are other kinds of mathematical-computer modeling, prominent among which is *discrete modeling*. This type of modeling is used in the study of different aspects of transport, such as telephone traffic and shipping port congestion problems, making much use of probability distributions. It may also be applied in medicine to problems of patient flow in the doctor's office, the intensive care ward or the operating room. Languages (such as GPSS and Simscript) have been devised for computer simulation of discrete system models (Gordon-69), and others have been designed for the modeling of systems that combine continuous and discrete characteristics (Oren-77).

The use of the seemingly approximate but effective methods that human experts use in problems ranging from aircraft control to medical diagnosis has been called the *expert system* approach (Starr-86). It has been included as a discipline in what is known as *artificial intelligence* (*AI*), which is an important area of practical application with its own body of theory and computer modeling programs. The initial theoretical approach to expert systems in AI seems to have originated in 1965 in the work of Lofti Zadeh on "fuzzy sets" (Zadeh-73). Medical applications of AI will not be discussed in any detail here, but may be found in various sources (Chokhani-81), Szolovits-82, Carson-85, Rennels-88); such methods have been given particular attention in the field of anesthesiology (Rennels-88).

A new kind of computer modeling is *neural modeling* in which the computer elements are interconnected in a manner suggested by the human central nervous system; such a computer can "learn" when exposed to suitable information (Anderson-88). Efforts are now being made to combine such neural-based models with languages such as ACSL.

1.4 DEFINITIONS OF TERMS: NOMENCLATURE

Bioengineers must learn two sets of scientific nomenclature, one from engineering science and the other from medicine. One special difficulty is with those terms that have the same name but different meanings in these two disciplines. An example is the word *parameter,* which in engineering usually refers to the physical constants of a system but in medicine may refer to such quantities as blood pressure or cardiac output. These quantities are called *system variables* (or short-term averages of such variables) in engineering parlance. A closer examination of many system parameters in engineering will reveal that they are not really constant, but are still referred to as parameters because they vary slowly or because they are externally controlled. An example of such a parameter is the slowly varying mass of a rocket as it burns up its fuel.

Another problem with nomenclature is that different names may be used for a given quantity or effect. For instance, in engineering, the term *regulation* is used in automatic control to refer to the operation of a control system with an input that is usually constant; thus we speak of temperature regulation in a home heating system that has an input setpoint that is usually fixed. In physiological systems the term often used is *homeostasis* (Cannon-29), and it refers to the various means (mostly using negative feedback) for maintaining the internal environment of the body constant as regards such quantities as temperature and pH.

Both medical dictionaries and up-to-date engineering handbooks can help bioengineers bridge the gap between the two disciplines. Here are a few important and basic definitions that require special attention will be discussed:

A *system* is an intercoupled set of elements that can perform some function (see Section 1.0).

Dynamic systems are time-varying systems; most physiological systems fall into this category. These systems are usually described by differential equations, often partial differential equations.

Lumped system models are obtained from the initial descriptions of systems (such as blood vessels) in terms of partial differential equations (PDEs) with time and one, two, or three space dimensions as independent variables. If we assume that finite steps may be taken in the space dimensions, then ordinary differential equations (ODEs) may be used to describe the system, and the system may be drawn graphically in *compartments* or *sections* (or segments or lumps!).

Small individual parts of a section of a lumped model (such as the resistance in the equivalent circuit for a segment of artery) are called *components*.

Other definitions appear in later chapters. The index at the end of this book will help by indicating the first occurrence of important terms, where a definition or meaning might be expected.

Terminology is constantly being changed, but it is also becoming better and better defined, and standards are being set up: thus the papers on mass transport terminology by Bassingthwaighte *et al* and by Brownell is recommended reading in connection with Chap. 3 (Bassingthwaighte-86, Brownell-68).

Problems appear in nomenclature in equations, especially in equations that are to be solved by computer programs, which do not accept subscripts and superscripts. It is helpful to follow some orderly procedure in naming variables and parameters so that programs are easier to read and to repair or modify. Here we designate quantities first by a letter indicating the *kind* of quantity, *P* for pressure, *V* for volume, *F* for flow, *R* for resistance, and so on. These may be followed by what would be a subscript ordinarily, but cannot be in present computer parlance; thus, for a system with many pressures, two additional letters may be desirable, such as AO for aortic (PAO), AT for atrial (PAT), and so on. Another letter may be needed if some other qualification is needed, such as L for left or R for right. It is further desirable to use the same number of subscripts for the same kind of quantities throughout.

REFERENCES

ALMASI, G. S. AND A. GOTTLIEB, (Eds.) *Highly Parallel Computing,* Redwood City, CA: Benjamin/Cummings Pub. Co.; 1989.

ANDERSON, J. A. AND E. ROSENFELD, *Neurocomputing: Foundations of Research,* Cambridge, Mass.: MIT Press; 1988.

APTER, JULIA T., "Biosystems modeling," Chap. 5 in *Biomedical Engineering Systems,* M. Clynes and J. H. Milsum, (Eds.); New York: McGraw-Hill; 1978.

BASSINGTHWAIGHTE, J. B., "Using computer models to understand complex systems," *The Physiologist,* Vol. 28, No. 5, pp. 439–42; 1985.

——— ET AL, "Terminology for mass transport and exchange," *Am. J. Physiol.* 250 (*Heart Circ. Physiol.* 19): H539–H545; 1986.

BEKEY, G. A., "Models and reality: some reflections on the art and science of simulation," *Simulation,* pp. 161–64; Nov. 1977.

BELTRAMI, EDWARD, *Mathematics for Dynamic Modeling,* Boston: Academic Press, Inc.; 1987.

BENEKEN, JAN E. W., "A mathematical approach to cardiovascular function," (PhD thesis, University of Utrecht) 1965.

———, "Some computer models in cardiovascular research," Chap. 5 in *Cardiovascular Fluid Dynamics* D. H. Bergel, Ed., New York, Academic Press, 1972.

BROWNELL, G. L., ET AL, "Nomenclature for tracer kinetics," *Intl. Jl. of Appl. Radiation and Isotopes,* Vol 19, pp. 249–62; 1968.

CANNON, W. B., "Organization for physiological homeostasis," *Physiol. Rev.* Vol. 9, pp. 399–431; 1929.

CARSON, E. R. AND D. G. CRAMP (Eds.), "*Computers and Control in Clinical Medicine,*" New York: Plenum Press; 1985.

CHOKHANI, S., "Correspondences between biomathematical and causal models for clinical decision-making," *J. Med. Systems,* Vol. 5, p. 249; 1981.

COLEMAN, T. G. (Ed.), *Simulation of Biological Systems,* La Jolla, CA: The Society for Computer Simulation; 1977.

DICK, D. E., "A Hybrid Computer Study of Major Transients in the Canine Cardiovascular System," (PhD thesis, University of Wisconsin); 1968.

DICKINSON, C. J., "A digital computer model to reach and study gas transport and exchange between lungs, blood, and tissue (MACPUF)," *J. of Physiology* (London), Vol. 224, 7P–9P; 1972.

———AND E. P. SHEPARD, "A digital computer model of the systemic circulation and kidneys ('MACPEE')," *J. Physiol.* (London), Vol. 216, 11P–12P; 1972.

DICKINSON, C. J. ET AL., "MACMAN: a digital computer model for teaching some basic principles of hemodynamics," *J. Clinical Computing,* Vol. 2, pp. 42–50; 1973.

FUKUI, YASUHIRO, "A study of the human cardiovascular-respiratory system using hybrid computer modeling," (Ph.D. thesis, University of Wisconsin). 1971.

——— AND N. TY SMITH, "Interactions among ventilation, the circulation, and the uptake and distribution of halothane; I. The basic model," *Anesthesiology,* Vol. 54: pp. 107–18, 1981a.

———, "Interactions among ventilation, the circulation, and the uptake and distribution of halothane, II. Spontaneous ventilation and the effect of CO2," *Anesthesiology*: Vol. 54, pp. 119–24; 1981b.

GARFINKEL, DAVID, "Computer modeling, complex biological systems and their simplifications," *Am. J. Physiol.* Vol. 239 (*Regulatory Integrative Comp. Physiol.* 8): R1–R6, 1980.

GORDON, G., "*System Simulation,*" Englewood Cliffs, NJ: Prentice Hall; 1969.

GRODINS, F. S., "Integrative cardiovascular physiology: a mathematical synthesis of cardiac and blood vessel hemodynamics," *Quart. Rev. Biol.,* Vol. 34, pp. 93–116; 1959.

______ AND S. M. YAMASHIRO, *Respiratory Function of the Lung and its Control,* New York: Macmillan. 1978.

GROTH, T., "The role of formal biodynamic models in laboratory medicine," *Scand. J. Clin. Lab. Investigation,* Vol. 44 (Supp. 169); 1984.

HARMON, L. D. AND E. R. LEWIS, "Neural modeling," in "*Advances in Biomed. Eng. and Med. Physics*" Vol. 1, Interscience Pub.; 1968.

HARVEY, WILLIAM, "An anatomical disquisition on the motion of the heart and blood in animals," 1628; pp. 19–79 in "*Classics of Cardiology*" Vol. 1; New York: Dover Publications, Inc., F. A. Willius and T. E. Keys, Eds.; 1941.

HAUSNER, ARTHUR, "Analog and Analog/Hybrid Computer Programming," Englewood Cliffs, NJ: Prentice Hall, 1971.

HIMMELSTEIN, K. J. AND R. J. LUTZ, "A review of the applications of physiologically based pharmacokinetic modeling," *J. Pharmacokinetics and Biopharmaceutics,* Vol. 7, No. 2, pp. 127–45, 1979.

HINDS, C. J. AND C. J. DICKINSON, "The potential of computer modelling techniques in intensive care medicine," in "*Computing in Anesthesia and Intensive Care*" The Hague: Martinus Nijhoff; 1983.

JACKSON, A. C. AND T. T. MILHORN, "Digital computer simulation of respiratory mechanics," *Comp. Biomed. Res.,* Vol. 6, pp. 27–56; 1973.

JAGER, G. N., "Electrical Model of the Human Arterial Tress," (Ph.D. thesis, University of Utrecht). 1965.

JONES, RICHARD W., "System theory and physiological processes," *Science,* Vol. 140, No. 3566 pp. 461–64; 1963.

LAMPARD, D. G. ET AL, "Electronic digital computer control of ventilation and anaesthesia," *Anaesth. Intensive Care,* Vol. 1, p. 382; 1973.

MCLEOD, J., "PHYSBE . . . a physiological simulation benchmark experiment," *Simulation,* Vol. 7, No. 6, p. 324; Dec. 1966.

MAPLESON, W. W., "Circulation-time models of the uptake of inhaled anaesthetics and data for quantifying them," *Brit. J. Anaesth.,* Vol. 45, p. 319; 1973.

MILHORN, T. G. (Ed.), *Simulation of Biological Systems,* La Jolla, CA: Society for Computer Simulation; 1974.

NOORDERGRAAF, A., "Development of an analog computer for the human systemic circulatory system," in *Circulatory Analog Computers,* Amsterdam: North-Holland, 1963.

OREN, T. I., "Software for the simulation of combined continuous and discrete systems: a state-of-the-art review," *Simulation,* pp. 33–45; 1977.

PHILIP, J. H., "Model for the physics and physiology of fluid administration," *J. Clin. Monitor.,* Vol. 5, No. 2, pp. 123–134; 1989.

RANDALL, JAMES E, *Microcomputers and Physiological Simulation,* Raven Press; 1987.

RENEAU, D. D., D. F. BRULEY AND N. N. KNISELY, "A mathematical simulation of oxygen release, diffusion and consumption in the capillaries and tissues of the human brain" pp. 135–241 in *Chemical Engineering in Medicine and Biology,* New York: Plenum Press, 1967.

RENNELS, G. D. AND P. L. MILLER,"Artificial intelligence research in anesthesia and intensive care," J. Clin. Monit., Vol. 4, pp. 274–289; 1988.

RIDEOUT, V. C., "Simulation in life sciences," pp. 39–46 in *Simulation of Systems* L. Dekker (Ed.), Amsterdam: North-Holland Publ. Co.; 1976.

ROSENBLUETH, A. AND N. WIENER, "The Role of Models in Science," *Philosophy of Science,* Vol. 12, No. 4; Oct. 1945.

SARGENT, R. G. "Verification and validation of simulation models," Chap. 9, in *Progress in Modeling & Simulation,* F. E. Cellier (Ed.), New York, Academic Press; 1982.

SCHILS, F. J., "A Study of Servoanesthesia," (Ph.D. thesis, University of Wisconsin); 1983.

———, F. J. SASSE, AND V. C. RIDEOUT, "Automatic control of anesthesia using two feedback variables," *Ann. Biomed. Eng.,* Vol. 15, pp. 19–34; 1987.

SCHWID, H. A.,"A flight simulator for general anesthesiology training," *Computers & Biomed. Res.,* Vol. 20, pp. 64–75; 1987.

SCHWID, H. A., C. WAKELAND, AND N. TY SMITH, "A simulator for general anesthesia," *Anesthesiology,* Vol. 65, No. 3A, p. A475; Sept. 1986.

SKALAK, RICHARD, "Synthesis of a complete circulation," Chap. 19, pp. 341–376 in *Cardiovascular Fluid Dynamics,* Vol. 2, D. H. Bergel, (Ed.), New York, NY: Academic Press; 1972.

SLENT G. S., "Cellular communication," *Scientific American,* Vol. 22; Sept. 1972.

SNYDER, M. F. AND V. C. RIDEOUT, "The study of human venous system dynamics using hybrid computer modeling," NASA Contractor Report, NASA CR-2084; July, 1972.

STARR, P. J., AND J. B. ANDERSON, "Application of expert systems technology to the modeling of continuous systems," pp. 39–43 in F. D. Cellier, *Languages for Continuous System Simulation,* San Diego, CA: SCS; 1986.

SZOLOVITS, P. (Ed.), *Artificial Intelligence in Medicine,* Boulder, CO: Westview Press; 1982.

THAM, ROBERT Q., "A Study of the Effects of Halothane on the Canine Cardiovascular System and Baroreceptor Control," (Ph.D. thesis, University of Wisconsin); 1987.

WARNER, HOMER R., "Use of analog computers in the study of the control mechanism in the circulation," *Fed. Proc.,* Vol. 21, pp. 87–96; 1962.

YAMAMOTO, W. S. AND ELLEN S. WALTON, "On the evolution of the physiological model," *Ann. Rev. Biophysics Bioeng.,* Vol. 4, pp. 81–102; 1975.

ZADEH, LOFTI A., "Outline of a new approach to the analysis of complex systems and decision processes," *IEEE Trans. on Syst., Man and Cybern.,* Vol. SMC-3, No. 1; January 1973.

2

The Tools of Modeling

2.0 INTRODUCTION

It is often said that modeling is more of an art than a science. This may mean that it belongs in the "expert system" category discussed in Section 1.3. Certainly, the choice of what to include in a physiological model (and what to exclude) is an important matter that modelers do not often say much about. Thus, a model of the cardiovascular system that excludes the respiratory system cannot easily be used to study effects of exercise in which the oxygen supply to the heart is important; arguments for the inclusion of the thermoregulatory system might be presented, but adding this complication would probably not be justified unless body temperature, sweating, and thermoregulatory system control of blood flow (Chapter 7) were of direct concern.

Attempts have been made to set up systematic schemes for modeling (Sage-77, Vansteenkiste-83, Spriet-82), but the difficulties are great for physiological modelers, just as they are for economic modelers. A short list of important areas of knowledge for the modeler (or modeling team) is as follows:

1. Physiology (and anatomy)
2. Biochemistry (and biophysics)
3. Instrumentation and measurement
4. Applied mathematics (including statistics and automatic control)
5. Computer hardware and software

These five general areas are briefly discussed in the sections that follow; references are cited at the end of the chapter to aid those who want to delve more deeply. Also, an attempt is made to indicate a methodology for physiological modeling.

2.1 PHYSIOLOGY AND BIOCHEMISTRY: SOURCES FOR MODELERS

Many excellent textbooks in physiology (Ganong-89, Stryer-88) and biochemistry (Berne-88) are available; perhaps the modeler will find that the work of physiologists who are also modelers is most useful (Guyton-86, Noordergraaf-80, Dedrick-73). The medical dictionary is also an important tool (Stedman-82, Dorland-88), as are various handbooks such as the Handbook of Physiology (Shepherd-83). The up-to-date modeler will also need to refer to both recent papers and the "classics"; both kinds of references are cited as they are needed in later chapters.

2.2 INSTRUMENTATION AND MEASUREMENT: DATA SOURCES

Perhaps the most difficult part of modeling is to determine the numerical values of all important parameters and the range of values of each system variable. There is no "average" human, and even if there were, it would not be possible to measure many of the important numbers needed without causing undue stress or impermissible invasion of the body. The modeler cannot give up but must sift through the physiology literature to find what data are available. Some helpful sources, in addition to the references above, are (Barratt-58, and Wade-62) for cardiovascular data, and (Cassels-62 and 66, Emmanouilides-70, Goudsouzian-87, and Katz-87) for the hard-to-find infant and fetal data.

The serious modeler will almost invariably find that some needed data cannot be located in the available literature, and animal experiments or new clinical observations will be necessary. Measurement techniques are important in seeking new data; Webster and others have discussed such matters in (Webster-78).

In Section 2.7 scaling and the use of allometric graphs and equations are discussed. These are relationships that permit the approximate determination of human data from animal measurements, as well as from humans of a different size.

2.3 APPLIED MATHEMATICS FOR MODELING AND SIMULATION

The models developed and discussed in this book are all in the form of sets of ordinary differential equations (ODEs) (with initial conditions), usually in first-order form but with associated algebraic equations shown separately. These equations originate from the partial differential equations (PDEs) that describe diffusion

$$\frac{\partial \phi}{\partial t} = k_1 \frac{\partial^2 \phi}{\partial x^2} + k_2 \frac{\partial^2 \phi}{\partial y^2} + k_3 \frac{\partial^2 \phi}{\partial z^2} \tag{2.3.1}$$

or wave motion

$$\frac{\partial^2 \phi}{\partial t^2} = K_1 \frac{\partial^2 \phi}{\partial x^2} + K_2 \frac{\partial^2 \phi}{\partial y^2} + K_3 \frac{\partial^2 \phi}{\partial z^2} \tag{2.3.2}$$

The coefficients k_i and K_j may in some cases be functions of time and/or space rather than constants.

Typically only one or at the most two dimensions in space must be considered, and the right-hand side of either equation is converted to difference form. Thus, if only the x-dimension need be considered in (2.3.1), for example, it becomes

$$d\phi_n/dt = k_1(\phi_{n+1} + \phi_{n-1} - 2\phi_n)/(\Delta x)^2 \tag{2.3.3}$$

if k_1 is constant or a function of t, and similarly for (2.3.2). Thus the PDEs in flow and diffusion problems may often be converted to ODEs. But because a digital computer is used, the time derivatives are also, in effect, dealt with using finite differences.

Another way of dealing with problems described by partial differential equations is the finite element method. This method is particularly useful for elasticity problems, as well as electromagnetic and fluid-flow field problems, especially those with irregular boundaries (Vemuri-81, Vichnevetsky-81).

Because few physiological systems can be represented by linear sets of equations, the numerical solution of ODEs has received much attention in recent years, and a variety of integration algorithms has been developed and compared (Lapidus-71). There are two principal classes of such algorithms; the multipoint schemes (such as Adams-Moulton) and the self-starting single-point Runge-Kutta methods; a number of integration algorithms of each type is usually provided in ODE-solving languages (Mitchell-86). For many ordinary problems in biosimulation using ACSL, the second-order Runge-Kutta (RK-2) algorithm is preferred. Note, however, that the predict-correct methods and the RK-Fehlberg methods enable the time step to be altered as the problem proceeds in order to maintain the integration error below some set limit.

Statistics is of interest to modelers of biosystems because probability distributions are needed to describe the variations of any parameter in a typical population. If these distributions are known or can be guessed at, they may be used to vary one or more parameters in a model as repeated runs are made, and the resulting averages or ranges of response can be noted (these are called Monte Carlo studies). Such applications of modeling and probability are not given as specific examples in this book, but those readers with some knowledge of probability can easily proceed with such studies (Johnson-87).

Automatic feedback control is also important in many of the models discussed here and in other related models that might be set up. An elementary introduction to negative feedback systems and their modeling is given in Appendix C, and applications are discussed in Section 4.5 and in Chapter 8. Important references include (Jones-69, Houk-88, and Mitamura-87).

2.4 COMPUTERS: HARDWARE AND SOFTWARE

The study of models such as those described in this book requires a computer with at least the power of the IBM AT, with a hard disk and math chip and a dot-matrix or laser printer; a Mac II can also be used. More powerful computers, including such workstations as the Sun and Hewlett-Packard, are preferable for anyone with problems that have outgrown those discussed here. Essential software for the dynamic systems modeler is a differential equation–solving language, such as ACSL, CSMP, or CSSL-IV; most of these languages are designed to be used with a compiler language, such as Fortran or C. ACSL and its use are introduced in Appendix A; other such languages are referenced there.

2.5 MODELING TECHNIQUES

Techniques important to biosystem modelers are discussed in a number of books and papers without attempting to set forth formal modeling techniques (Beneken-72, Doebelin-80, Spriet-82, Moller-83). Sage has suggested formal methods for setting up models, but these seem better suited to economic than physiological models (Sage-77). Sargent's study of the problems of model verification and validation is of importance to modelers in any field (Sargent-82).

In the modeling described in this book, and in the work of many of the authors cited, the approach is to start with simple submodels and work toward a more complete system model by adding components to submodels and combining them. Thus, in Chapter 4, a segment of artery or vein is first modeled, then several such segments are combined with valves and a variable compliance ventricle to produce the left heart and systemic system. Next the right heart and pulmonary system are set up and added to the first system to give a complete loop. Then barocontrol is added, and later, in Chapters 5 and 6, the combination of such a pressure-flow model and a transport model is discussed. Throughout its development, the model is checked for verification and validation. It is the author's hope that the submodels presented here will serve as modules that will better enable modelers to build up the computer simulations of interest to them.

2.6 SYSTEMS OF UNITS

The metric system used in most scientific work was originally used in the CGS (centimeter-gram-second) form, but beginning about 1935 there was a change to the MKS (meter-kilogram-second) system. In 1950, the MKS system was replaced by the MKSA (meter-kilogram-second-ampere) system, which provides convenient relationships between mechanical and electrical units. An expanded modification of the MKSA system, the SI (Système International d'Unités), was defined and given official status by the Eleventh General Conference on Weights and Measures in Paris in 1960 (Mechtly-64); the U.S. National Bureau of Standards adopted this system in 1962, and the Metric Conversion Act of 1975 (U.S. Public Law 94-168) calls for its general adoption.

The SI system has seven units, defined for seven basic quantities, as shown in Table 2.6.1.

In the past, the medical profession in the United States has used the CGS system with some added units. Blood pressure, for example, is measured in terms of mm Hg (millimeters of mercury), and so is dependent on the force of gravity, which varies with the distance from the center of the earth. The SI units, particularly with the introduction of the use of the mole for amount of substance, should lead to important changes in clinical laboratory measurements. European scientists are beginning to use the SI system in their clinical and published work, but adoption is slower in the United States (Goldman-81) and particularly so in the field of medicine. There are sound reasons for making some effort to proceed with a changeover, and in this book the new units will be shown along with the old in at least some typical applications.

Table 2.6.2 provides a list of derived SI units with special names and

TABLE 2.6.1

Quantity	Name	SI Symbol
length	meter	m
mass	kilogram	kg
time	second	s
temperature	kelvin	K
amount of substance	mole	mol
electric current	ampere	A
luminous intensity	candela	cd

TABLE 2.6.2

Quantity	Derived Unit	Name	SI Symbol
area	m^2		
volume	m^3		
velocity	m/s		
acceleration	m/s^2		
density	kg/m^3		
force	$kg*m/s^2$	newton	N
pressure	N/m^2	pascal	Pa
work, energy, heat	N*m	joule	J
power	J/s	watt	W
quantity of electricity	A*s	coulomb	C
electric potential	W/A	volt	V
capacitance	C/V	farad	F
resistance	V/A	ohm	Ω
conductance	A/V	siemens	S
magnetic flux	V*s	weber	Wb
magnetic flux density	Wb/m^2	tesla	T
inductance	Wb/A	henry	H
frequency	1/s	hertz	Hz
electric field strength	V/m	volt per meter	
electric charge density	C/m^3	coulomb per m^3	
electric flux density	C/m^2	coulomb per m^2	
permittivity	F/m	farad per meter	
permeability	H/m	henry per meter	
dynamic viscosity	Pa*s	pascal second	
moment of force	N*m	newton meter	
surface tension	N/m	newton per meter	
power density or heat flux density	W/m^2	watt per m^2	
heat capacity, entropy	J/K	joule per kelvin	
specific heat capacity or specific entropy	J/(kg*K)	joule per kg kelvin	
specific energy	J/kg	joule per kg	
thermal conductivity	W/(m*K)	watt per m kelvin	
energy density	J/m^3	joule per cubic meter	
molar energy	J/mol	joule per mole	
molar entropy, molar heat capacity	J/(mol*K)	joule per mole kelvin	

symbols. This list does not include derived units relating to radioactivity, X-ray dosage, and related quantities.

Table 2.6.3 shows alternate units which are not officially a part of

TABLE 2.6.3

Quantity	Symbol	Units
time	t	minute (min), hour (h), day (d), year (a)
temperature	T	degree Celsius (°C)
plane angle	Θ	degree (°), minute ('), second (")
volume	V	liter (L), milliliter (ml)
mass	m	gram (g or gm), millikg
pressure	p	bar (bar), special name for 10^5*Pa
flow rate	x, f	milliliters per second (ml/s) or liters per minute (L/min)
solute flow rate		g/sec or millimoles/sec
fluid flow resistance	R	g/(cm^4*sec) (CGS units)
flow inertance	L	g/cm^4 (CGS units)
vessel compliance	C	cm^4*sec^2/g (CGS units)
pressure	P	dynes/cm^2 = g/(cm*sec^2) (CGS units)

TABLE 2.6.4

Factor	Prefix	Symbol
10^9	giga	G
10^6	mega	M
10^3	kilo	k
10^2	hecto	h
10	deka	da
10^{-1}	centi	c
10^{-3}	milli	m
10^{-6}	micro	μ
10^{-9}	nano	n
10^{-12}	pico	p

TABLE 2.6.5

Quantity	Name	Symbol	One unit = SI units
length	inch	in	$2.54*10^{-2}$ m
length	angstrom	Å	10^{-10} m
mass	pound	1b	0.4536kg
force of gravitation	kg-force	kgf	9.8066 N
pressure	mm Hg	mm Hg	133.32 Pa
atmospheric pressure	torr	Torr	1.0 mm Hg
heat energy	British thermal unit	Btu	1055 J
thermochemical energy	calorie	cal	4.184 J

SI, but are recognized as allowable because of convenience and widespread use.

Note that Q is often used for average blood flow rate in the medical literature. In this book we will use q for variable fluid volumes and Q for fixed volumes, or quantities, while using f or F for flow rate. Thus we might express cardiac output (CO) as either F or $\dot{Q} \equiv dQ/dt$.

Note also that the derived units in the two lists may be expressed in terms of SI base units, which may be important when checking equations for consistency. For example, thermal conductivity, given as watts per meter kelvin has the base units m*kg/K*s^3. We will use this and other SI unit expressions to check units in thermal diffusion equations in Chapter 7.

Important prefixes are used with SI units to keep numerical values within convenient ranges. Some of these prefixes are defined in Table 2.6.4.

Some conversion factors from non-SI to SI units are given in Table 2.6.5.

2.7 SCALING IN PHYSIOLOGICAL SYSTEM MODELING

A common problem in physiological modeling is the determination of a system parameter (e.g., metabolic rate or cardiac output at rest) for some human or other mammal, assuming that we know the numerical value of this parameter for some standard or average individual. The parameter may be a function of weight or age, and knowledge of the relationship should permit us to find at least its approximate value. Experiment has shown that such *scaling* is often possible; an example is the relationship between metabolic rate, M, and body weight, B, which is linear when plotted on a logarithmic scale not only among humans but for all mammals (Kleiber-47, Dickinson-77, Boxenbaum-82, Sackner-74). Thus, for a log-log plot, the experimental values determined for 26 mammals from a mouse to a cow may be shown to lie close to the straight line, as determined by regression (see Section 9.1):

$$\log M = 1.83 + 0.756 \log B \pm 0.05 \tag{2.7.1}$$

where M is in kilocalories per day, B is in grams, and the factor 0.05 refers to the standard deviation. Ignoring the standard deviation and changing to the units kilocalories per hour for M and kilograms for B, we can put the equation into the form

$$\begin{aligned} \log M - \log B^{0.756} &= \log 522.0, \qquad \text{whence} \\ M &= 522.0 * B^{0.756} \end{aligned} \tag{2.7.2}$$

Such equations are called *allometric* equations. They have been determined experimentally for mammals for a number of properties that vary with body weight B (in kilograms), including the two shown in Fig. 2.7.1, and the following (Adolph-49):

$$\begin{aligned} \text{Oxygen uptake (ml/min), } V_{O_2} &= 10.0*\mathrm{B}^{0.75} \\ \text{Ventilation rate (L/min), } \dot{V} &= 0.266*\mathrm{B}^{0.74} \\ \text{Heart weight (kg), } W_h &= 0.00575*\mathrm{B}^{0.98} \\ \text{Brain weight (kg), } W_{br} &= 0.0103*\mathrm{B}^{0.7} \\ \text{Total blood weight (kg), } W_{bl} &= 0.0589*\mathrm{B} \\ \text{Creatinine output } (\mu\text{g/hr}), \dot{N} &= 0.586*\mathrm{B}^{0.90} \\ \text{Cardiac output (L/min), } \dot{Q} &= 0.2*\mathrm{B}^{0.75} \\ \text{Cardiac output (ml/s), } \dot{Q} &= 3.33*\mathrm{B}^{0.75} \end{aligned} \tag{2.7.3}$$

These relationships may be of some assistance in setting up models in which data from a dog experiment or clinical data from humans of different sizes are to be used. Note that for the important cardiac output equation (and also for basal metabolism and ventilation rate), the body weight appears raised to the three-quarters power (approximately). Because this is close to a two-thirds power, and because surface area of a sphere varies as the two-thirds power of the volume, it was once thought that there was some physiological reason for such quantities as basal metabolism, cardiac output, and ventilation rate to be directly proportional to skin area. Of course most of our bodies are not too spherical, and a better formula for skin area in the human (Dubois-27) was devised:

$$S = 0.007184*B^{0.425}*L^{0.725} \qquad \mathrm{m}^2 \tag{2.7.4}$$

where B is (human) body weight (kg) and L is body length (cm).

It is common medical practice to calculate S using the Dubois formula for patients who are to undergo surgery and to use it in determining the cardiac index, CI, which is the measured cardiac output $\dot{Q}$ (or CO) in L/min divided by S:

$$\mathrm{CI} = \dot{Q}/S \qquad \mathrm{L/(min*m^2)} \tag{2.7.5}$$

This index serves as a guide in administration of anesthesia and the various pharmaceuticals required in surgical procedures. But for our modeling purposes, and certainly to estimate equivalent human parameters from dog experiment results, the formulas based on weight only may be used.

Modelers should be aware that these allometric equations are not very useful for determining parameters for human infants under about two years of age (Goudsouzian-87), and fetal modeling is still more difficult (Waisman-70). Similarly, the modeler must be cautious in the use of allometric equations for elderly humans or animals because of the significant decline in many physiological quantities with age (Evans-73, Ste-

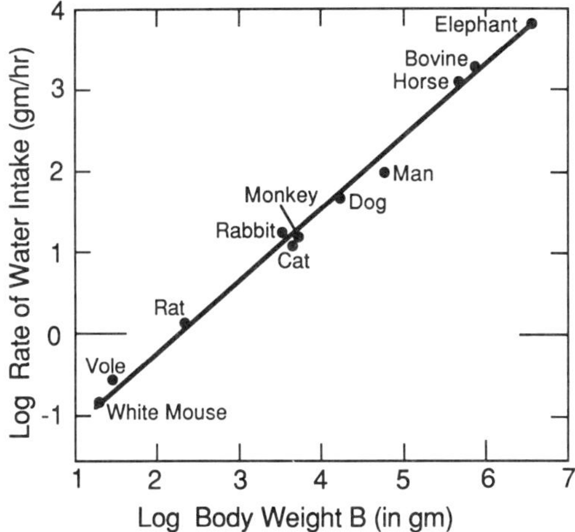

Figure 2.7.1. (a) Rate of water intake in relation to body weight among mammals. (From Adolph-49 with permission).

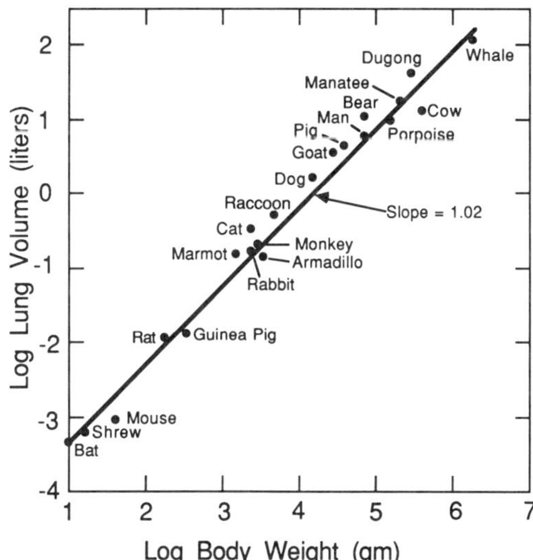

(b) Lung volume in relation to body weight among mammals. (From Tenney-63 with permission).

phen-86, McLeskey-86); thus the cardiac index may be reduced at age 75 to 70 percent of what it is at age 30, while the elimination half-life of the drug diazapam may be more than doubled. It should also be noted that obesity may have a different effect from other kinds of size change in humans.

PROBLEMS

2.1 In linear pressure-flow modeling (see Chapter 4), equations for the series elements in a cylindrical vessel segment are $p_R = Rf$ and $p_L = Ldf/dt$, corresponding to $e_R = Ri$ and $e_L = Ldi/dt$ in a series $R-L$ electrical circuit. The equation for a compliance is $f = Cdp/dt$, corresponding to $i = Cde/dt$ for an electrical compliance.

(a) Verify the units of the fluid-flow R, L, and C against those given in Table 2.6.3.

(b) Compliance in a fluid circuit may also be obtained using the integral of $f = Cdp/dt$, $q - q_U = Cp$, where q_U is the volume in the segment when the average pressure p is zero. Use this expression to find the units of C and check against the results in (a).

2.2 **(a)** Write and use an ACSL (see Appendix A) or other computer program to plot surface area, S, versus body weight, B, for three values of body length, L, using Equation [2.7.4]

(b) Change axis scales to plot log S versus log B.

2.3 If a dog has a cardiac output of 25 ml/sec, use allometric equations to estimate its oxygen uptake, ventilation rate and heart weight. (Answer: 75 ml/min 0_2, 1.94 L/hr, 0.08 Kg.)

2.4 If a man has a blood volume of 5 liters, use allometric equations to estimate his body weight. (Note, average blood density is 1.05 gm/ml).

2.5 Describe a person most likely to have a high cardiac index, considering only the factors of weight and height. Verify your answer with Equations [2.7.3, 4, and 5].

2.6 Ventilation rate is equal to the tidal volume of the lungs times the rate of breathing (see Section 5.1). A scaly anteater weighing 10 kg is resting after a large meal in the tropics of Africa. Estimate its tidal volume if the anteater normally breathes at the rate of 15 breaths per minute. (Answer: $V_T = 0.097$ liters)

REFERENCES

ADOLPH, E. F., "Quantitative relations in the physiological constitution of mammals," *Science,* Vol. 109, pp. 579–585; June 10, 1949.

BARRATT-BOYES, B. G. AND E. H. WOOD, "Cardiac output and related measurements," *J. Lab. Clin. Med.,* Vol. 51, pp. 72–90; 1958.

BASSINGTHWAIGHTE, J. B., "Using computer models to understand complex systems," *The Physiologist,* Vol. 28, No. 5, pp. 219–21; 1985.

BENEKEN, J.E.W., "Some computer models in cardiovascular research," in D. H. Bergel, (Ed.), *Cardiovascular Fluid Dynamics*; London: Academic Press; 1972.

BERNE, R. M. AND M. N. LEVY, *Physiology,* (2nd Ed.); St. Louis: C. V. Mosby Co.; 1988.

BOXENBAUM, HAROLD, "Interspecies scaling, allometry, physiological time and the ground plan of pharmacokinetics," *J. Pharmacokin. Biopharm.*, Vol. 10, pp. 201–27; 1982.

CASSELS, D. E. (Ed.), *The Heart and Circulation of the Newborn Infant,* Springfield, IL: Grune & Stratton, 1966.

CASSELS, D. E. AND M. MORSE, *Cardiopulmonary Data for Children,* Springfield, IL: Thomas; 1962.

DEDRICK, R. L., "Animal scale-up," *J. Pharmacokin. Biopharm.*, Vol. 10, No. 5, pp. 435–61; 1973.

DICKINSON, C. J., "Adjustment of model parameter to sex, age, height and weight," Chap. 21 in *A Computer Model of Human Respiration,* Baltimore, MD: University Park Press; 1977.

DOEBELIN, E. O., *System Modeling and Response,* New York, NY: John Wiley & Sons; 1980.

DORLAND, *Dorland's Illustrated Medical Dictionary,* 27th Ed., Philadelphia, PA: W. B. Saunders; 1988.

DUBOIS, E. F., *Basal metabolism in health and disease,* Philadelphia: 1927.

EMMANOUILIDES, G. C. ET AL, "Cardiac output in newborn infants," *Biol. Neonate,* Vol. 15, pp. 186–97; 1970.

EVANS, T. I., "The physiological basis of geriatric general anesthesia," *Anaesth. Intensive Care,* Vol. 1, p. 319; 1973.

GANONG, W. F., *Review of Medical Physiology,* (14th Ed.) Los Altos, CA: Appleton & Lange; 1989.

GOLDMAN, DAVID T., "The metric system: its status and future," *IEEE Spectrum,* pp. 60–63, April 1981.

GOUDSOUZIAN, N. G., "Anatomy and physiology in relation to pediatric anesthesia," Chap. 1 in *Anesthesia and Uncommon Pediatric Disease,* Jordan Katz and D. J. Steward, Eds., Philadelphia: W. B. Saunders Co.; 1987.

GUYTON, A. C., *Textbook of Medical Physiology,* (7th Ed.) Philadelphia: Saunders; 1986.

HOUK, JAMES C., "Control strategies in physiological systems," *Faseb J.* Vol. 2, pp. 97–107; 1988.

JOHNSON, R. AND G. BHATTACHARYA, *Statistics: Principles and Methods,* New York: Wiley; 1987.

JONES, RICHARD W., "Biological control mechanisms," Chap. 2 in *Biological Engineering,* H. P. Schwan, (Ed.); New York: McGraw-Hill; 1969.

KATZ, JORDAN, *Anesthesia and Uncommon Pediatric Diseases,* Philadelphia, PA: W. B. Saunders; 1987.

KLEIBER, MAX, "Body size and metabolic rate," *Physiol. Rev.,* Vol. 27, No. 4, Oct. 1947.

LAPIDUS, LEON, AND J. H. SEINFELD, *Numerical Solution of Ordinary Differential Equations,* New York: Academic Press; 1971.

MCLESKEY, C. H., "Anesthesia for the elderly patient," *Anesthesia* and *Analgesia,* pp. 133–138; April 1986.

MECHTLY, E. A., "The International System of Units," NASA SP-7012 Washington DC: NASA Sci. and Tech. Information Div.; 1964.

MITAMURA, Y., "Control aspects of the circulatory system," pp. 34–52 in *Control Aspects of Biomedical Engineering,* M. Nalecz, (Ed.), Oxford: Pergamon Press; 1987.

MITCHELL & GAUTHIER ASSOCIATES, *ACSL Reference Manual,* Concord, Mass.: Mitchell and Gauthier Assoc.; 1986.

MOLLER, D., D. POPOVIC, AND G. THIELE, *Modeling, Simulation and Parameter Estimation of the Human Cardiovascular System,* Braunschweig, West Germany: Vieweg & Sohn; 1983.

NOORDERGRAAF, A., AND J. MELBIN, "The development of recognition of component significance in closed-loop cardiovascular control," *Ann. Biomed. Eng.,* Vol. 8, pp. 391–404; 1980.

SACKNER, M. A., ET AL, "Pulmonary arterial blood volume and tissue volume in man and dog," *Circ. Res.,* Vol. 34, pp. 761–69; June, 1974.

SAGE, A. P. *Methodology for Large-Scale Systems,* New York: McGraw-Hill; 1977.

SARGENT, R. G., "Verification and validation of simulation models," in F. E. Cellier, (Ed.), *Progress in Modeling and Simulation,* New York: Academic Press; 1982.

SHEPHERD, J. T. AND F. M. ABBOUD (Eds.), "Handbook of Physiology" Sec. 2, Part 1, Vol. III, *The Cardiovascular System*; Bethesda, MD: American Physiol. Soc., 1983.

SPRIET, J. A. AND G. C. VANSTEENKISTE, *Computer-aided Modelling and Simulation,* London and New York: Academic Press; 1982.

STEDMAN, T. L., *Stedman's Medical Dictionary,* (24th Ed.) Baltimore: Williams & Wilkins; 1982.

STEPHEN, C. R., AND R.A.E. ASSAF, *Geriatric Anesthesia: Principles and Practice,* Boston, Mass.: Butterworth; 1986.

STRYER, L., *Biochemistry of Physiology,* (3rd Ed.); New York: W. H. Freeman & Co.; 1988.

TENNEY, S. M. AND J. E. REMMERS, "Comparative quantitative morphology of the mammalian lung: diffusing area,: *Nature,* Vol. 197, No. 4862, pp. 54–56; 1963.

VANSTEENKISTE, G. C. AND P. C. YOUNG (EDS.), *Modelling and Data Analysis in Biotechnology and Medical Engineering,* Amsterdam: North-Holland Pub. Co.; 1983.

VEMURI, V. AND W. J. KARPLUS, *Digital Computer Treatment of Partial Differential Equations,* Englewood Cliffs, NJ: Prentice-Hall; 1981.

VICHNEVETSKY, R., *Computer Methods for Partial Differential Equations,* Englewood, Cliffs, NJ: Prentice Hall; 1981.

WADE, O. L. AND J. M. BISHOP, *Cardiac Output and Regional Blood Flow,* Philadelphia: F. A. Davis Co.; 1962.

WAISMAN, H. A. AND G. R. KERR, *Fetal Growth and Development,* New York: McGraw-Hill; 1970.

WEBSTER, J. G. (ED.), *Medical Instrumentation: Application and Design,* Boston, Mass.: Houghton Mifflin; 1978.

3

Mass Transport: Compartment Modeling

3.0 INTRODUCTION

The uptake, transport, and elimination of a wide range of substances in the body are of great importance in both research and clinical work. Substances may be carried by *flow* and by *diffusion* processes in body tissue (Bird-60), (Jacquez-72).

Flow transport of substances such as oxygen or pharmaceutical agents may occur in the body in a number of ways, including

1. *Blood flow* in the cardiovascular system
2. *Airflow* in the respiratory system
3. *Flow of food and digestive juices* in the gastrointestinal system
4. *Urine flow* in the renal and urinary system

The modeling of flow transport in physiological systems is discussed in some detail in Sections 3.2 to 3.5.

The diffusion of substances through membranes that separate blood from tissue or from air in the lungs can also occur in a number of ways (Cooney-76), (Friedman-86), including the following:

1. *Passive diffusion,* in which the substance is driven by the difference in concentration of the substances on either side of the membrane, in accordance with Fick's first law. Such diffusion may be facilitated by various effects that modify the diffusion constants.

2. *Active transport,* in which processes (not always well understood) may use up energy in forcing flow in a direction opposite to that of passive diffusion.
3. *Passive diffusion of ionized atoms or radicals,* or electrolytes, in which the electrical properties of the membrane contribute to flow.
4. *Osmosis,* in which the solvent moves through a membrane from a lower concentration of the total solute to a higher one.
5. *Pressure-induced flow,* as in the glomeruli of the kidneys, in which pressure differences cause a flow through the membrane of molecules smaller than the openings in the membrane.

Models have long been used to describe and to help study the movement of various substances in the body; some of these are the following:

1. *Indicator substances,* infused into the blood to measure cardiac output and blood volume (Zierler-66, Bassingthwaighte-77) and to study heart defects noninvasively (Zimmerman-60). Originally, inert dyes, which attach to red blood cells and are rather slowly eliminated from the circulation, were used. An infusion of chilled saline solution (Roselli-75) may be used in place of dye for some purposes, such as measuring cardiac output (see Section 3.4). Radionuclide angiocardiography is also used to avoid the need for catheterization (Flaherty-67).
2. *Pharmaceutical* substances, introduced either into the veins in liquid form by intravenous injection or drip or into the lungs in gaseous form. Introduction of drugs into the body by way of the gastrointestinal system, by diffusion through the skin, or by injection into tissue is also used. The term *pharmacokinetics* is used to describe the kinetics of such transport (Gibaldi-82, Friedman-86, Teorell-74); the term *pharmacodynamics* is used to describe the dynamics of the action of a drug upon the body.
3. *Natural substances,* such as proteins, oxygen, or sodium ions, being carried by blood flow or air flow in the lungs.
4. *Radioactive tracers,* which have become a part of some substances whose kinetics are to be studied.
5. *Heat energy* is also transported by air or blood flow and by diffusion in tissue. Its modeling is somewhat like that for the types of substances listed above, but there are many differences, and the modeling of thermoregulation and heat flow in the body is discussed in Chapter 7.

3.1 DIFFUSION: EQUATIONS AND MODELING

In physiology we are much concerned with the diffusion of solutes through semipermeable membranes, such as capillary walls. The passage of the solvent (usually water) through the membranes is also important. We will assume that the solute is a nonelectrolyte, so that electrical forces need not be considered. We will also assume the one-dimensional case, which is adequate in most biological applications. In such a case the free diffusion flux, or flow rate of solute per unit area, is given by Fick's first law (Bird-60) as

$$J_s = -D_s * d\gamma_s/dx + J_v * \gamma_s \qquad (3.1.1)$$

where J_s is solute and J_v the total flux. In the first term on the right side of (3.1.1), D_s is the coefficient of mass diffusivity for solute s in the membrane, x is distance normal to the membrane, and γ_s (gm/cm^3) is the mass concentration of s in the solvent. The first term on the right side of (3.1.1) is what is usually referred to as the diffusant flux of solute; the second term is the solute carried by the volume flux J_v, and is usually negligible where diffusion through membranes is being considered (however, in transport of solute along veins and arteries, the second term is the important one).

The flow of solute s through a uniform membrane of area A and thickness Δ_x, neglecting volume flux, is

$$f_s = J_s * A = -(A * D_s/\Delta x) * \Delta\gamma \qquad \text{(gm/s)} \qquad (3.1.2)$$

For the single-compartment system shown in Fig. 3.1.1, concentration γ_1 is assumed to be uniform. (The M in the upper left corner of the compartment indicates that it is assumed to be a "perfect mixing cham-

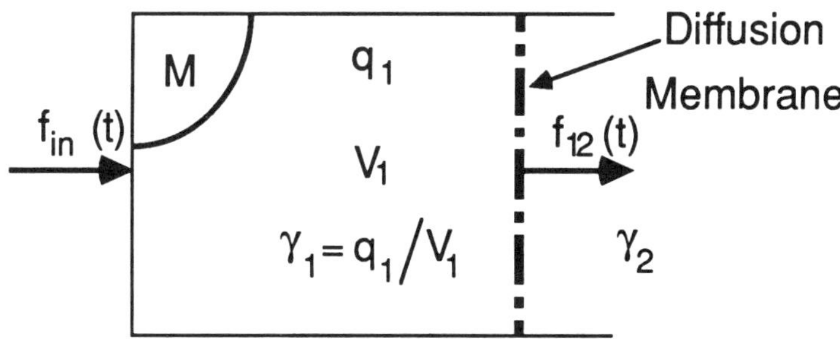

Figure 3.1.1. A one-compartment system, characterized by perfect mixing, a known rate of input flow of solute, and diffusion output to a region of known solute concentration, γ_2.

ber" in which mixing is instantaneous.) An inflow rate $f_{\text{in}}(t)$ of solute is also assumed, so that the net inflow of solute, by (3.1.2), is

$$f_{in} - f_{12} = f_{\text{in}} + K_1*(\gamma_2 - \gamma_1) \tag{3.1.3}$$

where $K_1 = A_1*D_s/\Delta x_1$, and γ_2 is the concentration outside the compartment (or in the next compartment). Note that we have dropped the subscript for substance s to prevent confusion, since subscripts referring to compartment number had to be introduced.

If γ_2 is essentially zero, and q_1 is the quantity of solute in the compartment, then

$$dq_1/dt = f_{\text{in}} - K_1*\gamma_1 \tag{3.1.4}$$

or, in integral form

$$q_1 = \int_0^t (\mathrm{f}_{\text{in}} - K_1*\gamma_1)dt + q_1(0)$$

where $q_1(0)$ is the initial mass of solute s in the compartment.

If a two-compartment diffusion system is set up, as shown in Fig. 3.1.2, and if γ_2 is the nonzero concentration in a second compartment, equations for compartments 1 and 2 may be written as

$$dq_1/dt = f_{\text{in}} - K_1*(\gamma_1 - \gamma_2) \tag{3.1.5}$$

$$dq_2/dt = K_1*(\gamma_1 - \gamma_2) + K_2*\gamma_2 \tag{3.1.6}$$

where $\mathrm{K}_2 = A_2*D_s/\Delta x_2$, and concentration outside compartment two is zero (or membrane two only permits one-way flow).

It is desirable to work with equations with only one kind of dependent variable, and the best choice in equations such as (3.1.5) and (3.1.6) is to use concentrations. If we divide these equations by the compartment volumes V_1 and V_2 and use $q_1/V_1 = \gamma_1$ and $q_2/V_2 = \gamma_2$, then

$$V_1*d\gamma_1/dt = f_{\text{in}} - K_1*(\gamma_1 - \gamma_2) \tag{3.1.7}$$

$$V_2*d\gamma_2/dt = K_1*(\gamma_1 - \gamma_2) - K_2\gamma_2 \tag{3.1.8}$$

The method of modeling used in the study of mass (and energy)

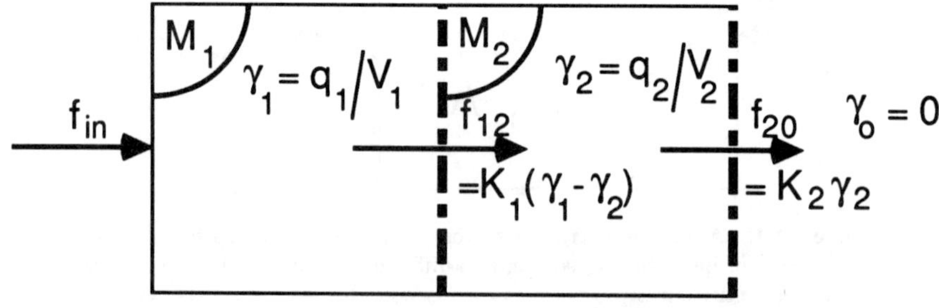

Figure 3.1.2. Two-compartment diffusion system.

transport in the body is based on *compartmentalization* of those parts of the body that the substance enters in nonnegligible amounts. It is possible to set up *continuous models* of, for example, the arterial circulation, but the detail of the kinetic descriptions soon becomes unmanageable because of the complexity of its branchings. Assemblages of blood vessels, portions of lungs, or tissue beds may be selected as compartments, interconnected by fluid flow or the diffusion through tissue or vessel walls. Selection of the size and number of compartments needed is a major initial problem in any modeling effort and will be referred to repeatedly in the examples that follow.

Some initial assumptions will be made regarding the system and its modeling; later on, some of these assumptions will not be needed as the models are improved. These initial assumptions are as follows:

1. The system may be divided into compartments that are either "perfect mixing compartments," in which the mixing of the entering blood (and the substance it carries) with the original contents of the compartment is instantaneous and complete, or "delay compartments," in which transport delay occurs with no mixing and the time course of concentrations is the same at the output as it is at the input, except for this delay.
2. The flow of blood between compartments is unidirectional, constant, and nonpulsatile. Later on, we can deal with varying and pulsatile flows, using multiple models (see Chapter 6).
3. The flow of any substance carried by the blood is so much smaller than the blood flow that it does not appreciably add to the total flow. Thus we can assume that the equations for blood flow, pressure, and volume (considered in Chapter 4) are not directly influenced by the introduction of the substance. In the case of substances carried by air, such as oxygen, the transported substance may be an appreciable part of the total, and will have to be considered in setting up pressure-flow equations (see Section 5.3).
4. It will also be assumed at first that the substance does not chemically interact with blood. Later on, we will have to consider the reversible combination of a substance, such as oxygen with red blood cells, as being equivalent to an increased solution of oxygen in blood. It may also be necessary to consider substances that interact with one another, metabolize, bind to receptors or proteins, and the like.
5. Red blood cells form an appreciable part of any volume of blood (the hematocrit) and may not travel at the same rate as plasma. However, it will be assumed here that all components of blood travel at the same rate.

3.2 ONE-COMPARTMENT MODELS: LAPLACE AND NUMERICAL SOLUTIONS

It is often possible to treat the entire cardiovascular system as a single compartment. This is true, for example, if the solute is an inert, large molecule indicator, such as indocyanine green dye that has been infused into the blood, because this substance cannot diffuse into tissues and its elimination is slow. However, it is possible to study the slower kinetics of other drugs, even though they diffuse into tissue, if the drug concentration in the tissue may be assumed to follow that in the blood.

We are not much interested in such simple cases, but will choose one as a first example of the use of Laplace transform (see Appendix B) and of the ACSL differential equation–solving language (see Appendix A), keeping in mind that these methods also make it possible to study rather easily more complex, and hopefully better, models.

To analyze the one-compartment system of Fig. 3.1.1, let us begin by assuming that its kinetics may be described by the first-order differential equation (3.1.4), with q_1 replaced by $V_1 * \gamma_1$, the product of volume (a constant, V_1) and concentration, γ_1:

$$V_1 * d\gamma_1/dt = f_{in} - K_1 * \gamma_1 \tag{3.2.1}$$

where the initial condition is now $\gamma_1(0) = q_1(0)/V_1$.

If f_{in} is a step function of input flow of amplitude A

$$f_{in} = A * u(t) \tag{3.2.2}$$

and its Laplace transform (see Appendix B) is A/s. Taking Laplace transforms throughout (3.2.1) gives

$$V_1 * (s * \Gamma_1 - \gamma_1(0)) = A/s - K_1 * \Gamma_1 \tag{3.2.3}$$

where lowercase γ_1 is replaced by uppercase Γ_1 to indicate the change in independent variable from t to s.

Solving for Γ_1 in (3.2.3) gives

$$\Gamma_1(s) = \frac{A/V_1}{s(s + K_1/V_1)} + \frac{\gamma_1(0)}{(s + K_1/V_1} \tag{3.2.4}$$

From the table of transforms (Appendix B)

$$\gamma_1(t) = (A/K_1) * (1 - e^{-t/T_1} + \gamma_1(0) * e^{-t/T_1} \tag{3.2.5}$$

where T_1, the characteristic time constant of this system, equals V_1/K_1. If the numerical values of the system parameters and initial condition are $A = 0.6$, $V_1 = 3.0$, $K_1 = 0.01$, and $\gamma_1(0) = 25.0$ (in some consistent set of units), then the response $\gamma_1(t)$ will be

$$\gamma_1 = 60 * (1 - e^{-t/300}) + 25 * e^{-t/300} \tag{3.2.5}$$

This response is made up of a first term that is an exponential rise to an amplitude of 60 in response to the input step, followed by an exponentially decaying term in response to the initial amplitude $\gamma_1(0) = 25$. The numerical values of these two response functions may be determined by a simple Fortran or Basic program, and are plotted in Fig. 3.2.1a, together with their sum, the total response $\gamma_1 \equiv C_1$.

Although the closed-form algebraic solution of this linear system as given in (3.2.4) is a valuable result of Laplace transform analysis, the determination of the graphical output for a given set of numerical values of parameters may be obtained quite easily from the original equation using ACSL differential equation–solving software. We will begin by writing (3.2.1) in integral form:

$$\gamma_1 = \int_0^t [(f_{in} - K_1 * \gamma_1)/V_1]\, dt + \gamma_1(0) \tag{3.2.6}$$

(a)
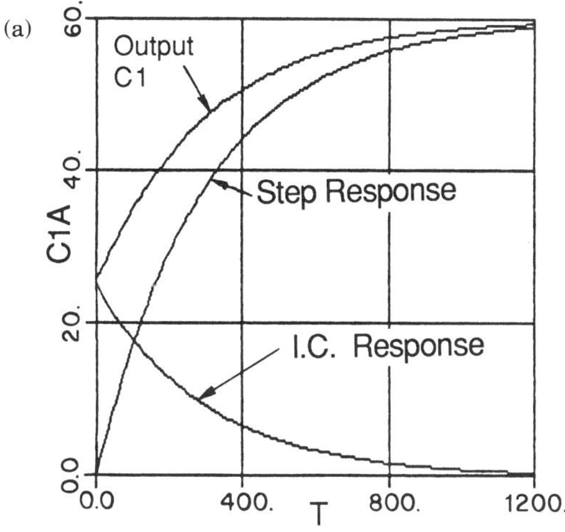

(b)
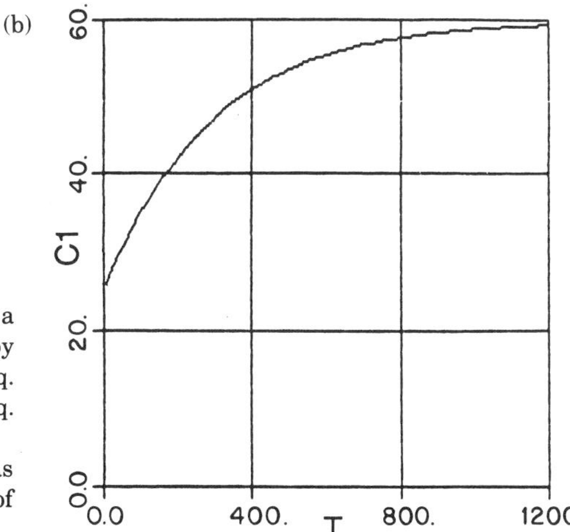

Figure 3.2.1. (a) Response $\gamma_1(t)$ of a one-compartment system obtained by Laplace transform solution of Eq. (3.2.1) and given numerically by Eq. (3.2.5).
(b) A plot of the system of Eq. (3.2.1) as determined by direct ACSL solution of the differential equation.

This can be expressed in ACSL form by using the integrate (INTEG) command (see Appendix A), with some changes in nomenclature:

$$C1 = \text{INTEG}((\text{FIN} - \text{K1}*\text{C1})/\text{V1}, \text{C1IC}) \tag{3.2.7}$$

This system equation has been incorporated into an ACSL program called COMPART1, as shown below, with the same numerical parameters used in (3.2.5).

```
PROGRAM COMPART1

 DYNAMIC
   Cinterval CINT=10.
   CONSTANT  TSTP=1200.     $'Final time is'
   TERMT (T .GE. TSTP)      $'chosen to be 4.*T1'

  DERIVATIVE
   Algorithm IALG=4         $'Second-order R-K'
   Nsteps    NSTP=1         $Maxterval MAXT=2.5
   Constant A=0.6, V1=3.0, K1=.01, C1IC=25.0
   C1 = INTEG ((FIN - K1*C1)/V1,C1IC)
   FIN = A              $'Input step in flow of amp. A'

  END                   $ 'of Deriv.'
 END                    $ 'of Dynamic'
END                     $ 'of Program'
```

This program may be solved, once it is translated and compiled, by using the *run-time commands*:

```
OUTPUT T,C1,'NCIOUT'=5
PREPAR T,C1,FIN
START
```

After the run is complete, a plot of output may be obtained by using the plot command:

```
PLOT C1
```

or, using plot commands to improve the scale somewhat over the automatic scaling provided in ACSL, Fig. 3.2.1b shows the ACSL plot using

```
PLOT 'XHI'=TSTP, C1, 'HI'=60.
```

A more interesting result may be obtained if we use a function switch to terminate the constant inflow of drug $f(t)$ at T = 500. This requires that TX = 500 be added to the list of constants and that the following commands be added to the program above in place of FIN = A:

```
FIN = FCNSW(Z,A,0.0,0.0)
Z = T - TX
```

Note that the value of Z will be negative for T < TX and FIN will therefore be equal to A for 0. < T < 500., and zero thereafter. This case is plotted in Fig. 3.2.2a, with TSTP set at 900 and C1IC set at 15. This result is replotted in Fig. 3.2.2b using the plot command

```
PLOT C1,'LOG'
```

for a logarithmic ordinate scale. Note that the exponential decay curve

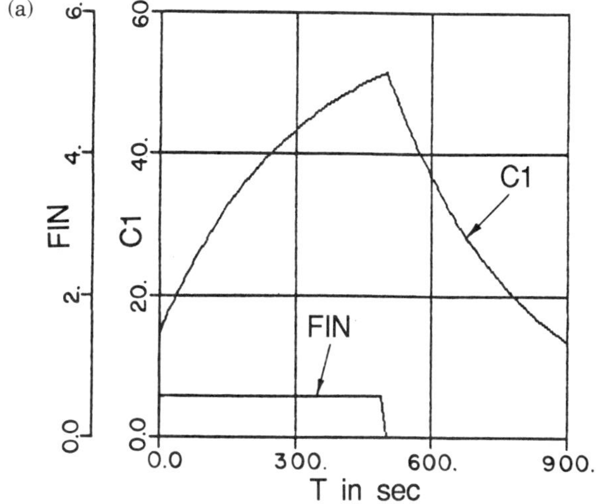

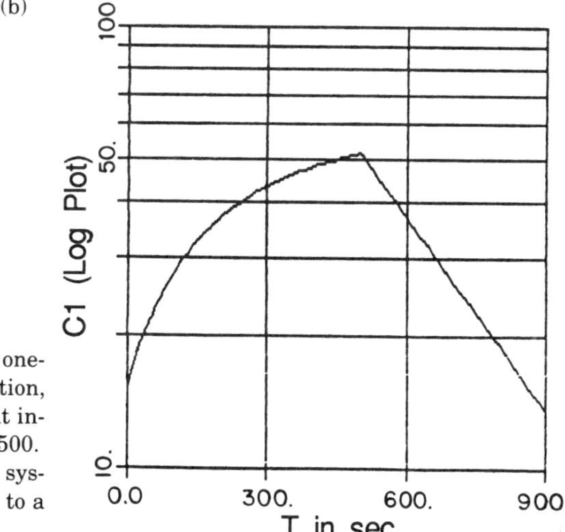

Figure 3.2.2. (a) ACSL plot of one-compartment system concentration, C1, for the case where the constant input FIN is reduced to zero at t = 500. (b) ACSL plot of C1 for the same system, but with the ordinate plotted to a log-scale.

after T = TX now becomes a straight line in the $\log_{10}$ plot, with a slope determined by the system time constant, $T_1 = V_1/K_1 = 300$.

It is often desirable to show a number of plots on one graph as a parameter is "swept" through a range of values (see Appendices A and C). Thus, in the case considered above, we may wish to sweep the initial condition, C1IC, through a range from zero to 60.0 in steps of 15.0; to do this, an Initial section and a Terminal section must be added to the program to give the equivalent of a do-loop. The result is shown in Fig. 3.2.3a.

Another interesting case (see Fig. 3.2.3b) is one in which the initial concentration, C1IC, is always zero but the input infusion is at a double rate for the first 50.*N units of time, with N running from zero to 5.0 in

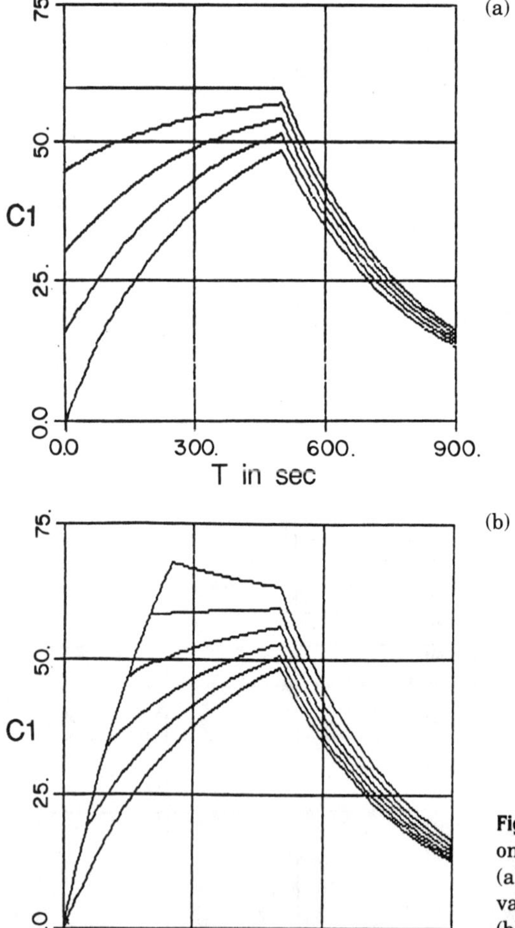

Figure 3.2.3. Concentrations in the one-compartment model
(a) with sweep of initial concentration values (Prob. 3-1).
(b) with sweep of the length of an initial double-rate infusion period. (Program COMPART2).

steps of 1.0; note that for the case of double-rate infusion lasting until T = 200., the concentration is constant at the final rate of $\gamma_1 = 60.0$ for 200. < T < 600. units of time. The sweep program, for the case of this initial double-rate infusion, is named COMPART2 and is shown below.

```
PROGRAM  COMPART2
 INITIAL
  Constant T2=0.,DT2=50.,DTN=255.
   L1..CONTINUE
 END          $ 'of Initial'

 DYNAMIC
    Cinterval CINT=10.
    TERMT (T .GE. TSTP)
    Constant TSTP=900.

 DERIVATIVE
    Algorithm IALG=4
    Nsteps    NSTP=1
    Maxterval MAXT=2.5
    Constant A=0.6, V1=3.0, K1=.01, T1=500.,C1IC=0.0
    C1 = INTEG ((FIN - K1*C1)/V1, C1IC)
    Z = T-T1 $ Y = T-T2
    FIN = FCNSW(Z, B, 0.0, 0.0)
    B = FCNSW(Y, 2.*A, A, A)
   END        $ 'of Deriv.'
  END         $ 'of Dynamic'

  TERMINAL
    CALL LOGD(.TRUE.)
    T2 = T2 + DT2              $'The original T2 is fixed'
    IF (T2 .LT. DTN) GO TO L1 $'but is outside the do-loop'
  END         $ 'of Terminal'
END           $ 'of Program'
```

Run-time commands are as in COMPART1, except that a retrace elimination command (SET FTSPLT = .T.) must be included. Note that although commands in DERIVATIVE are nonprocedural, this is not true in INITIAL or TERMINAL. Thus T2 is given its initial value of zero above the "top" of the do-loop.

A nicer way of providing the commands for a pulse FIN of length T1 with an initial double amplitude (out to T2) is to use the Real-Switch, replacing the last four commands in DERIVATIVE in COMPART2 by

```
FIN = RSW(T .LT. T1, B, 0.0)
B = RSW (T .LT. T2, 2.0*A, A)
```

Alternatively, two PULSE commands could be set up and summed.

3.3 MASS TRANSPORT BY FLUID FLOW

Before examining more detailed models related to diffusion, we will study the modeling and simulation of fluid-flow transport, the principal scheme that nature has evolved for moving nutrients, enzymes, oxygen, and other substances to the places where they are needed in the body or where diffusion processes can take over the distribution. Medical clinicians take advantage of this delivery scheme in administering pharmaceuticals. Here we will examine the modeling of flow transport schemes and then consider diffusion transport through membranes and tissue in more detail than in Sections 3.1 and 3.2, as well as combined transport (diffusion and flow) in following sections. Initially, transport by blood flow in the cardiovascular system will be considered, with some initial assumptions (listed at the end of Section 3.1) being made regarding the system and its modeling. As the models are improved, many of these assumptions will no longer be needed.

As blood flows along an artery, even in a smooth, laminar fashion, the blood near the walls of the vessel moves more slowly than that in the center. Both lateral and longitudinal diffusion within the flowing liquid will tend to even out the peaks and valleys in input concentration at points farther downstream. Turbulence, if it occurs, will increase mixing, as will the different lengths of parallel paths, as in capillary beds, and blood pulsatility. The series combination of perfect mixing chambers and plug-flow compartments of the right number and size will usually serve as a satisfactory model of any part of a blood flow or air flow system for pharmacokinetic or other transport studies. These modeling elements are relatively easy to depict mathematically and to use in computer studies. We will now consider how to set up computer simulations and observe responses.

Consider a segment of artery or vein, as shown in Fig. 3.3.1a, with average blood flow F (ml/s), and let us assume that flow is uniform across the diameter of the vessel and that any pulsatility in F is small and may be neglected. Suppose that the input flow pulse of solute f_0 and the resultant output f_2 from the segment are known to be as shown in Fig. 3.3.1b. The input and output concentrations will also be known and will have the same waveforms as the solute flows, since

$$\gamma_0(t) = f_0(t)/F \qquad \text{and} \qquad \gamma_2(t) = f_2(t)/F \tag{3.3.1}$$

If a lumped model of the segment is to be devised, we might begin by using a series combination of one perfect mixing compartment M and one delay compartment D, as shown in Fig. 3.3.1c. Transport in these compartments may be described mathematically as follows.

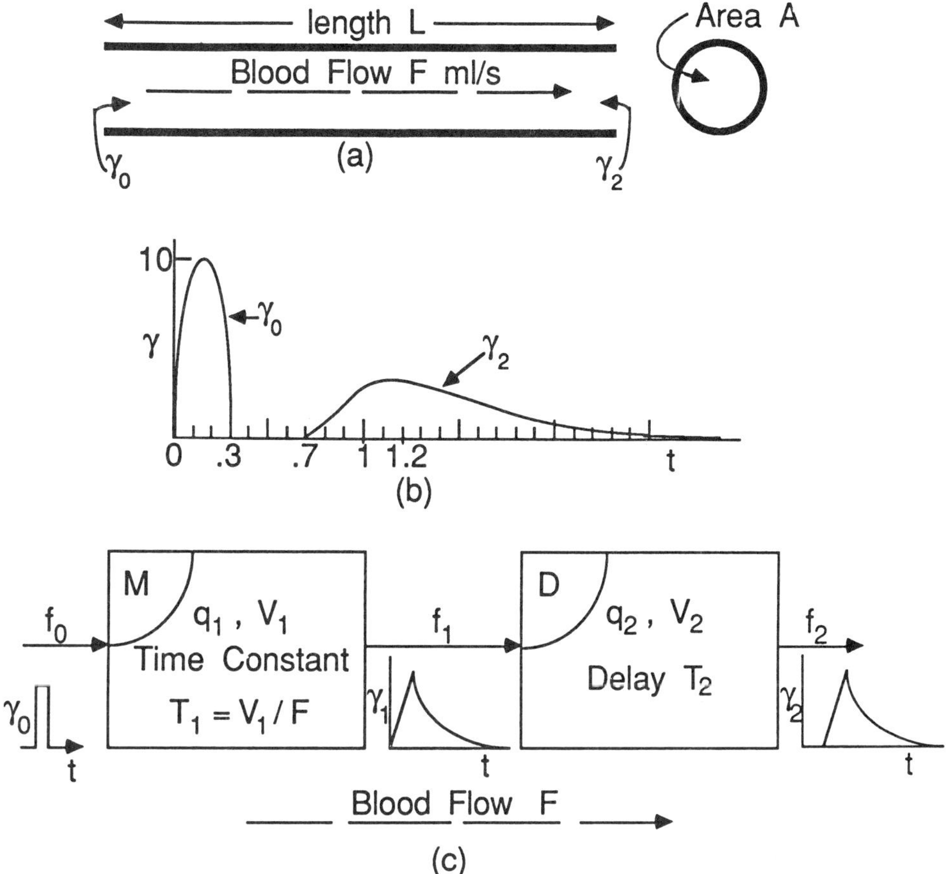

Figure 3.3.1. (a) Blood vessel of known volume V and constant cross-section, assumed to have constant blood flow F and observed input and output concentration curves γ_0 and γ_2.
(b) Known input and output concentrations versus time, γ_0 and γ_2.
(c) Assumed model with a mixing compartment, M, and a delay compartment, D, in series. These compartments have volumes V_1 and V_2, where $V_1 + V_2 = V$. Sketches of expected waveforms of γ_0, γ_1, and γ_2 are shown.

The quantity of solute $q_1(t)$ in M, by mass balance, is

$$q_1 = \int_0^t (f_0 - f_1)\, dt + q_1(0) \tag{3.3.2}$$

where $q_1(0)$ is the initial quantity (zero, in this case). (Note that in this equation and in much of what follows we will often omit the indication that the variables are functions of time, and write q_1 in place of $q_1(t)$, etc.)

The use of concentrations as independent variables is preferred, so using $\gamma_1 = q_1/V_1$, $f_0 = F*\gamma_0$, $f_1 = F*\gamma_1$ in (3.3.2)

$$\gamma_1 = \frac{F}{V_1} * \int_0^t (\gamma_0 - \gamma_1)dt + \gamma_1(0) \qquad (3.3.3)$$

where $\gamma_1(0) = q_1(0)/V_1$.

In (3.3.3), V_1/F is the characteristic time constant of mixing chamber M, which we will call T_1. We can use T_1 in writing (3.3.3) in differential equation form:

$$d\gamma_1/dt = (\gamma_0 - \gamma_1)/T_1 \qquad (3.3.4)$$

The flow f_1 of solute of concentration γ_1 is the input to the delay compartment in our model. Its output is

$$f_2(t) = f_1(t - T_2) \qquad (3.3.5)$$

Here the input flow must be known for t equal to or greater than $-T_2$; fortunately, it is zero for $-T_2 < t < 0$ in this case.

The output concentration equation, from (3.3.5), is

$$\gamma_2(t) = \gamma_1(t - T_2) \qquad (3.3.6)$$

Here we may again use Laplace transforms (see Appendix B) to find the form of the solution. Taking the transform of each side of (3.3.4) and using the uppercase symbol $\Gamma(s)$ in place of $\gamma(t)$ after transformation into the s domain, we will obtain

$$s\Gamma_1 - \gamma_1(0) = (F/V_1)*(\Gamma_0 - \Gamma_1)$$

From this equation, using $V_1/F = T_1$,

$$\Gamma_1(s) = \frac{\Gamma_0(s) + T_1\gamma_1(0)}{1 + sT_1} \qquad (3.3.7)$$

We can now guess at an approximation for $\gamma_0(t)$ and then substitute its transform $\Gamma_0(s)$ into (3.3.8) to find a model in Laplace form. The measured input γ_0 looks like a half-sinusoid, but we will initially choose a square-topped pulse of amplitude 8.0 and length 0.3 as an easier input to study. This will give

$$\gamma_0(t) = 8.0*u(t) - 8.0*u(t - 0.3)$$

After Laplace transformation

$$\Gamma_0(s) = 8.0/s - (8.0/s)e^{-0.3s} \qquad (3.3.8)$$

Substituting this in (3.3.8) and noting that $\gamma_1(0) = 0.0$ gives

$$\Gamma_1 = \frac{8.0}{s(1 + sT_1)} - \frac{8.0*e^{-0.3s}}{s(1 + sT_1)} \qquad (3.3.9)$$

This expression may be transformed to give

$$\gamma_1 = 8.0*(1 - e^{-t/T_1})*\mu(t) - 8.0*(1 - e^{-(t-0.3/T_1)})*\mu(t - 0.3) \qquad (3.3.10)$$

The output $\gamma_2(t)$ may be obtained from (3.3.10) by delaying everything by T_2. We can estimate $T_1 = 0.5$ and $T_2 = 0.7$ from Fig. 3.3.1b and use hand or machine computation to find the waveform of the estimated output γ_2, as shown in Fig. 3.3.2. This waveform is not a very good match because we took the easy approximation of a square-topped pulse input, and the response peak occurs too soon and is too high. However, the Laplace approach is rather awkward if we want only numerical answers and is very unsuitable if there is any future possibility that nonlinearities must be considered. Therefore, an ACSL programming approach will be used to reexamine the modeling of this system.

The modeling procedure used here is an elementary kind of system *structural identification* (in this case, the choice of one perfect mixing and one ideal delay compartment, in series), as well as some *parameter estimation*. These determinations began here with an educated guess and continued using "eyeball" methods. Needless to say, there are many highly developed mathematical methods for formal system identification and parameter estimation; some of these are introduced in Chapter 9, with problems relating to this section.

The ACSL program FLOTRAN1 shown below uses a better (half-sine wave) representation of the input γ_0, here called C0, and a REALPL, or simple lag, followed by a DELAY to give γ_2, followed in turn by a second lag.

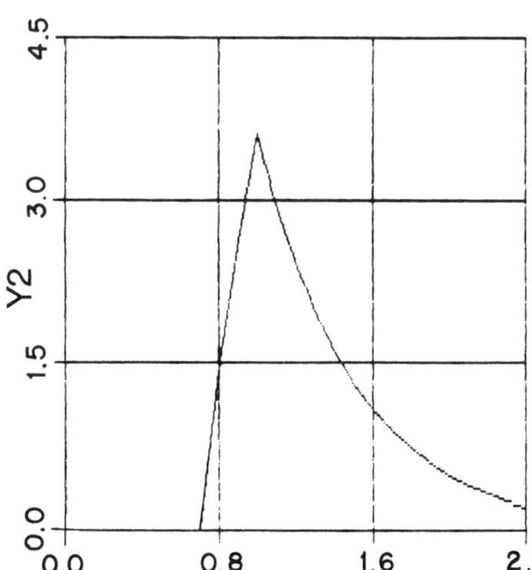

Figure 3.3.2. Waveform of the response of the Laplace approximation for $\gamma_2(t)$ from Eq. (3.3.10), delayed by $T_2 = 0.7$.

```
PROGRAM    FLOTRAN1         $ 'Flow Transport'
    Constant    PI = 3.141592, TPULS= 0.3

 INITIAL
    FREQ = 1.0/(2.0*TPULS)     $'Calculate frequency in hertz'
    W = 2.*PI*FREQ             $'and W in Rad./Sec. of a'
                               '0.3 sec. half-sine-wave'
 END $ 'of Initial'

 DYNAMIC
    Cinterval CINT=.02
    Constant TF = 2.4
      DERIVATIVE
    Algorithm IALG = 4  $ 'Runge Kutta 2'
    Maxterval MAXT = .002
    Nsteps NSTP = 1
  'System Equations'
    X = T- TPULS
    Y = 10.*SIN(W*T)
   Constant T1 = 0.25, T2 = 0.7
    C0 = FCNSW(X, Y, 0.0, 0.0)      $'Generates a half-sinusoid'
    C1 = REALPL(T1, C0, 0.0)        $'First simple lag'
    C2 = DELAY (C1, 0.0, T2, 2000) $'Time delay'
    C3 = REALPL(T1, C2, 0.0)        $'Second simple lag'
  END $ 'of Deriv.'

    TERMT (T .GE. TF)
 END $ 'of Dynamic'
END  $ 'of Program'
```

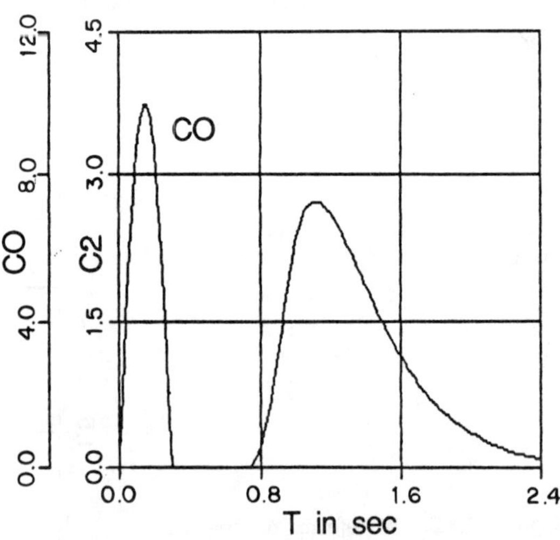

Figure 3.3.3. Response, C2, of the model in the FLOTRAN1 program to a half-sine input, C0. (compare with Fig. 3.3.1(b)).

The input C0 and output C2 obtained with this program are shown in Fig. 3.3.3; note that the output is better because the simulation of the input is improved. However, more improvement resulted because one simple lag of 0.5 sec was replaced by two, each of 0.25 sec, as shown.

3.4 INDICATOR DILUTION: MODELING AND COMPUTER SIMULATION

Indicators such as cool saline solutions or inert dyes may be introduced into the cardiovascular system to determine the cardiac output (CO) or average blood flow (F) or to study heart defects (Zierler-63; Bassingthwaighte-74,77). A common procedure is to introduce a bolus of cold saline into the right ventricle by means of a catheter, after which thermocouple measurements are made to determine the concentration versus time of the cold liquid in the blood of the radial artery (Roselli-75). An inert dye was formerly used for these measurements; radio-opaque dyes are still used, together with X rays, to analyze coronary artery and other heart defects. Radionuclide substances are often used (Flaherty-67) to study heart defects such as ventricular septal defects that give rise to left-to-right shunts.

Computer simulation of indicator transport in the cardiovascular system may be important in studying indicator techniques. It should be noted that because the transients of interest encountered in indicator dilution are much faster than those in most pharmacokinetic (PK) studies, models of indicator dilution must be more detailed. Thus, if a satisfactory model of indicator dilution can be set up, it should be satisfactory as a basis for design of PK models.

Simulation study of indicator dilution can be accomplished with a model that combines delay and perfect mixing compartments as described for simple cases in Section 3.3; the compartments in this case must be connected in a complete loop, corresponding to the cardiovascular loop. Figures 3.4.1a and 3.4.1b show typical measured concentrations for radial artery output, with input to the right heart. Note that the measured concentration in the normal case (Fig. 3.4.1a) shows a small second peak, corresponding to a recirculation of the original bolus around the cardiovascular loop; it also shows an initial zero response up to the "appearance time" when response is first seen. With a VSD, or ventricular septal defect (an opening between the ventricles), particularly for the larger defect (Fig. 3.4.1c), a fast recirculation through the VSD and the right ventricle and lungs gives rise to a new peak just after the initial pulse. Also, the main recirculation peak is flattened and delayed.

In order to set up a compartment model using only delay and mixing compartments, it is necessary to know the following data:

1. *Total transport time* T_t around the loop. This time, which is about 39 sec in the healthy human adult, is approximately given by the peak-to-peak time, (if the second peak can be distinguished).
2. *Appearance time* T_a around the loop. This time, about 13 sec in the human adult, may be represented by delay compartments, leaving approximately $T_t - 13 = 27$ sec for the total of the time constants of the mixing compartments.
3. *Cardiac output* or average loop flow F.
4. *Blood volumes* in the principal parts of the CV system.

Knowledge of these data will not tell us how many compartments of each kind are needed. However, some experimentation will show that too few mixing chambers will cause the simulated thermal dilution curves to be too low and flat, whereas too many will cause them to be too sharply peaked.

Because the plug flow simulated by delay compartments is distributed throughout the cardiovascular system, some detailed simulations might require a number of such delays, perhaps one for each mixing compartment. Here we will compromise by arbitrarily assigning one delay compartment to the approximate 5 sec of appearance time delay in the pulmonary circulation, and one of 8 sec in the systemic circulation.

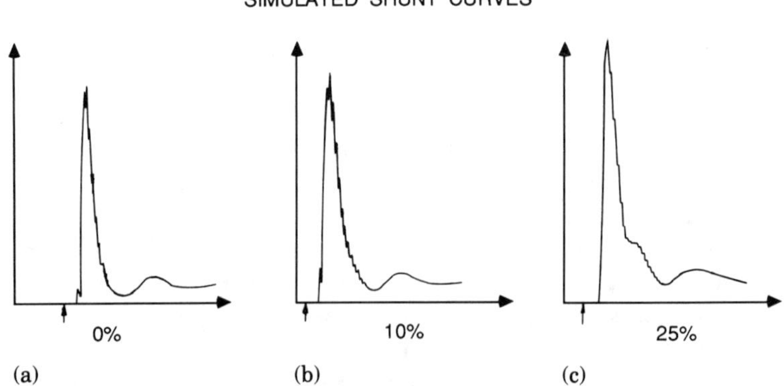

Figure 3.4.1. Canine indicator curves measured at the femoral artery (from (Castillo-66), with permission).
(a) Normal heart
(b) With 10% ventricular septal defect (simulated by injecting the major amount of dye into the left ventricle and the indicated fraction into the right ventricle simultaneously).
(c) With 25% ventricular septal defect, also simulated.

These values may be obtained from an assumed delay compartment volume of 500 ml in the pulmonary and 800 ml in the systemic system, according to the following equations:

$$T_p = V_p/F = 500/100 = 5 \text{ sec}$$
$$T_s = V_s/F = 800/100 = 8 \text{ sec} \tag{3.4.1}$$

where the cardiac output is $F = 100$ ml/sec.

Experimentation has shown that eight mixing compartments in addition to the two delay compartments give a fair match to the observed thermal or dye dilution curves in the healthy adult human. Let us select one mixing compartment for each of the ventricles and assign other compartments, as shown in Fig. 3.4.2 and Table 3.4.1. Note that the total blood volume is 4000 ml, corresponding, for $F = 100$, to a total delay time of 40 sec.

Figure 3.4.2 shows a complete model of the cardiovascular system using ten compartments, and includes an input flow, FD (of dye or cold saline), to the pulmonary artery compartment. It includes a ventricular septal defect (VSD), with left-to-right average blood flow shunt, F_{VSD}. This defect will not be present, in effect, if F_{VSD} is set to zero.

A third kind of compartment that slightly skews the response has sometimes been included in other simulation studies but is not used here.

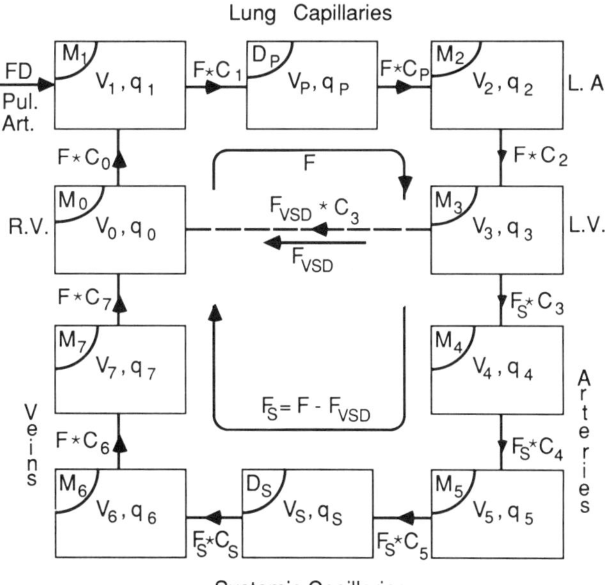

Figure 3.4.2. Ten-compartment model used to study indicator transport in the cardiovascular system.

Also, the loop is rather simple with no parallel paths. If parallel paths were used in a more detailed model, some skewing and flattening of the output peak would result if the parallel paths were of different lengths.

Before writing a simulation program for the model of Fig. 3.4.2, we must adapt the compartment equations developed in Section 3.2 to the needs of this model. Beginning with compartment 1 (pulmonary artery), into which the bolus of indicator is injected, (3.3.3) with indicator input flow included becomes

$$q_1 = \int_0^t (f_0 - f_1 + f_d)\, dt + q_1(0) \tag{3.4.2}$$

In terms of concentrations, as in (3.3.3)

$$\gamma_1 = (F/V_1)*\int_0^t (\gamma_0 - \gamma_1 + f_d/F)\, dt + \gamma_1(0) \tag{3.4.3}$$

where F/V_1 is $1/T_1$, the reciprocal of the time constant of compartment 1. Thus, in the ACSL program nomenclature

```
C1 = INTEG ((C0 - C1 + FD/F)/T1, 0.0)
```
(3.4.4)

if the initial condition is zero.

A simple ACSL program for the model of Fig. 3.4.2 may now be written for the case of no VSD (flow FVSD = 0.0), using the typical time constants for an adult male given in Table 3.4.1; this program, IND-DIL1, is shown here.

TABLE 3.4.1

Compartment No.	Kind	Anatomy Represented	Volume (ml)	T_n (sec) (for F = 100 ml/s)
0	(M)	Right ventricle	125	1.25
1	(M)	Pulmonary artery	250	2.5
P	(D)	Pulmonary capillaries and veins	500	5.0
2	(M)	Left atrium	125	1.25
3	(M)	Left ventricle	125	1.25
4	(M)	Aorta, large arteries	750	7.5
5	(M)	Small arteries	200	2.0
S	(D)	Systemic capillaries and small veins	800	8.0
6	(M)	Systemic veins	1000	10.0
7	(M)	Right atrium	125	1.25
		Totals	4000 ml	40 sec

```
  PROGRAM  IND-DIL1
   DYNAMIC
     Cinterval CINT=0.2
      Constant TF=80.0

    DERIVATIVE
     Maxterval MAXT = .02        $ Nsteps NSTP = 1
     FD = A*PULSE(0.0,1.E6,PW)  $'Single pulse, Amp. A, width PW'
      Constant A = 0.5, PW = 0.5
     C1  =  INTEG  ((CO  +  FD/F  -  C1)/T1,0.0)  $'Pulm.  Art.'
Constant F=100., T1=2.5
     CP = DELAY (C1, 0.0, TP, 1000)        $'Pulm. delay'
      Constant  TP=5.
     C2 = INTEG ((CP - C2)/T2, 0.0)        $'Pulm. veins,L.atrium'
      Constant  T2=1.25, T3=1.25, T4=7.5, T5=2.0
     C3 = INTEG ((C2 - C3)/T3, 0.0)        $'L. ventricle'
     C4 = INTEG ((C3 - C4)/T4, 0.0)        $'Aorta, large Arts.'
     C5 = INTEG ((C4 - C5)/T5, 0.0)        $'Small arteries'
     CS = DELAY (C5, 0.0, TS, 1600)        $'Systemic delay'
      Constant  TS=8.0
     C6 = INTEG ((CS - C6)/T6, 0.0)        $'Small veins'
      Constant  T6=10., T7=1.25, TO=1.25
     C7 = INTEG ((C6 - C7)/T7, 0.0)        $'Large veins,Rt.atrium'
     CO = INTEG ((C7 - CO)/TO, 0.0)        $'Rt.  ventricle'
    END    $ 'of Deriv'
     TERMT (T .GE. TF)
   END     $ 'of Dynamic'

  END     $ 'of Program
```

The waveforms obtained with this program (see Fig. 3.4.3) resemble those obtained from normal adult humans; closer resemblance might require the use of many more compartments in the model. But it should be more than adequate for most pharmacokinetic simulations with their narrower-band frequency content, as pointed out in Section 3.3.

Note that the peak-to-peak time in C5 is about 37 sec, which is close to the sum (40 sec) of all time constants given in program IND-DIL1. With some checks of this sort and evidence of self-consistency in the model, we can go ahead and use it to give at least approximate answers for the effects of various defects on the indicator curves. Note that although "eyeball" checks are encouraging and helpful, the fine-tuning of a model to fit real data better may require formal parameter estimation methods (see Chapter 9).

A single defect (a VSD, as shown in Fig. 3.4.2) will be included in the next study. In order that the size of the VSD can be conveniently

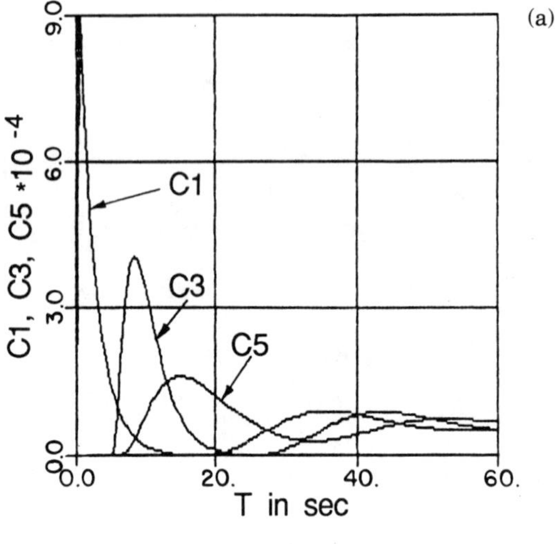

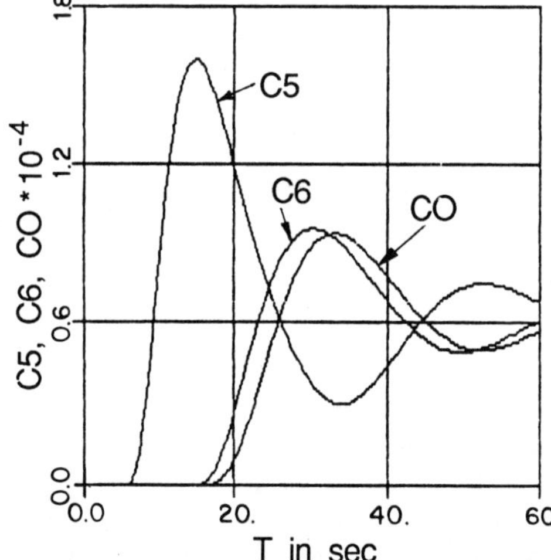

Figure 3.4.3. Indicator dilution (concentration) waveforms for C1, C3, C5, C6 and C0 obtained with program INDDIL1, simulating the model of Fig. 3.4.2; note the recirculation peaks and the smoothing (lowering and widening) of all peaks after passage through mixing compartments.

changed from run to run, F_{VSD} will now be included in the system constants. The systemic flow F_S is given in (3.4.5), and is used in place of F in the equations for C_4 through C_7 in the systemic circuit.

$$F_S = F - F_{\text{VSD}} \tag{3.4.5}$$

The equation for compartment zero with its two inflows is based on

$$q_0 = \int_0^t (f_7 + \gamma_3 {*} F_{\text{VSD}} - f_0)\, dt + q_0(0)$$

$$= \int_0^t (\gamma_7 {*} F_S + \gamma_3 {*} F_{\text{VSD}} - \gamma_0 {*} F) dt + q_0(0)$$

The concentration in this compartment is γ_0/V_0; therefore

$$\gamma_0 = (F/V_0)*\int_0^t (\gamma_7*F_S + \gamma_3*F_{VSD} - \gamma_0*F)dt + \gamma_0(0) \qquad (3.4.6)$$

It will now be interesting to examine the effects of the VSD in this compartment model; in order to do this, a better program has been written that includes not only the VSD effects but also the determination of time constants in the INITIAL part of the program, so that new time constants are automatically determined when blood flow F or F_{VSD} is changed. Two convenient constants are defined and calculated in INITIAL,

$$K_7 = F_S/F \text{ and } K_3 = F_{VSD}/F \qquad (3.4.7)$$

The program, entitled IND-DIL2, is shown below (except for run-time commands). In Fig. 3.4.4 are shown various model output concentration curves versus time, with and without a VSD.

```
PROGRAM  IND-DIL2
  Constant F=100.,FVSD=0.0,V1=250.,...
  V2=125.,VP=500.,V3=125. ,V4=750.,...
  V5=200.,VS=800.,V6=1000.,V7=125.,...
  V0=125.

 INITIAL
  FS= F-FVSD $ T1= V1/F    $ TP=VP/F
  T2=V2/F    $ T3=  V3/F   $ T4=V4/FS
  T5=V5/FS   $ TS=  VS/FS  $ T6=V6/FS
  T7=V7/FS   $ T0= V0/F    $ K7=FS/F
  K3=FVSD/F
 END   $ 'of Initial'

 DYNAMIC
  Constant TF=80.
  Cinterval CINT=0.5

  DERIVATIVE
   Algorithm IALG= 4
   Maxterval MAXT= 0.25
   Nsteps NSTP= 1
  Constant PW = 0.5, A = 0.5
   FD= A*PULSE(0.0,1.E6,PW)
   C1= INTEG((C0+FD/F-C1)/T1,0.)
   CP= DELAY(C1,0.,TP,1000)
   C2= INTEG((CP-C2)/T2,0.)
   C3= INTEG((C2-C3)/T3,0.0)
   C4= INTEG((C3-C4)/T4,0.0)
   C5= INTEG((C4-C5)/T5,0.0)
```

```
          CS= DELAY(C5,0.,TS,1600)
          C6= INTEG((CS-C6)/T6,0.0)
          C7= INTEG((C6-C7)/T7,0.0)
          CO= INTEG((K7*C7+K3*C3-CO)/TO,0.)
         END $'of Derivative'

         TERMT (T.GE.TF)
        END $ 'of Dynamic'

       END $ 'of Program'
```

The effects of the VSD, as shown in Fig. 3.4.4, again give concentration waveforms that have a fair resemblance to corresponding waveforms obtained clinically. Particularly noteworthy is the early peak of C0 due to VSD flow. The model can also be used to give approximate indicator-dilution responses for various other defects, such as an atrial septal defect, patent ductus arteriosus, or combinations of such defects (see the problems at the end of this chapter).

It is not easy to study the effects of a VSD by comparing the case of no VSD to a single case with a VSD of assumed size, so a program has been written using a parameter sweep scheme (see Appendix A) to show the effect of varying FVSD from 0 to 30 in 6 ml/s steps. This required that the program be modified by removing the constant FVSD and introducing three new constants, plus a modified Initial and a new Terminal portion, in program IND-DIL2, as shown below:

```
'New Initial program and Constants for FVSD sweep'

CONSTANT FVSDI=0.,DFVSD=6.,MFVSD=30.

 INITIAL
   FVSD=FVSDI    $ T1=V1/F   $ TP=VP/F
   T2=V2/F       $ T3=V3/F   $ TO=VO/F
   L1..CONTINUE

   FS = F-FVSD    $   K3 = FVSD/F
   T5=V5/FS $  TS=VS/FS     $ T6=V6/FS
   T7=V7/FS $  T4=V4/FS     $ K7=FS/F
 END $'Of Initial'

 'New Terminal program (after End of Dynamic) for sweep'
 TERMINAL
   CALL LOGD(.TRUE.)
   FVSD=FVSD+ DFVSD
   IF(FVSD .LE. MFVSD) GO TO L1
 END $'Of Terminal'
```

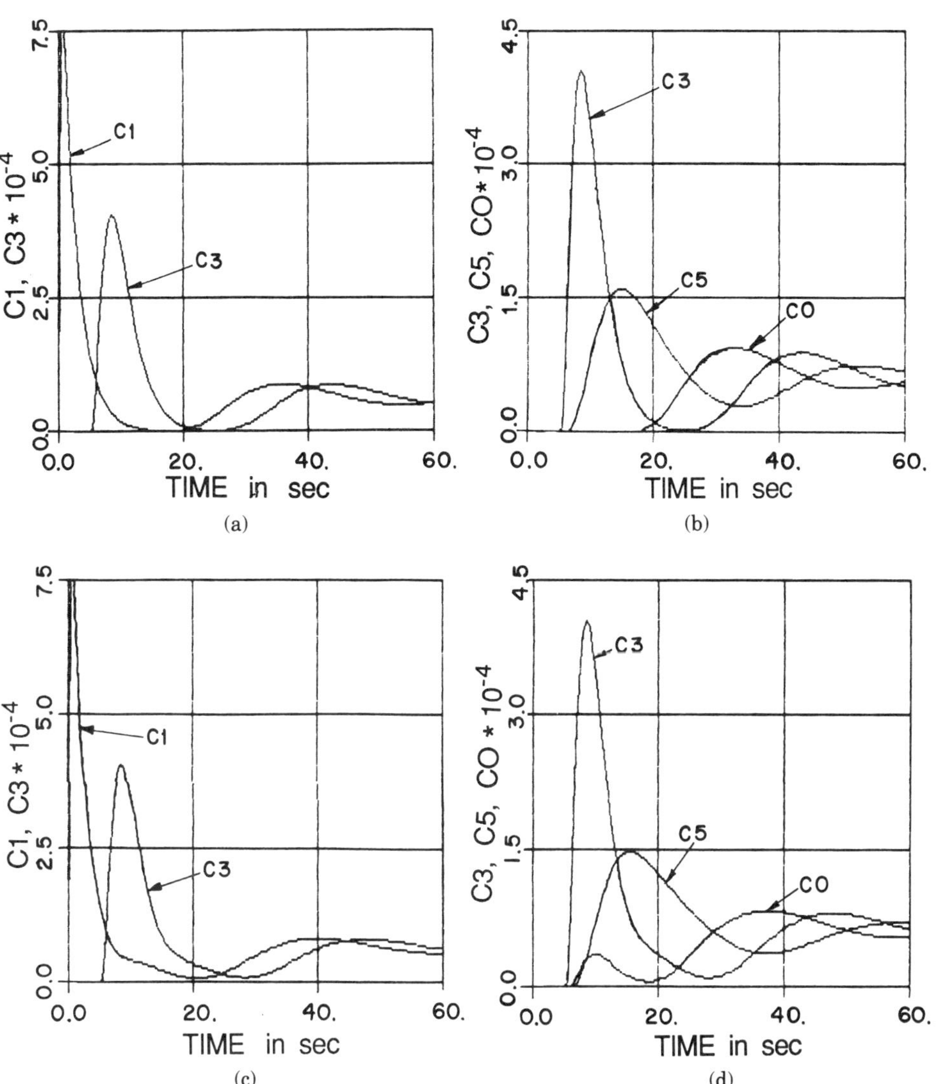

Figure 3.4.4. (a) Plots of concentrations C1 and C3 for the case of no VSD in response to an input pulse FD of length 0.5 sec.
(b) Plots of C3, C5, and C0 (no VSD). Note the new ordinate scale.
(c) Plots of C1 and C3 with VSD, for FVSD = 10.
(d) Plots of C3, C5, and C0 with VSD. Note that the early VSD recirculation pulse is quite evident in C0 but is more difficult to detect in C1 and C3 in (c). Its only visible effect on C5 is to delay the second peak.

The results of using this parameter sweep program (which will be named IND-DIL3) are as shown in Fig. 3.4.5 for concentrations C3, C7, and C0. Note that the concentration curves tend to have lower peaks that occur later in time as the VSD aperture size and flow increase. These effects are caused by the larger time constants in the systemic circuit as FS gets smaller, and by the later addition of the peak due to the VSD flow to the original first peak caused by indicator injection.

The single-loop model of Fig. 3.4.2 used in the programs given above is more than adequate for reproduction of transients in pharmacokinetic studies, in which the drug is introduced into the blood stream rather slowly, and is taken up still more slowly by diffusion into tissues. The

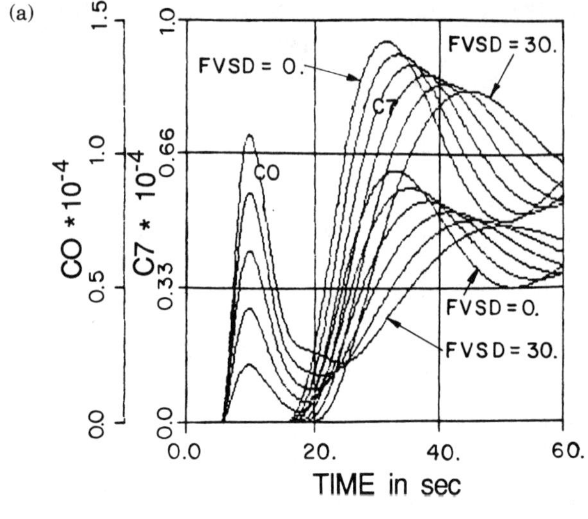

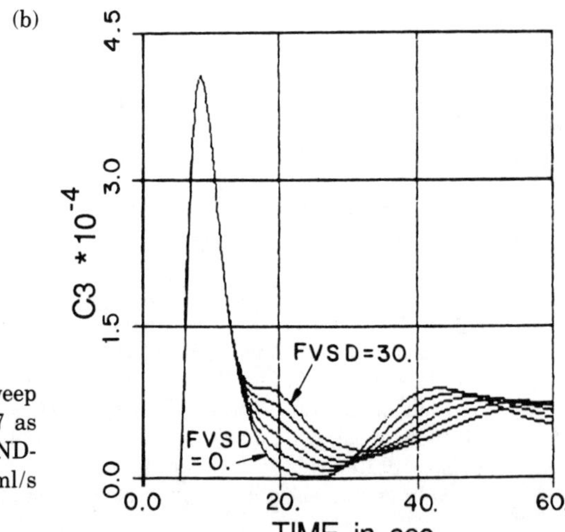

Figure 3.4.5. (a) Parameter sweep plots of concentrations C0, and C7 as FVSD is varied (in Program IND-DIL3) from zero to 30 ml/s in 6 ml/s steps.
(b) Plots of C3 during the same sweep.

physical, or structural, models used by such modelers as Bischoff and Dedrick do not require as many compartments in the main loop, but may need several systemic compartments in parallel to represent tissue beds in various organs (Bischoff-66,71, Dedrick-68, and Morrison-75). The combination of flow and diffusion transport required in pharmacokinetic studies is discussed in Section 3.5.

The transport model of Fig. 3.4.2 may also be used to simulate and study the use of indicator-dilution methods for measurement of cardiac output and system volume (Zierler-63,62, Bassingthwaighte-74,77). If a chain of compartments is not connected in a loop or if the effects of recirculation can be subtracted off in some way, then by conservation of mass

$$Q_I = F*\int_0^\infty \gamma_{AO}(t)dt = F*\int_0^\infty \gamma_n(t)dt \tag{3.4.8}$$

where F is cardiac output and Q_I is the total indicator volume injected into the right heart. This assumes that γ_{AO} (in the aorta) equals γ_n anywhere in the arterial system, because complete mixing has occurred in the left ventricle before the blood divides into its various channels. Thus the average cardiac output or blood flow F from the left heart is the total amount Q_1 of indicator injected divided by the integral of concentration in any compartment n in the arterial system:

$$F - Q_I \div \int_0^\infty \gamma_n(t)\, dt \tag{3.4.9}$$

This is the Stewart-Hamilton expression for cardiac output, widely used clinically for cardiac output (CO) measurement, particularly with cold saline indicator (Roselli-75). The ACSL model IND-DIL2 given earlier in this section (now to be called IND-DIL4) may be used to illustrate the use of (3.4.9) by first eliminating recirculation altogether in the model and then examining methods for eliminating its effects in model or living subject tests. Recirculation elimination in the model becomes quite simple if a constant X, which may be set at zero or one, is introduced into the recirculation term in the C1 equation in the program referred to above, as follows:

```
C1 = INTEG((C0*X + FD/F - C1)/T1, 0.0)
```
(3.4.10)

Recirculation will be normal if X is set to unity at run time, but if it is set to zero, it will be eliminated.

In addition to using this new equation for C1 in the indicator program, we also need to add to the Derivative section the integral required in (3.4.9), which we will choose to determine for compartments 4 and 0; in ACSL form these are

```
INT4 = INTEG (C4, 0.0)
INT0 = INTEG (C0, 0.0)
```
(3.4.11)

Because we need only the final values of these integrals, we choose some adequate length of run, TF = 100., and add to the program a Terminal section, using ACSL versions of (3.4.9) to find estimates of average flow *F*, such as FM4 and FM0, as follows:

```
TERMINAL
'Cardiac output may be found using integrals of C4 and CO'
  FM4 = QI/INT4                                              (3.4.12)
  FMO = QI/INTO
End  $ 'Of Terminal'
```

With these additions in IND-DIL4, the run-time commands will yield various concentration and other curves of interest and will give the cardiac output as determined by sampling output concentration at compartment 4 (FM4) and compartment 0 (FM0). The initial run-time commands are

```
SET TF=100., X=0.0
OUTPUT T,INT4,INTO, 'NCIOUT'=20
PREPAR T,C4,CO,INT4,INTO
START
```

As the run is in progress, the output can be checked to see that TF is adequately long by noting if INT4 and INT0 reach steady maximum values. It is then possible to call for plots of C4, INT4, C0, and INT0, as shown in Fig. 3.4.6. Also, we can make a run-time display command (DISPLY) that calls for the final values; this command and the resultant values are shown below:

```
DISPLY T,QI,C4,CO,INT4,INTO,FM4,FMO
T= 100.000000        QI= 0.25000000       C4=2.3838E-09
CO=4.5492E-07        INT4=0.00247582      INTO=0.0024711
FM4=100.97700        FMO=101.166000
```

Here the relatively small final values of C0 and C4 indicate that apparently our choice of TF = 100.0 is an adequate integration time. However, the estimates of cardiac output, FM0 and FM4, are about 1 percent off; this results because the concentration integrals INT0 and INT4, which should equal $Q_I/F = 0.0025$, are about 1 percent off.

To determine cardiac output in a living subject the recirculation "tail" of the concentration must be eliminated. One way of doing this is to fit a decaying exponential to the falling concentration curve just before recirculation appears, and to use this in place of the continuing tail of the complete curve. Two points on the concentration curve will serve to define an exponential as to initial value and time constant.

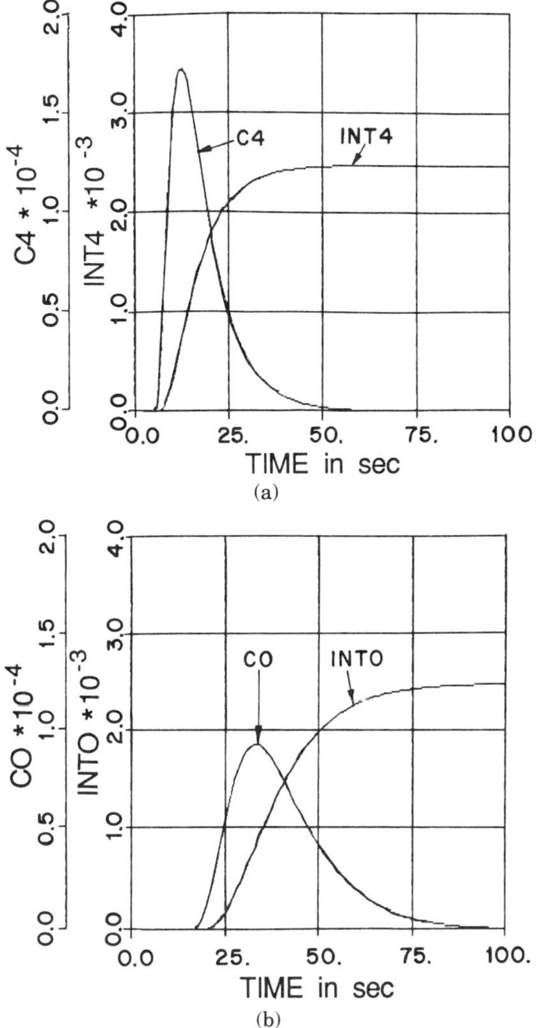

Figure 3.4.6. (a) Concentration γ_4 (C4 in ACSL) and its integral, INT4. (b) Concentration C0 and INTO.

Some other interesting and important quantities may be determined from indicator-concentration curves; these include average transit times between any two compartments and blood volume for any compartment or sequence of compartments. These quantities are most conveniently determined using the transport function, defined as

$$h_n(t) = F*\gamma_n(t)/Q_I \tag{3.4.13}$$

This function contains the instantaneous flow of solute $F*\gamma_n$, which, when divided by the total input of solute Q_I, gives the fraction of solute arriving at the output of compartment n per unit of time. The equations for this transport function in ACSL form for compartments 4 and 0 are

```
H4 = F*C4/QI
                                        (3.4.14)
H0 = F*C0/QI
```

If the input FD is a true impulse, and if recirculation is somehow removed, then any $h_n(t)$ for the resultant open-loop case is the unit impulse response at the output of compartment n. Plots of H4 at the end of four compartments and H0 at the end of all eight compartments for the near impulse input used in IND-DIL4 are shown in Fig. 3.4.7a.

The average time of transit from compartment 0 to any compartment, n, may be determined by using the transport function in the integral

$$t_n = \int_0^t t*h_n\ t)\ dt \tag{3.4.15}$$

or, in ACSL notation, for compartment 4

```
TA4 = INTEG(T*H4, 0.0)
```

If (3.4.14) and (3.4.15) are included in the Derivative section of IND-DIL2, the final values of the average transit times TA4F and TA0F may be determined by calling for the values of TA4 and TA0 using the DISPLY command after the run is completed. (Here their values will be found to be TA4F = 17.7423 and TA0F = 39.9598; note how close the latter is to the sum of all the time constants in the model.)

The volume of blood in the system may be determined by using the command

```
V = FM0*TA0                             (3.4.16)
```

which is the product of estimated average flow and average transit time. Use of DISPLY will then show that the total volume V is 4042.57, which is close to the exact value for Fig. 3.4.2 of 4000 ml. For the first four compartments, calculation of volume using V4 = FM4*TA4 will give 1791.55, which is close to the calculated model volume V1 + V2 + VP + V3 + V4 = 1750 ml.

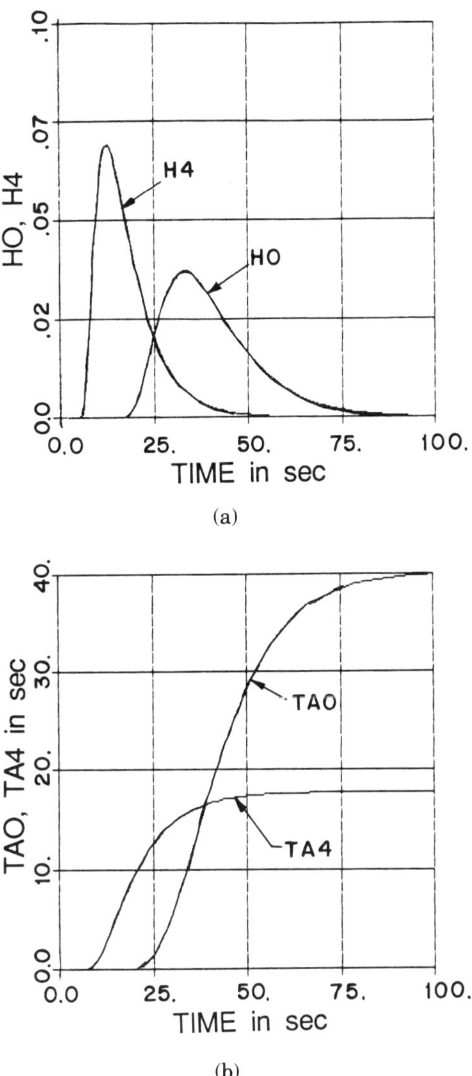

Figure 3.4.7. (a) Plots of transport functions γ_4 and γ_0 (H4 and H0). (b) Plots of transport times TA4 and TA0.

3.5 TRANSPORT BY FLOW AND DIFFUSION IN COMPARTMENT SYSTEMS

The transport of solutes by diffusion transport was discussed for simple one- and two-compartment models in Sections 3.1 and 3.2 and flow transport was examined in Sections 3.3 and 3.4 in both simple models and models that had some relationship to physiological form. However, only flow transport for large molecule inert substances such as indicator dyes was considered; since these substances do not readily diffuse into tissue and are not important when they do, their kinetics are mostly in the bloodstream and do not offer the complexity of the vast range of therapeutic drugs that can diffuse through vascular and cell walls and react with other substances in the blood. Natural substances, such as oxygen, carbon dioxide, and hormones, may diffuse into or out of tissue, and the modeling of such transport may be of considerable interest. Here we will examine various aspects of diffusion and of transport by combined effects of diffusion and flow for a wider range of substances (Bischoff-66, Wagner-75, Himmelstein-79).

It is helpful to begin by re-examining the two-compartment model for diffusion transport (shown in Fig. 3.1.2) in order to establish nomenclature and to add some important features to the models we consider, relating to solubility and protein binding. Initially, we will neglect these effects and rewrite Eqs. (3.1.7) and (3.1.8) for the slightly more general case where the coefficient of diffusivity K_1 has a forward value of k_{12}, and a value of k_{21} in the reverse direction, as follows:

$$V_1 * \frac{d\gamma_1}{dt} = f_1 - k_{12} * \gamma_1 + k_{21} * \gamma_2$$

$$V_2 * \frac{d\gamma_2}{dt} = k_{12} * \gamma_1 - k_{21} * \gamma_2 - k_{20} * \gamma_2 \qquad (3.5.1)$$

where $\gamma_1 = q_1/V_1$ and $\gamma_2 = q_2/V_2$, and $k_{20} * \gamma_2$ is a term expressing loss of the solute from the system, perhaps by metabolism into another chemical, the kinetics of which might need to be modeled by another, similar set of equations.

The system represented by (3.5.1) is shown in Fig. 3.5.1a, and is referred to as a diffusion-limited system. Note that it is easily possible to add other tissue segments coupled by diffusion to the main "blood pool" in Fig. 3.5.1a. Diffusion-limited models have been used to model the pharmacokinetics of substances that do not rapidly equilibrate between capillary blood and tissue, such as salicylate (Chen-79) and actinomycin-D.

The system shown in Fig. 3.5.1b is a flow-limited system with a simple blood circulation loop containing a single mixing chamber M_1. The equation for the blood pool is

$$V_1 * \frac{d\gamma_1}{dt} = f_I - F * (\gamma_1 - \gamma_2) \qquad (3.5.2)$$

where $\gamma_v = \gamma_2$ because equilibrium is assumed to have been reached between the solute concentration in the venous end of the capillaries and

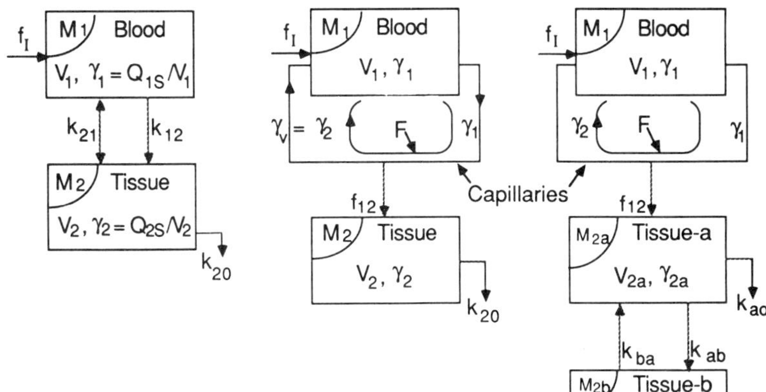

Figure 3.5.1. (a) Compartment modeling of diffusion-limited transfer of solute between blood pool and tissue.
(b) Modeling of flow-limited transfer of solute between capillaries and tissue.
(c) Modeling of a combination of flow and diffusion limiting of solute transfer to (or from) tissue.

that in the tissue bed in flow-limited (or perfusion-limited) systems. The solute outflow in this case from capillaries to tissue is

$$f_{12} = F*(\gamma_1 - \gamma_2) \tag{3.5.3}$$

In the tissue bed, with inflow f_{12} and outflow determined by an elimination diffusion constant k_{20},

$$V_2* \frac{d\gamma_2}{dt} = f_{12} - k_{20}*\gamma_2 = F*(\gamma_1 - \gamma_2) - k_{20}*\gamma_2 \tag{3.5.4}$$

Note that Eqs. (3.5.2) and (3.5.4) are much the same as Eq. (3.3.3), except that the latter is in integral form.

Various modeling schemes may be used if blood-to-tissue transport is not completely flow limited. One method is shown in Fig. 3.5.1c, where the tissue bed is split into one part of volume V_{2a}, which is near the capillaries, and another part of volume $V_{2b} = V_2 - V_{2a}$, with diffusion transport between the two tissue beds. In some early papers the blood in the capillaries is assigned to one or more lumped compartments coupled by diffusion to interstitial space which is in turn coupled to intracellular space (Bischoff-66).

Solubility may be different in tissue than in blood, and as a result, the effective volume of tissue may need to be changed, or partition coefficients may be used. Typically, a tissue/blood partition coefficient, defined as the ratio at equilibrium of concentration of solute in tissue to that in blood, is used:

$$\lambda_{tb} = \gamma_t/\gamma_b \tag{3.5.5}$$

This partition coefficient should be used in the tissue equation (3.5.4) for the flow-limited case in Fig. 3.5.1b, as follows:

$$V_2 * \frac{d\gamma_2}{dt} = F*\gamma_1 - F*\gamma_2/\lambda_{tb} - k_{20}*\gamma_2 \tag{3.5.6}$$

If there are other tissue compartments in parallel with the single tissue compartment of Fig. 3.5.1b, the equation for each would need to be modified to include the appropriate tissue/blood partition coefficient (Kety-51, Chen- 79). The partition coefficients are particularly important in models of the pharmacokinetics of gaseous anesthetics because they may be quite large; thus, for halothane in fatty tissue λ_{bg} may be over 50, indicating possible serious problems with storage of dissolved halothane in body fat. Modeling of the uptake of such gaseous substances is considered in Chapters 5 and 6.

An important nonlinear term should often be included in pharmacokinetic model equations in which elimination of a substance by enzyme catalysis takes place. This is the Michaelis-Menten term (Bartolomy-62, Niazi-79), which is derived and discussed in more detail in Section 3.6. It gives an added rate of concentration change:

$$V * \frac{d\gamma}{dt} = -\frac{v_m * \gamma}{K_m + \gamma} \tag{3.5.7}$$

Here K_m is called the Michaelis constant and v_m (also called V_{max}) is the maximum rate of decrease, as shown by

$$V*d\gamma/dt = -v_m \quad for\ \gamma >> K_m \tag{3.5.8}$$

For small concentrations, ($\gamma << K_m$)

$$V*d\gamma/dt = -(v_m/K_m)*\gamma \tag{3.5.9}$$

Equation (3.5.9) is linear and may be used in place of Eq. (3.5.7) when γ is small compared to K_m.

The action of Michaelis-Menten elimination is by metabolism of the transported substance to some other form. Modeling of the transport of this new substance may require that another model be set up, a kind of multiple modeling (see Chapter 6). A similar modeling problem arises when a given substance is carried in the blood in two forms—bound (usually to proteins in the blood) and free. Here, too, one model may be used for the bound substance and one for the free; or a single model may be used (Dedrick-73) in which, for example, the total concentration of a substance in compartment n is

$$\gamma_n = \alpha * \gamma_{nf} + (1 - \alpha) * \gamma_{nb} \tag{3.5.10}$$

where the first term is the free and the second is the bound concentration.

3.6. ENZYME SYSTEMS AND MODELS

The form and importance of simple enzyme systems were pointed out in Section 3.5. The nonlinearities in such systems result because an enzyme reacts with a substrate (which may be a pharmaceutical substance) in proportion to the product $C_E{*}C_S$ of enzyme and substrate concentrations, C_E and C_S, in a region treated as a compartment (we will first consider a closed system, with no inflow or outflow). The study of enzyme systems, or of larger systems in which they appear, usually requires computer simulation because of the strong nonlinearities resulting from these product terms (Hayashi-86).

It is interesting to examine the model of a simple single-enzyme system (Gold-77, Gibaldi-82), following what is referred to as the Michaelis-Menten kinetics. The concentration relationships in such a system may be expressed by

$$E + S \underset{k_2}{\overset{k_1}{\rightleftharpoons}} X \overset{k_3}{\rightharpoonup} E + P \tag{3.6.1}$$

in which E is the enzyme, S the substrate, X the enzyme-substrate complex (often called ES), and P the product or metabolite; k_1, k_2, and k_3 are rate constants.

In the rate equations corresponding to (3.6.1), the concentrations C_E, C_S, C_X, and C_P appear, together with the compartment volume V and the rate constants:

$$\begin{aligned} V{*}(dC_E/dt) &= -k_1{*}C_E{*}C_S + (k_2 + k_3){*}C_X \\ V{*}(dC_S/dt) &= -k_1{*}C_E{*}C_S + k_2{*}C_X \\ V{*}(dC_X/dt) &= \quad k_1{*}C_E{*}C_S - (k_2 + k_3){*}C_X \\ V{*}(dC_Pdt) &= \quad k_3{*}C_X \end{aligned} \tag{3.6.2}$$

Because the first and third equations in (3.6.2) are identical except for sign, and because C_P appears only in the fourth equation, the system can be solved using only the first two equations. Here the mass balance relationships at zero time are used with initial conditions $C_X(0)$ and $C_P(0)$ assumed to be zero, giving

$$\begin{aligned} C_X &= -(C_E - C_E(0)) \\ C_P &= \int_0^t (k_3/V)*C_X \, dt + 0.0 \end{aligned} \tag{3.6.3}$$

The equations for the system, from the first two equations of (3.6.2), are, in integral form

$$\begin{aligned} C_E &= \int_0^t (-k_1*C_E*C_S + (k_2 + k_3)*C_X)/V \, dt + C_E(0) \\ C_S &= \int_0^t (-k_1*C_E*C_S + k_2*C_X)/V \, dt + C_S(0) \end{aligned} \tag{3.6.4}$$

An ACSL program may be used to solve (3.6.3) and (3.6.4) for all concentrations; such a program is shown below. However, it is interesting first to examine the derivation and form of the Michaelis-Menten (MM) approximation for this system. If dC_X/dt may be assumed to be zero (a quasi-steady-state assumption), then from (3.6.2) and (3.6.3)

$$\begin{aligned} C_X &= \frac{C_E(0)*C_S}{(k_2 + k_3)/k_1 + C_S} \\ dC_S/dt &= \frac{-k_3*C_E(0)*C_S}{(k_2 + k_3)/k_1 + C_S} \end{aligned} \tag{3.6.5}$$

Using $dC_P/dt = k_3*C_X$, (3.6.5) yields the "velocity" of product formation v_p and of substrate disappearance v_s:

$$\begin{aligned} v_P &\equiv dC_P/dt = V_{max}*C_S/(K + C_S) \\ v_s &\equiv dC_S/dt = -V_{max}*C_S/(K + C_S) \end{aligned} \tag{3.6.6}$$

where $V_{max} = k_3*C_E(0)$ is the maximum rate in both cases, and $K_m = (k_2 + k_3)/k_1$ is the MM (Michaelis-Menten) constant. If C_S is small compared to K_m in the denominators, then it may be neglected, giving linear relationships in place of (3.6.6). If C_S is large, then K_m may be neglected in the denominators of (3.6.6), and the constant V_{max} appears.

Program ENZ-MM1 for (3.6.3) and (3.6.4) enables us to find ACSL solutions for all concentrations in the system for some assumed parameter values. The MM approximation for the first equation in (3.6.6), DCPA, is also calculated, as is the approximate value of the product concentration, CPA.

```
PROGRAM ENZ-MM1
   Constant K1=10.,K2=0.1,K3=10.,V=1.,CSIC=6.0,CEIC=0.1

 INITIAL
   KM = (K2+K3)/K1          $'MM Constant'
   VMAX = V*K3*CEIC         $'Max velocity of dCP/dt'

 DYNAMIC
   Cinterval CINT=0.1
   Nsteps NSTP=1
   Constant TF=10.

  DERIVATIVE
   Maxterval MAXT = .01

   CE =INTEG((-K1*CS*CE + (K2+K3)*(CEIC-CE))/V,CEIC)
   CS =INTEG((-K1*CS*CE + K2*(CEIC-CE))/V,CSIC)
   CP =INTEG((K3*(CEIC-CE)), 0.0)
   CX =-(CE - CEIC)

   DCPA= VMAX*CS/(KM+CS) $'MM Approx. to dCP/dt'
   CPA = INTEG(DCPA, 0.) $'MM Approx. to CP'
   CPE = CP-CPA          $'Error of MM approx. to CP'
  END
   TERMT(T .GE. TF)
 END
END
```

If this system is solved for concentrations C_E, C_S, C_P, and $C_X = -C_E + C_E(0)$ for the case in which C_S is initially equal to 6.0, the resulting curves are as shown in Figs. 3.6.1a and 3.6.1b; this is repeated for $C_S(0) = 0.6$ in parts c and d of the same figure. Note the sharp initial transient in C_X and C_E in both cases; this corresponds to a very large amplitude of the derivative of these quantities for a short initial period. This is neglected in the MM approximation. However, an examination of CPA as compared to CP from this program will show that in the cases considered the error in using the MM approximation is less than 1 percent.

In the solution of a system with widely varying time constants, such as this enzyme model, a variable-step algorithm, or even the Gear algorithm available in most languages such as ACSL, may be desirable rather than the Runge-Kutta routines that have been used in all other programs in this chapter.

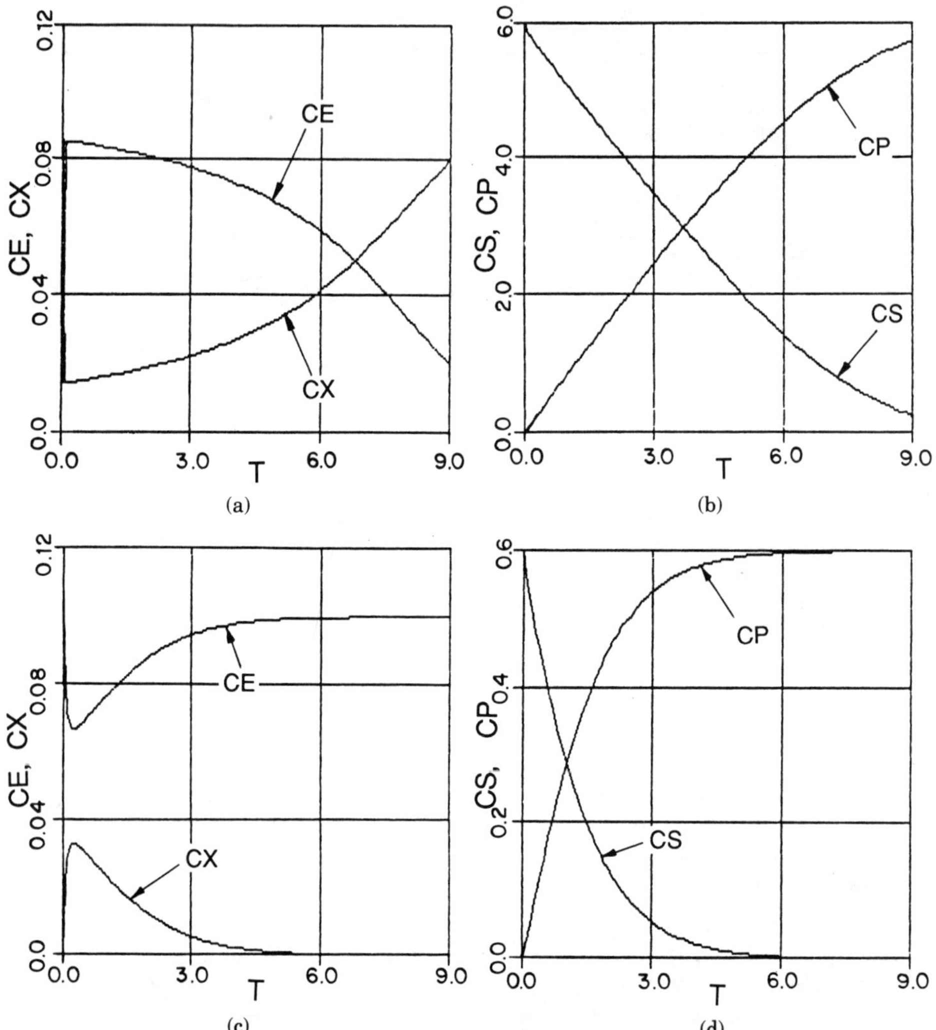

Figure 3.6.1. (a) Concentration of enzyme C_E and enzyme-substrate complex C_X in a closed system, plotted versus time with an impulse input of substrate (with $C_S(0) = 6.0$).
(b) Concentration of substrate C_S, and of product C_P.
(c,d) Runs and plots of (a,b) repeated with an initial substrate concentration $C_S(0) = 0.6$.

Enzyme modeling is often important in body models set up to study the elimination of drugs in the kidneys or their conversion to other forms in the liver.

PROBLEMS

3.1. The one-compartment system of Fig. 3.1.1 is used in Section 3.2 as an introduction to ACSL.

(a) Try running the program COMPART1 given in Section 3.2 and compare your results with those shown in Fig. 3.2.1(b).

(b) Repeat (a) for a pulse of length 500 time units using:

```
FIN = FCNSW(Z, A, 0., 0.)
Z = T - TX
Constant TX = 500.
```

or, using the pulse command (with a very long repetition interval),

```
FIN = A * PULSE(0.0, 1.E6, TX)
Constant TX = 500.
```

Compare your results with those in Fig. 3.2.3(a).

(c) Repeat (b) for a sequence of inflow pulses of period R, using:

```
FIN = A* PULSE (0., R, TX)
Constant TX = 50., R = 100.
```

Discuss the results obtained compared to those in (b). Note that this kind of input is often used to maintain an approximate concentration level, using an injection pump that is either ON or OFF. Discuss the programming of a larger initial pulse in the model so that the desired average concentration is reached more quickly.

3.2. A program COMPART2 which sweeps through a range of input pulse lengths is given in Section 3.2;

(a) Try program COMPART2 as given, and compare your results with those of Fig. 3.2.3(b).

(b) Use a pulse sequence input as in Problem 3.1(c), and sweep the pulse length from 10 to 70 in steps of 10.

3.3. **(a)** Run ACSL program IND-DIL1 for indicator transport in a complete cardiovascular loop (Fig. 3.4.2, Section 3.4), for the case of no VSD. Check the concentration curves against those shown in Fig. 3.4.3.

(b) Note that the indicator concentration curves in Fig. 3.4.3 all converge to the value $0.6*10^{-4}$. Explain and verify this value.

(c) Repeat (a) using the improved program IND-DIL2 for FVSD = 0.0 (Section 3.4) with F = 100., and F = 60. Explain the changes in the concentration curves when F is reduced.
(d) Run IND-DIL2 for the case of a VSD (use F = 100., FVSD = 10.) and check results against Fig. 3.4.4(c) and (d). Repeat for F = 60.

3.4. (a) Run the parameter-sweep (of FVSD) program IND-DIL3, and check results against Fig. 3.4.5.
(b) Rewrite program IND-DIL3 for the system of Fig. 3.4.3 with an atrial septal defect (ASD) between compartments M2 and M7); plot and explain results for concentration curves if FASD = 10.
(c) Repeat (b) for a patent ductus arteriosus (PDA) existing between ascending aorta and the pulmonary artery (between M4 and M1 in Fig. 3.4.1).

3.5. Program IND-DIL4 is the same as IND-DIL2 with commands (3.4.11) and (3.4.12) included. Set up IND-DIL4 and study the determination of cardiac output and total blood volume using TF = 200.

3.6. Set up the enzyme program ENZ-MM1 with a sweep of $C_S(0)$ from 0.6 to 6.0 and check the results shown in Fig. 3.6.1.

REFERENCES

BARTOLOMY, A. F., "Enzymatic reaction-rate theory; a stochastic approach," *Ann. N.Y. Acad. Sci.,* Vol. 96, art. 4, pp. 897–912; March, 1962.

BASSINGTHWAIGHTE, J. B., "The measurement of blood flows and volumes by indicator dilution," in *Medical Engineering* Part III, C. C. Ray (Ed.), Year Book Medical Publ.; 1974.

———. "Physiology and theory of tracer washout techniques," *Prog. Cardiovascular Diseases,* Vol. XX, No. 3; 1977.

BIRD, R. B., W. E. STEWART AND E. N. LIGHTFOOT, *Transport Phenomena.* New York: Wiley & Sons; 1960.

BISCHOFF, K. B. AND R. G. BROWN, Drug Distribution in Mammals," *Chem. Eng. Progr. Symp. Series No. 66,* Vol. 62, pp. 33–45; 1966.

BISCHOFF, K. B., R. L. DEDRICK, D. S. ZAHARKO AND J. A. LONGSTRETH, "Methotrexate pharmacokinetics," *J. Pharmaceut. Sci.,* Vol. 60, No. 8, pp. 1128–1123; Aug. 1971.

BROWNELL, G. L., MONES BERMAN AND J. S. ROBERTSON, "Nomenclature for tracer kinetics," *Intl. J. Appl. Radiation and Isotopes,* Vol. 19, pp. 249–262; 1968.

CASTILLO, C. A. ET AL, "Simulated Shunt Curves," *Amer. J. Cardiol.,* Vol. 17, pp. 691–694; May 1966.

CHEN H-S. AND J. F. CROSS, "Estimation of tissue-to-plasma partition coefficients used in physiological pharmacokinetic models," *J. Pharmacokinetics and Biopharm.,* Vol. 7, No. 1, pp. 117–125; 1979.

COONEY, DAVID O., *Biomedical Engineering Principles: An Introduction to Fluid, Heat and Mass Transport Processes,* New York: Marcel Decker; 1976.

DEDRICK, R. L. AND K. B. BISCHOFF, "Pharmacokinetics in applications of the artificial kidney," *Chem. Eng. Prog. Symp. Series 84,* No. 64; 1968.

FLAHERTY, J. ET AL, "Use of externally recorded radioisotope dilution curves for quantitation of left-to-right shunts," *Amer. J. Cardiol.,* Vol. 20, p. 341; 1967.

FRIEDMAN, M. H. *Principles and Models of Biological Transport,* New York: Springer-Verlag; 1986.

GIBALDI, MILO AND DONALD PERRIER, *Pharmacokinetics,* Second Edition, New York: Marcel Dekker, Inc.; 1982.

GOLD, H. J., *Mathematical modeling of biological systems,* New York: Wiley & Sons; 1977.

HAYASHI, K. AND N. SAKAMOTO, *Dynamic Analysis of Enzyme Systems,* New York: Springer-Verlag; 1986.

HIMMELSTEIN, K. J. AND R. J. LUTZ, "A review of the applications of physiologically based pharmacokinetic modeling," *J. Pharmacokin. Biopharm.,* Vol. 7, No. 2, pp. 127–145; 1979.

JACQUEZ, J. A. *Computational Analysis in Biology and Medicine: Kinetics of Tracer-Labeled Materials,* New York: Elsevier; 1972.

KETY, S. S., *Methods of Medical Research*; 1951.

MORRISON, P. F., T. L. LINCOLN AND J. AROESTY, "Disposition of Cytosine Arabinoside and its Metabolites: A Pharmacokinetic Simulation," *Cancer Chemother. Rpts.,* Vol. 59, No. 4; 1975.

NIAZI, S., *Textbook of Biopharmaceutics and Clinical Pharmacokinetics,* Englewood Cliffs, NJ: Prentice Hall; 1979.

ROSELLI, R. J., L. TALBOT AND J. A. ABBOTT, "Evaluation of the thermal indicator technique for the measurement of steady and pulsatile flows," *J. Biomechanics,* Vol. 8, pp. 157–66; 1975.

TEORELL, T., R. L. DEDRICK AND P. G. CONDLIFFE, EDS., *Pharmacology and Pharmacokinetics,* New York: Plenum Press; 1974.

WAGNER, JOHN G., "Do you need a pharmacokinetic model, and, if so, which one?", *J. Pharmacokin. Biopharm.* Vol. 3, No. 6, pp. 457–78; 1975.

ZIERLER, K. L., "Theory of use of indicators to measure blood flow and volume," *Circ. Res.* Vol. XII, pp. 464–71; May, 1963.

———. "Circulation times and the theory of indicator-dilution methods for determining blood flow and volume," Chap. 18, in *Handbook of Physiology—Circulation.*Vol. 1, Baltimore: Williams and Wilkins; 1962.

ZIMMERMAN, H. A. (ED.), *Intravascular Catheterization,* Springfield, IL: C. C. Thomas; 1966.

4 Pressure-Flow Modeling of the Cardiovascular System

4.0 INTRODUCTION

Blood flow is essential to the body as the means for carrying substances such as oxygen, nutrients, and hormones to the tissues where they are needed and for bringing waste products such as carbon dioxide and uric acid to the lungs or kidneys to be eliminated. The modeling of the transport of substances in the cardiovascular system was examined in Chapter 3 for the case where blood flow was assumed to be constant and nonpulsatile. In this chapter, *pressure-flow* modeling of the cardiovascular system at various levels of detail is considered, in both pulsatile and nonpulsatile forms. The modeling of air flow in the lungs is covered in Chapter 5, and then the methods learned in Chapters 3, 4, and 5 are used in Chapter 6 to set up the multiple models in which a pressure-flow model "drives" the transport models needed to simulate the uptake and kinetics of gases, or to study more advanced problems in pharmacokinetics. (Note that the term *pressure-flow modeling*, a short form of *pressure-flow-volume modeling,* is used here to distinguish what we are doing from compartment modeling.)

Some discussion was included in Section 1.2 on the history of cardiovascular simulation; the names of some of the people important in the development of this difficult area of modeling may be found in the references at the end of this chapter. Early cardiovascular system modelers in the United States and Holland whose work is referred to here include Grodins-59, Warner-62, Beneken-65,72, Jager-65, and Noordergraaf-63,78. Other modelers, some of them more recent, are also referenced (Skalak-72, Dickinson-73 and Brubakk-78). This author has also depended on the work done in collaboration with his many graduate students and others (Dick-68, Snyder-68,69, and 72, Fukui-72, Katra-66, Gianunzio-69, Blackstone-77 and 82, Rideout-67,69,72 and 80, Tham-88).

The entire cardiovascular system is such that blood flows in a continuous loop with many parallel branches, as shown in Fig. 4.0.1a. In the diagram the system has been simplified by showing only the most important vessels and capillary beds; other parallel vessels and beds are not omitted but are included in the system parameter determinations. Thus the many parallel paths in each leg are combined, and the legs themselves are combined. The large veins (vena cavae) return the blood to the right heart from the various capillary beds, which then pumps the blood through the pulmonary capillaries of the lungs. The heart with its four valves is shown in cross section; Fig. 4.0.2 provides a more detailed diagram.

The circuit shown in Fig. 4.0.1b represents a typical lumped model of the fluid-flow system in 4.0.1a, where each storage element (L or C) corresponds to a first-order differential equation. This model, used in venous studies (Snyder-69), includes some valves in the leg veins. Note that these valves, as well as the important heart valves, are represented by diode symbols.

In modeling studies of fluid motion such as blood flow in the cardiovascular (CV) system and gas flow in the respiratory system, we are concerned with the variables *pressure, flow,* and *volume*. Important basic parameters in addition to vessel dimensions are the *elasticity* of vessel walls and of the fluid, *density* of the fluid under standard conditions, and *viscosity*. These parameters and those derived from them (such as *resistance, inertance,* and *compliance*) are simpler for fluids like blood than for gases in the respiratory system (see Chapter 5), because blood, unlike air, may be assumed to be incompressible, and fluid density may be assumed constant. We can usually assume that blood is a Newtonian fluid (Charm-72), and can use linear analysis of the CV system except for the action of valves in the heart and in veins. However, relatively slow variations in CV vessel wall elasticity and dimensions may occur for various reasons (Gow-72).

In the cardiovascular system approximate linearity holds in the arterial system, but vessel wall collapse may occur under certain conditions in the veins, causing strong nonlinearities. The heart valves cause the entire system to be quite nonlinear, but under steady-state conditions we can sometimes assume piecewise linearity.

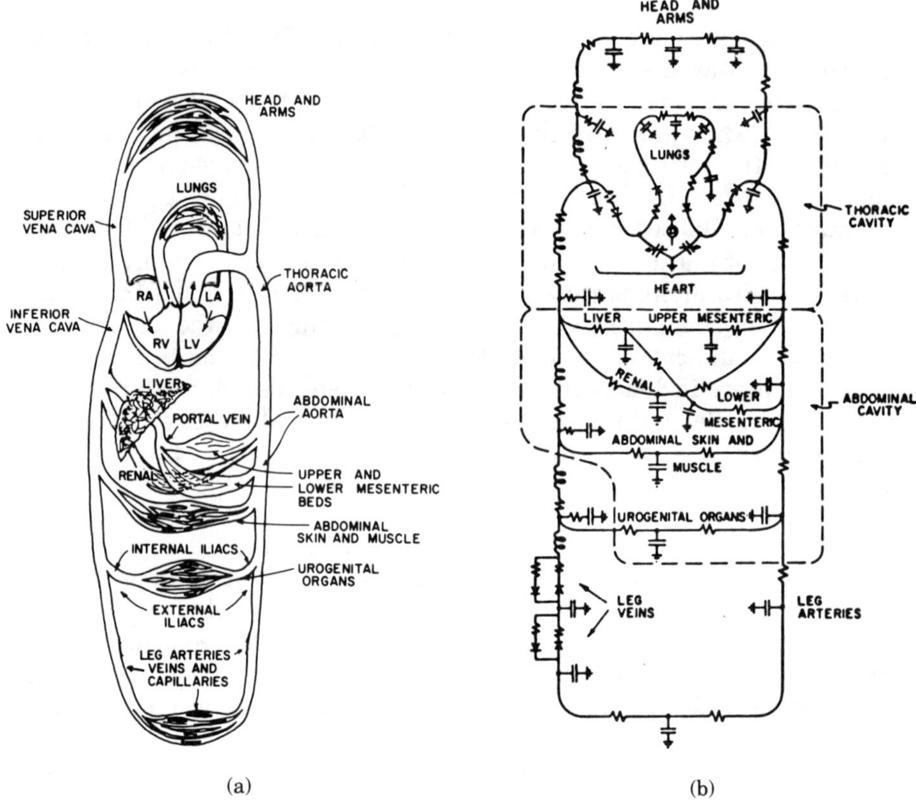

Figure 4.0.1 (a) A simplified diagram of the human cardiovascular system. (b) A fluid-flow circuit diagram corresponding to (a).

Some important early work on the mathematical relationships of pressure and blood flow in cylindrical vessels was done by Womersley, who considered sinusoidal variables in linearized versions of the basic Navier-Stokes equations (Womersley-57, Fry-64, Cox-68). More effective solutions that take into account the changes in vessel wall dimensions with pressure have more recently been obtained by (Hung-82). It is not too easy to incorporate these results into overall models. To overcome such difficulties a differencing scheme has been proposed (Rideout-67) that requires discrete "lumping" along both the longitudinal and radial dimensions in the assumed cylindrical vessels. This scheme makes it possible to include nonlinearities (Rideout-83a), whether they originate in the Navier-Stokes equations or in vessel wall elasticities.

In Section 4.1, a simple method of derivation of the pressure-flow equations is used that gives results corresponding to the double differencing scheme referred to above (Rideout-67) for the case where only two discrete divisions are used in the radial dimension. Such modeling, with adequately short longitudinal differencing and inclusion of the more important branchings, has been shown (Snyder-68) to give very satisfactory pulsatile simulation for the complete cardiovascular system. Models of this sort, together with extension to nonlinear cases involving venous collapse and certain square law resistance effects, are discussed later in this chapter. Note that the fluid-flow circuits presented here resemble electrical circuits. This is a convenient way to express graphically the form of cardiovascular systems, particularly because their components obey equations very much like those for simple R-L-C circuits.

The heart, which is shown in more detailed cross section in Fig. 4.0.2a, has been modeled very simply (Snyder-69) in an otherwise detailed CV model and has also been modeled in considerable nonlinear detail (Beneken-65, Dick-68). Figure 4.0.2b shows a circuit representation of the heart modeled in detail intermediate between these simulations.

4.1 PRESSURE-FLOW MODELING IN ARTERIES AND VEINS

As discussed, arteries and veins may be assumed to be made up of cylindrical vessels with linearly elastic walls, and to a good approximation the blood that flows in them may be regarded as an incompressible fluid with simple Newtonian characteristics. An ideal segment of this kind is shown in Fig. 4.1.1a. Let us initially assume that the vessel walls are rigid, that the input and output pressures are p_a and p_b, and the flow is f, as shown. Let the internal radius of the cylinder be R (with corresponding cross-sectional area $A = \pi * R^2$), and let the segment length be Δz.

The force moving the blood in the segment is assumed to be given by the product of the pressure difference between its ends and the area, $(p_a - p_b) * A$. Here we assume that the pressures are uniform across the diameter of the vessel. This force is balanced by the effects of fluid-flow resistance and of fluid-mass acceleration.

We now assume that the resistance to flow is given approximately by the Poiseuille steady-state formula (Noordergraaf-78)

$$R = 8 * \pi * \mu * \Delta z / A^2 \tag{4.1.1}$$

where μ is fluid viscosity.

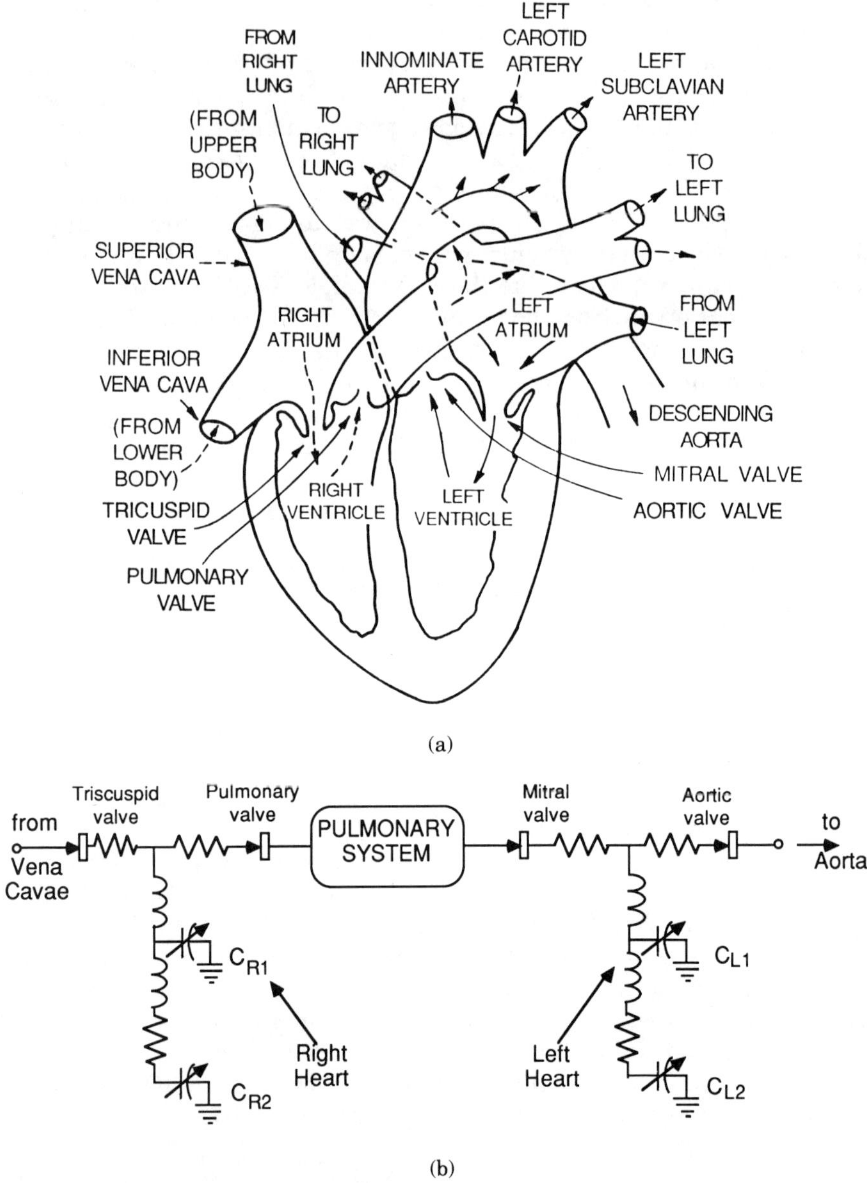

Figure 4.0.2. (a) Cross-sectional representation of the human heart. (b) Circuit representation of a model of the heart in medium detail.

(a)

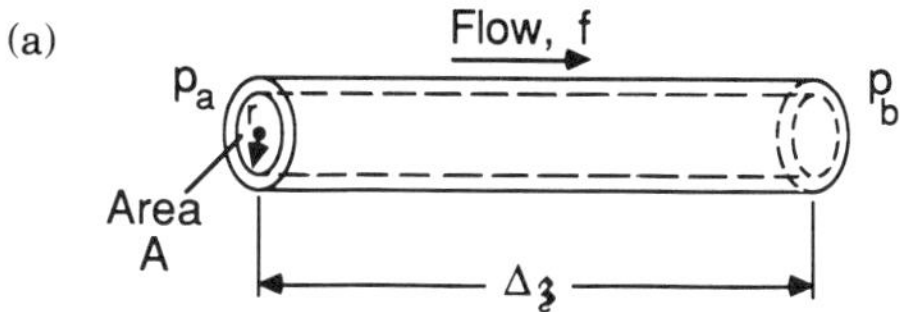

(b)

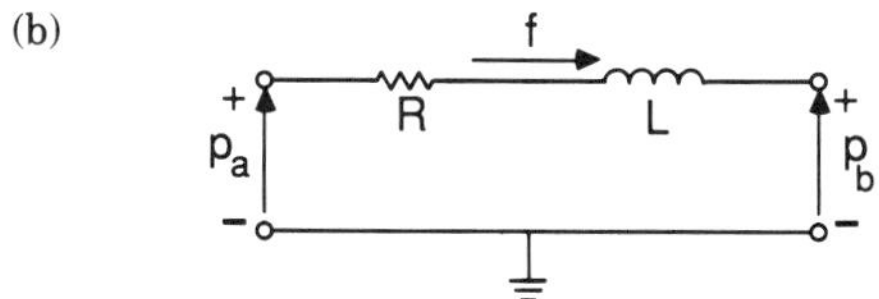

Figure 4.1.1. (a) Idealized segment of a vein or artery.
(b) Equivalent lumped fluid-flow circuit, ignoring wall compliance.

If it can be assumed that the flow is uniform across the diameter of the tube, the viscous resistance part of the pressure drop is given by

$$(p_a - p_b)\mid_{\text{vis}} = f*R \tag{4.1.2}$$

To find the pressure drop due to acceleration of the mass of the blood in the segment, we determine the mass to be

$$M = \rho*A*\Delta z \tag{4.1.3}$$

where ρ is blood density. If we assume that the blood flow is of uniform velocity v across the vessel radius, then the total flow is $f = v*A$. The force needed to balance acceleration of blood in the segment will be, by Newton's second law:

$$\begin{aligned} M\,dv/dt &= (\rho*A*\Delta z)*d(f/A)/dt \\ &= (\rho*\Delta z)*df/dt \end{aligned} \tag{4.1.4}$$

This acceleration force must equal the acceleration part of the pressure difference between the ends of the tube times its cross-sectional area, $(p_a - p_b)*A$. Using this on the left side of (4.1.4) and dividing through by A, we get the acceleration part of the pressure drop:

$$(p_a - p_b)\mid_{\text{accel}} = (\rho*\Delta z/A)*df/dt \tag{4.1.5}$$

The coefficient of the flow derivative in this equation may be called the inertance L (akin to the inductance in electric circuits):

$$L = \rho*\Delta z/A \tag{4.1.6}$$

The sum of the viscous resistance and mass acceleration pressure drops given by (4.1.2) and (4.1.5) gives the total pressure drop

$$p_a - p_b = R*f + L*(df/dt) \tag{4.1.7}$$

where R and L are given by (4.1.1) and (4.1.6).

A correction for the fact that the velocity is low near the walls of the vessel, with an overall parabolic cross section of flow velocities (in steady state), gives a slightly better value (Rideout-67) for the inertance L based on a two-radial-segment approximation,

$$L = 9*\rho*\Delta z/4*A = 9*\rho*\Delta z/(4*\pi*r^2) \tag{4.1.8}$$

So far, we have neglected the elasticity of the vessel walls. It can be shown (Jager-65) that the compliance C of a cylindrical vessel of radius r, length Δz, wall thickness h, and Young's bulk modulus of elasticity, E.

$$C = 3*\pi*r^3*\Delta z/2*E*h \tag{4.1.9}$$

where the wall material is uniform with a Poisson ratio $\sigma = ½$; however, the values of E and h are usually not available, and as a practical matter C may be determined as follows. For the vessel of Fig. 4.1.1a, if fluid velocity is zero and the pressure throughout the vessel is p_a

$$q = q_u + p_a*C \tag{4.1.10}$$

where q is the total volume of the segment and q_u is its unstressed volume, that is, the volume when transmural pressure is zero. (Although it might seem more reasonable in this case to use $(p_a + p_b)/2$ for the pressure, the choice of an endpoint makes sense when the equivalent *PI* or *T* sections are used, as shown in Fig. 4.1.3.) As a practical matter, C may be determined by varying p_a by Δp_a in (4.1.10), observing diameter and thus volume change, and finding C from

$$C = \Delta q/\Delta p_a \tag{4.1.11}$$

Thus the slope of p versus q curves such as those for veins in Fig. 4.1.2a may be used to find the reciprocal of the compliance, $1/C$, as volume is varied. Note also that this reciprocal term, called the stiffness S, is often easier to use than the compliance.

It may also be seen that C can only be regarded as a constant for a limited range of positive transmural pressures. Thus, if the volume is large, the vessel walls may begin to reach their limit of expansion, after which rupture may occur; if the volume is reduced below the unstressed volume q_u, collapse occurs with reduced slope (or increased C) until the vessel approaches zero volume, as shown by the sketches of its cross section. Large pressure excursions, which may occur in veins, may require the use of a function generator such as the four-section model of

Fig. 4.1.2b. If we generate the function in an ACSL program, a much smoother approximation curve may be set up using a function generation routine with a table of coordinate pairs of values of volume and pressure.

It is now possible to set up the complete lumped model for a segment of artery or vein by adding the appropriate compliance to the model in Fig. 4.1.1b. We will begin by assuming that the model always operates in a region where $q_u < q < q_m$ (see Fig. 4.1.2b) where C may be assumed constant.

The compliance C for the segment of Fig. 4.1.1a can be added to the center of the incomplete lumped circuit model by splitting R and L, as shown in Fig. 4.1.3a, or C may be divided into two equal parts and added to each end, as shown in Fig. 4.1.3b. These model forms are called T- and PI-sections, because of their graphical forms. If more segments are added in tandem, series $R/2$ and $L/2$ elements from adjacent arms must be combined if T-sections are used, or $C/2$ elements must be combined if PI-sections are used. Let us choose the latter, and examine some of the problems of tandem connections and branching. (Note that either T- or PI-sections may be split into two L-sections.)

Figure 4.1.4a shows a length of blood vessel that might be assumed to be part of the aorta, beginning on the left at the aortic valve, and

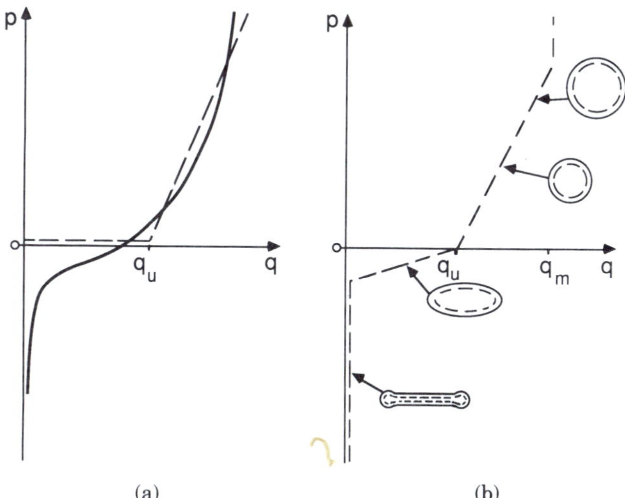

Figure 4.1.2. (a) Typical venous pressure-flow relation (solid line) and a two-section model fit (dashed line).
(b) Four-straight-line model fit for the venous pressure-flow relations of (a), from full collapse to vessel rupture.

including a single branch (segment 8). The vessel has been divided into longitudinal sections (indicated by solid lines), and it is assumed that the values of R_n, L_n, and C_n have been determined by use of (4.1.1), (4.1.6), and either (4.1.9) or (4.1.11). The unstressed volumes are also assumed known; typically, the unstressed volume q_u for a segment is N times the stressed volume at average normal pressure, $C{*}p_{\text{ave}}$, so that

$$q_u = N{*}C{*}p_{\text{ave}} \tag{4.1.12}$$

where $N = 4$ for arteries and $N = 7$ for veins, approximately (Beneken-65).

In the equivalent circuit model for Fig. 4.1.4a, as shown in Fig. 4.1.4b, the second compliance is $C_{01} = (C_0 + C_1)/2$; later on, we may replace the double subscript on compliances C_{01} etc. by something simpler.

The equations corresponding to the lumped model, for the second segment are as follows. First, for the total blood volume in the segment

$$q_{01} = \int_0^t (f_0 - f_1)\, dt + q_{01}(0) \tag{4.1.13}$$

where $q_{01}(0)$ is the total initial blood volume.

From (4.1.10), using the stressed volume, $q_{01} - q_{01}$, where q_{01} is the unstressed volume of the segment

$$p_{01} = (q_{01} - q_{u01})/C_{01} \tag{4.1.14}$$

(Note that $q_{01}(0)$ in (4.1.13) is usually set at $q_{u01} + q_{01}(\text{ave.})$.)

From (4.1.7)

$$p_{01} - p_{12} = L_1{*}df_1/dt + R_1{*}f_1$$

or, in integral form

$$f_1 = \int_0^t [(p_{01} - p_{12}) - R_1{*}f_1]/L_1\, dt \tag{4.1.15}$$

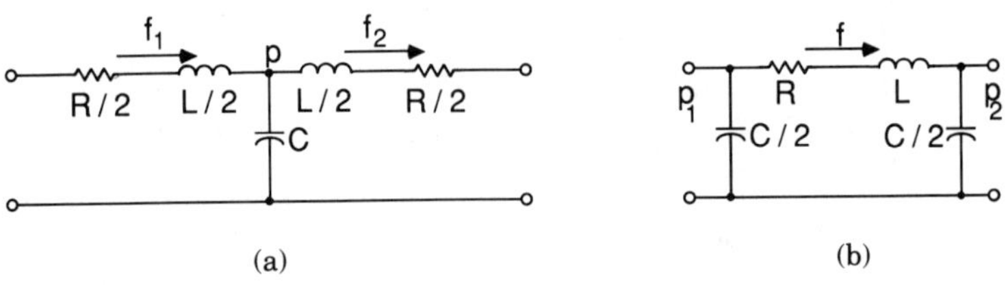

Figure 4.1.3. (a) T-section, and
(b) PI-section lumped-equivalent models of a blood vessel segment.

(a)

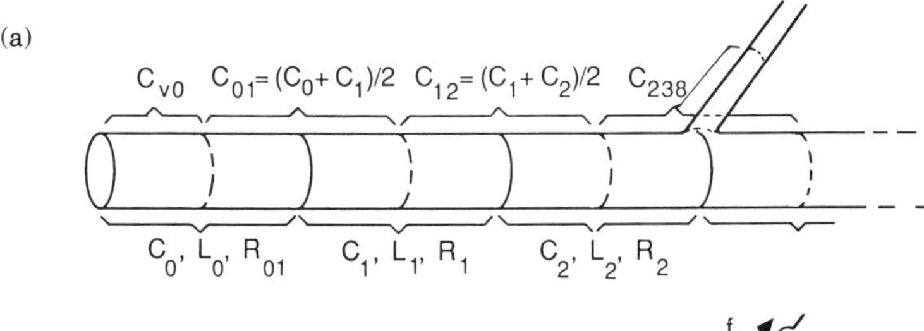

(b)

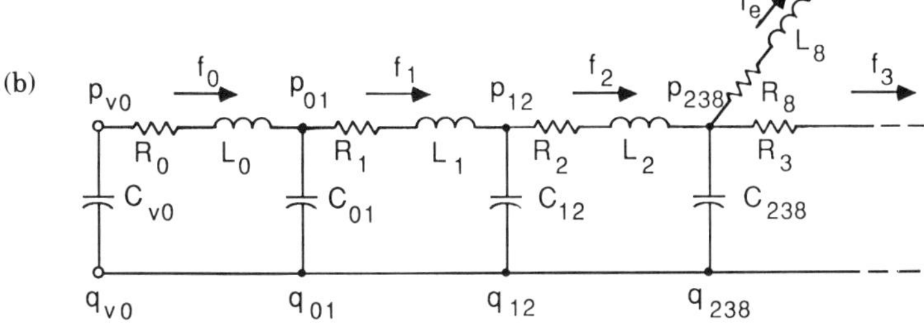

Figure 4.1.4. (a) A portion of the aorta (shown without curvature) including a branch, with division into segments shown by solid lines; dotted lines mark midpoints of segments.
(b) A lumped model of (a) shown in circuit form.

These equations may be thought of as characterizing the L-section made up of C_{01}, L_1, and R_1, and it can be seen from Fig. 4.1.4b that it is convenient to regard the ladder network obtained by combining PI-sections as a sequence of L-sections, with pressures, volumes, and flows determined by simultaneous solution of (4.1.13), (4.1.14), and (4.1.15) set up for each segment.

If a branch with flow f_8 is connected at the junction of segments 2 and 3, as shown in Fig. 4.1.4a, the equivalent lumped circuit model is easily set up. Note that $C_{238} = C_2/2 + C_3/2 + C_8/2$, and (4.1.13) becomes

$$q_{238} = \int_0^t (f_2 - f_3 - f_8)\, dt + q_{238}(0) \qquad (4.1.16)$$

Some discussion of units is important here. Consider the circuit of Fig. 4.1.1b with a compliance C added at the left side of the segment. Equations for the shunt (compliance) branch and the series (R-L) branch may be written in canonic first-order form as

$$\begin{aligned} C{*}dp_a/dt &= f_{\text{in}} - f \\ L{*}df/dt &= p_a - p_b - R{*}f \end{aligned} \qquad (4.1.17)$$

If we choose CGS units and include them in these equations, then (using force/cm^2 = gm*cm/(s^2*cm^2) = gm/(s^2*cm) for CGS units of pressure),

$$C[C_{\text{units}}] * \frac{dp_a}{dt} \frac{gm}{s^2 * cm} * \frac{1}{\text{s}} = (f_{\text{in}} - f) \frac{\text{cm}^3}{\text{s}}$$

$$L[L_{\text{units}}] * \frac{df}{dt} \frac{\text{cm}^3}{\text{s}} * \frac{1}{\text{s}} = (p_a - p_b) \frac{\text{gm}}{\text{s}^2 * \text{cm}} - R[R_{\text{units}}] * \text{f} \frac{\text{cm}^3}{\text{s}} \tag{4.1.18}$$

From these equations we can reconcile units and obtain the units of C, L, and R:

$$C_{\text{units}} = \text{cm}^4 * \text{s}^2/\text{gm}$$

$$L_{\text{units}} = \text{gm}/\text{cm}^4$$

$$R_{\text{units}} = \text{gm}/(\text{cm}^4 * \text{s}) \tag{4.1.19}$$

Note that the viscosity μ of normal blood is $\mu = 0.035$ poise (gm/cm s) and normal blood density is $\rho = 1.05$ gm/cm^3. Also, we have not used SI units here, but they can be introduced as needed, or related to the information given.

Many approximations have been made in developing the basic pressure-flow equations for cylindrical vessels in this section, (4.1.13), (4.1.14), and (4.1.15). These approximations may be reduced by using more sections radially, and also longitudinally, using methods based on the Navier-Stokes equations (Rideout and Dick 1967); they also permit some nonlinearities to be included. However, rather good cardiovascular system waveform reproduction is possible with the kind of linear model shown in Fig. 4.1.4, but with 25 segments used in the systemic arterial system (Snyder-68). Much simpler networks suffice for the many purposes that do not require too much precision in waveforms. Detailed descriptions of many aspects of cardiovascular modeling have been given (see Beneken-72, Noordergraaf-78, and Milnor-82).

4.2 SIMPLE MODELING OF THE LEFT HEART AND SYSTEMIC ARTERIES

The modeling method discussed in Section 4.1 is usually satisfactory for veins and arteries, but the valves in the heart provide strong nonlinearities (or are at best only "piecewise" linear), while the muscles in the ventricular wall that provide the pumping action make this part of the heart linear but time-varying. In this section we begin by developing a simple model of the left heart, consisting of mitral valve, ventricle, and aortic valve, with only a rudimentary systemic arterial load. Running this model and various improvements of it (Hillestad-66) will serve as a means for becoming better acquainted with techniques of modeling and the use of programming languages such as ACSL.

In the simple left heart model shown in lumped circuit form in Fig. 4.2.1a, the atrial pressure, PAT, is assumed to be fixed, as is the central venous pressure, PSV. (Note that the nomenclature here is that used in ACSL programs rather than the subscripted forms used in the diagram. Also, the variable quantities that are often expressed using lowercase letters also are in uppercase.)

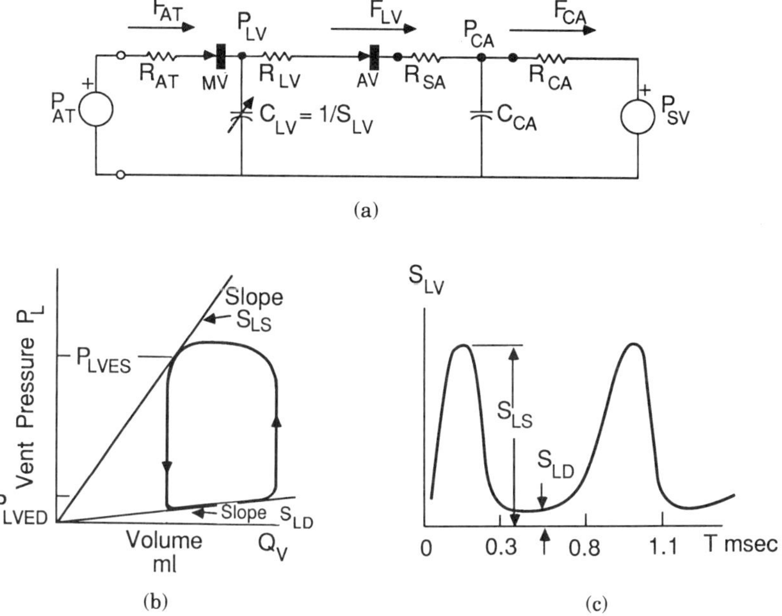

Figure 4.2.1. A simple lumped model of the left heart.
(a) Circuit representation of idealized left heart and systemic system load (in cgs units, except pressures in mmHg).
(b) A typical locus (or path) for one cycle of left ventricular pressure, PLV, plotted versus volume, QLV. Note that it lies between the lines whose slopes are the diastolic (minimum) muscle stiffness SLD and the systolic (maximum) stiffness, SLS. End systolic and end-diastolic pressures, PLVES and PLVED, are indicated.
(c) Time variations in stiffness, SLV, plotted versus time for two heart cycles. Initially these pulses will be assumed to be rectangular, and later on more realistic half-sinusoids will be used.

The blood inflow to the left ventricle (FAT) will occur during diastole, when the walls of this chamber are relaxed, and this flow can pass through the mitral valve (MV) and its associated flow resistance, RAT. The ventricle is modeled with a single varying compliance, corresponding to a muscle that is relaxed during the filling part of the heart cycle, or diastole, when stiffness SLV $\approx$ SLD, and strong during systole, when stiffness is high and SLV $\approx$ SLS. The variation of SLV with time is approximately as shown in Fig. 4.2.1c, but rectangular pulses will be used initially. The pulsing of SLV results in a counterclockwise locus in ventricular pressure-volume space, as shown by dotted line in Fig. 4.2.1b.

Outflow from the ventricle (FLV) occurs during systole when PLV increases, closing the mitral valve, and then with further increase causes the aortic valve (AV) to open. The resistance of the aortic valve (RLV) will be assumed to be zero because it is small and is in series with the larger resistances of the systemic load that follow.

The systemic arterial impedance or "load" consists of only two resistances and a compliance. The resistance (RSA) is the characteristic impedance of the aorta viewed as a transmission line, and RCA is the total resistance of all body (or systemic) capillary beds in parallel, while CSA is the total compliance of the systemic arterial system. This reduced model of the systemic arterial system is sometimes referred to as the "Westkessel" model (Westerhof-69) and is discussed in more detail in Section 4.4.

The ACSL program LH-PF-1 for simulation study of the left heart model of Fig. 4.2.1a is shown here. CGS units are used except for the applied input pressure, which is given in medical units (PATM = 6 mm Hg); note that this pressure and the systemic venous pressure (PVE) converted to CGS units in the INITIAL part of the program for use in the DERIVATIVE part. In similar fashion, the variable pressures PLV and PCA are converted from CGS to medical units (using PLVM = PV/1332, etc.) in the final part of the DYNAMIC section to make it convenient to plot pressures in the more familiar mm Hg units. It would also be possible to convert to pressures in kilopascals, or to flows in liters/min (see Section 2.6), if so desired.

In this model the parameters are roughly determined as follows. The diastolic filling period is assumed to last for 0.5 sec and the systolic period for 0.3 sec, for a heart period total of 0.8 sec, corresponding to 60/0.8 = 75 beats/min. The fixed pressure PAT at the entrance to the atrium causes FAT to flow through resistance RAT when the mitral valve is open during diastole, filling the ventricle. This resistance is assumed to be 5.0 CGS "fluid ohms," and in combination with the relaxed stiffness of the ventricle has a diastolic time constant of RAT*CLD, or 5/SLD; thus, for SLD = 67, as in the LH-PF-1 program, this time constant is

```
PROGRAM LH-PF-1
   'All quantities in DERIVATIVE are in cgs units'
   'some pressures elsewhere in Medical units, e.g. PATM'
INITIAL
    Constant PATM = 6.0,PVEM = 3.0
    PAT =PATM*1332.
    PVE =PVEM*1332.              $ 'Convert Medical to cgs units'
END $ 'of Initial'
DYNAMIC
  Cinterval CINT= 0.01
  Constant TF = 4.0
 DERIVATIVE
  Algorithm IALG = 4             $ 'Runge Kutta 2'
  Maxterval MAXT =0.005          $ Nsteps NSTP = 1

   'Differential Equations'
  Constant RAT=5.0
  FATX=(PAT-PLV)/RAT             $ 'Atrial flow with no valve.'
  FAT= BOUND(0.0,5000.,FATX)     $ 'Atrial flow with valve.'
  Constant QLVIC=120.,RSA=80.0
  QLV=INTEG((FAT-FLV),QLVIC)     $ 'Left ventricle volume.'
  PLV= QLV*SLV                   $ 'Left ventricle pressure.'
  FLVX=(PLV-PCA)/RSA             $ 'Left ventr. flow, no valve.'
  FLV= BOUND(0.0,1000.,FLVX)     $ 'L. ventr. flow, with valve.'
  Constant QCAIC=220.,CCA=.0022,RCA=1250.
  QCA=INTEG(FLV-FCA,QCAIC)       $ 'Volume, small arteries.'
  PCA= QCA/CCA                   $ 'Capillary entrance press.'
  FCA= (PCA-PVE)/RCA             $ 'Flow into capillaries.'

  Constant SLS=2500.,SLD=67.,TS=0.3,TH=0.8
   'Here TS is length of systole, and TH is the heart period'
  Logical XX
  X = T - ZOH(T,0.,0.,TH)        $ 'Creates sawtooth wave.'
  XX=(X .LE. TS)                 $ 'XX is True during systole.'
  SLV=RSW(XX,SLS,SLD)            $ 'Square-wave stiffness out.'
 END $ 'of Deriv.'

  TERMT (T .GE. TF)
  PLVM= PLV/1332.                $ 'Convert cgs output pressures'
  PCAM= PCA/1332.                $  'to medical units.'
 END $ 'of Dynamic'
END $ 'Of Program'
```

0.075 sec, which should allow adequate ventricular filling during diastole.

An average ventricular outflow (cardiac output) of 90 ml/s is assumed; at a heart period of 0.8 sec, this would correspond to a stroke volume of 90*0.8 = 72 ml. If the ejection fraction of the ventricle is 60 percent, then QLV would have a maximum volume of 72/0.60 = 120 ml and a minimum volume of 120 − 72 = 48 ml. From these volumes and assumptions as to pressures, the ventricular maximum and minimum stiffnesses may be determined. Thus, at the end of diastole

$$\begin{aligned} \text{SLD} &\approx \text{PAT} * 1332/\text{QLV(max)} = 6.0{*}1332/120 \\ &= 66.6 \end{aligned} \tag{4.2.1}$$

At the end of systole, if a ventricular pressure of PES = 90 mm Hg is assumed, the systolic (or maximum) stiffness is

$$\begin{aligned} \text{SLS} &\approx \text{PES} * 1332/\text{QLV(min)} = 90.0 * 1332/48 \\ &= 2497.5 \end{aligned} \tag{4.2.2}$$

Values close to these calculated normal values of ventricular stiffness, SLS = 2500 and SDS = 67, were chosen for model LH-PF-1, and initial volumes QLVIC = 120 and QCAIC = 220 were chosen after being adjusted to give small starting transients.

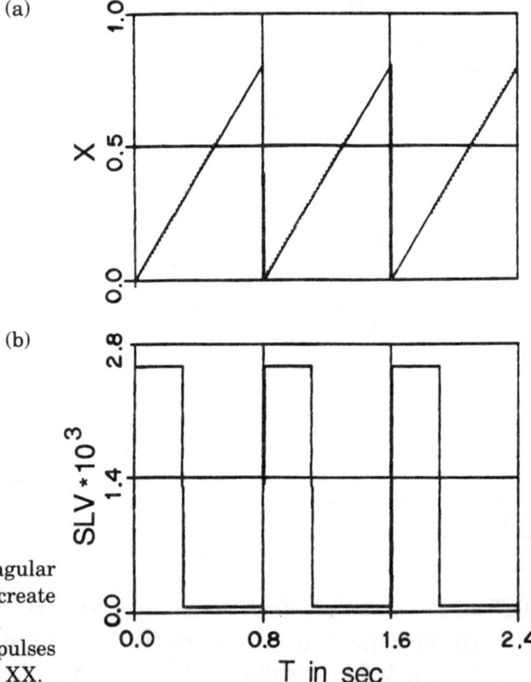

Figure 4.2.2. (a) Basic triangular waves, X, which can be used to create various ventricular wave shapes.
(b) Simple rectangular stiffness pulses SLV, obtained from a logic wave XX.

After the constants determined above were introduced into the model program LH-PF-1, various outputs were obtained and plotted using short run times of TF = 3.2 sec, or four beats, after some slight adjustments to give negligible starting transients. The first outputs shown (see Fig. 4.2.2) are for X (a succession of triangular waves of period

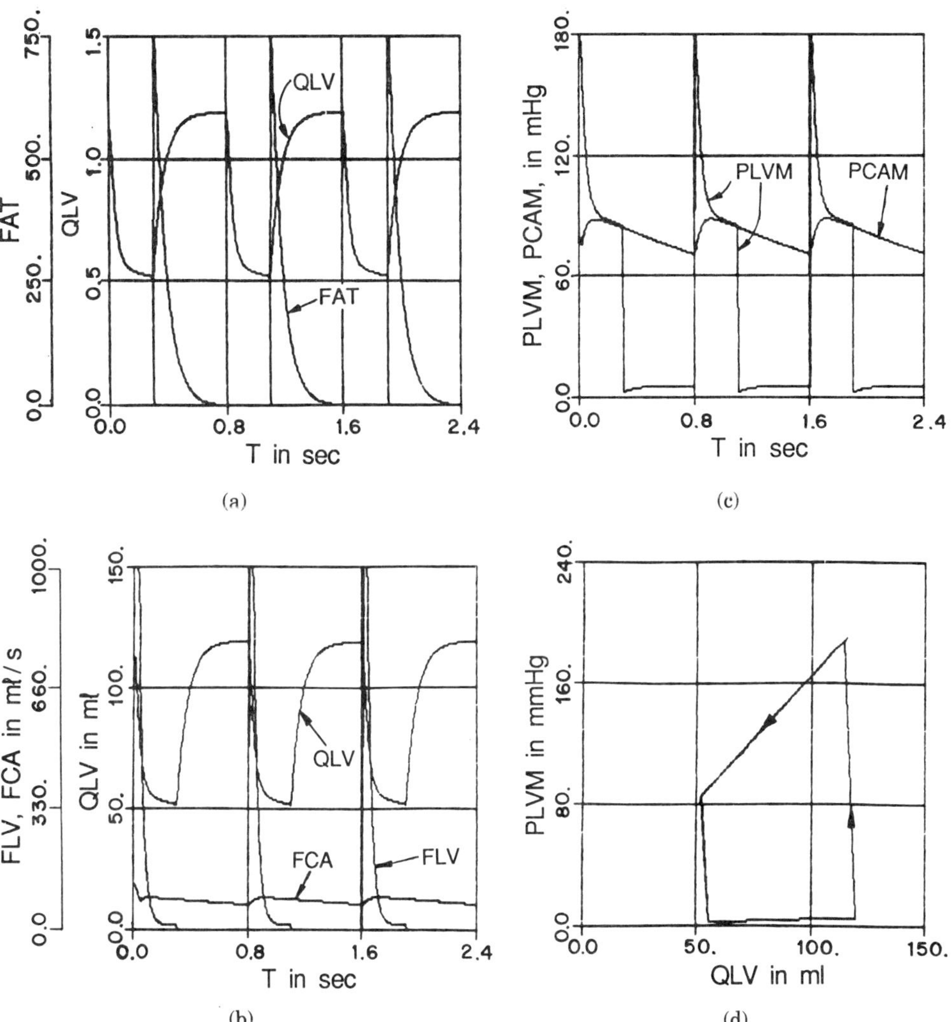

Figure 4.2.3. (a) Diastolic inflow, FAT, and ventricular volume, QLV.
(b) Systolic outflow, FLV, load flow, FCA, and QLV.
(c) Ventricular pressure, PLV, and arteriolar pressure, PCA, shown in medical units as PLVM and PCAM.
(d) Locus on the PLVM versus QLV plane.

0.8 sec.) and the square-wave ventricular stiffness SLV, obtained using the logic signal XX = (X .LE. TS).

The diastolic inflow, FAT, and the ventricular volume, QLV, are shown in Fig. 4.2.3a and the outflow, FLV, and QLV in Fig. 4.2.3b. The sharp rise to a peak and exponential drop in each flow pulse are not natural and will be replaced by more realistic waveforms when the model is improved with more rounded SLV pulses, and when inertances are included. Such an improved model is presented later in this section.

Figure 4.2.3c shows plots of the ventricular pressure, PLV, and the load pressure, PCA (located approximately in the arterioles). Note the slow exponential decay of PCA during diastole; the time constant here is TCA = RCA∗CCA = 2.75 sec, and thus during the 0.5 sec of diastole, the pressure may be approximated by

$$\begin{aligned} \text{PCA} &= \text{PES}*\text{Exp}(-\text{T}/\text{TCA}) \\ &\approx \text{PES}*(1.0 - \text{T}/2.75) \end{aligned} \tag{4.2.3}$$

where PES is the pressure at the end of systole. An examination of Fig. 4.2.3c shows that PES ≈ 84.5 and droops to about 71 at the end of diastole, which agrees fairly well with Eq. (4.2.3).

Another very important kind of plot is the locus of ventricular pressure (PLV) plotted versus volume (QLV), as shown in Fig. 4.2.3d; here the straight-line curves of slopes SLS and SLD may be seen as parts of the locus, and the counterclockwise direction of the locus has been indicated. Note that the width of this locus is the stroke volume. More realism would require rounded SLV pulses (as in Fig. 4.2.1c) and an upward curving diastolic stiffness curve for increasing QLV.

Because the system is piecewise linear, it is possible to use Laplace transform methods to obtain a numerical solution. This would require finding initial conditions and starting a new solution each time a valve opened or closed. Problems would mount up if detail were added to improve the model, and the addition of even one important nonlinearity would make Laplace solutions impossible. Thus a time-domain solution using a program such as ACSL is usually regarded as the best procedure for simulation study of system models, even at low levels of complexity.

Improvements will now be made in model LH-PF-1, and these changes will be incorporated in models of the complete cardiovascular loop. The first improvement is to change the actuating signal from a square-topped wave to a clipped half-sinusoid and to design this actuator to be one that can be used with the feedback systems of the body to change factors such as heart rate. This is achieved in the ACSL program shown below by again subtracting a zero-order hold (ZOH) from time T each TH seconds to generate a series of sawtooth waves (X) of unit slope, as in the simple generator of LH-PF-1. Then a logic signal XX is set to

TRUE whenever the repeating sawtooth X is of amplitude less than systolic time TS. The logic signal XX is used in an ACSL Real-Switch (RSW) to generate a spaced triangular wave (STW) during the systolic period. This wave, in turn, is used to generate spaced sine waves, (SSW).

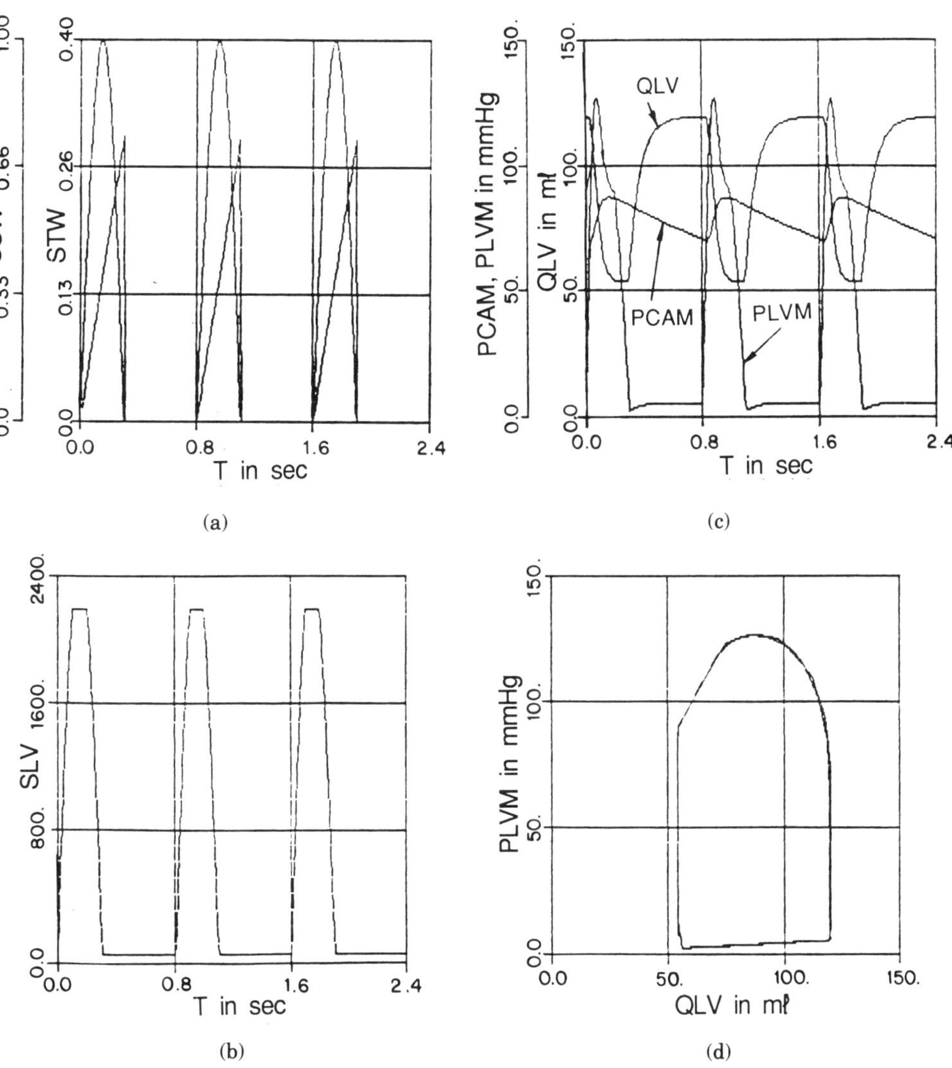

Figure 4.2.4. (a), (b) Waveforms in an improved activity generator.
(c) Ventricular and systemic pressures, PLVM and PCAM, and volume, QLV, with a half-sine-wave activity generator.
(d) Ventricular pressure-volume locus with an improved activity generator.

```
LOGICAL XX
Constant PI = 3.14159
X = T - ZOH(T,0.,0.,TH)
XX=(X .LE. TS)
STW=RSW(XX,X,0.0)
SSW=SIN(PI*STW/TS)
ACT=BOUND(0.,1.0,1.15*SSW)
SLV =SLD*(1.-ACT) + SLS*ACT
```

The spaced sine waves are amplified by 1.15, then clipped back to unity to give the activity function, ACT, which is used in turn to give a stiffness, SL, with near-half-sinusoid systolic pulse forms. These various waveforms may be obtained using the set of eight commands listed above in place of the last four commands in the DERIVATIVE section of LH-PF-1. This gives a new program that we will call LH-PF-2, which yields the waveforms shown in Figs. 4.2.4a and 4.2.4b.

This new actuator or activity generator may be modulated in period, systolic duration, and amplitude, and thus can be quite useful in a model that includes feedback control to maintain blood pressure levels when blood volume, flow resistances, or compliances change. Here these parameters are fixed, but it can be seen in Fig. 4.2.4c that ventricular pressure and flow waveforms have been improved. More impressive is the improvement in the shape of the ventricular pressure versus volume locus, as shown in Fig. 4.2.4d.

Two other improvements will now be made in the model, as shown in lumped circuit form in Fig. 4.2.5. These changes involve the introduction of inertance terms. One of these, L_{AO}, is included in a PI-section added between the aortic valve and the systemic load used in LH-PF-1; it also includes a resistance RAO and compliances CAO and CSA. This added section provides a better model of the first part of the aorta after the aortic valve. The equation for the flow through RAO and LAO is of the form given in (4.1.15). In ACSL notation this becomes

```
FAO = INTEG((PAO-PSA - RAO*FAO)/LAO, FAOIC)
```

(4.2.3)

The inertance LLV must be dealt with in a different way because it is in series with the aortic valve. It is not correct to use an integrator as in (4.2.3), followed by a separate limiter or BOUND command, because this might cut off the flow FAO when it should continue to appear due to inertial effects. To prevent this effect, often called "integrator windup," a combination integrator and limiter must be used, called the LIMINT command in ACSL. Thus FLV is now obtained by using

```
FLV= LIMINT((PAO-PSA -RAO*FAO)/LAO,FLVIC,0.0,5000.
```

(4.2.4)

Another small improvement in the spaced sine-wave SSW results because a small second-harmonic term is used to provide some "skew" in this waveform; this is also used in a following model, PF-1.

The complete ACSL program for the model LH-PF-3 shown in Fig. 4.2.5 is given next. Note that most constants are now included in the DERIVATIVE section, located near the point where they first appear for convenience.

```
PROGRAM LH-PF-3
    Constant PATM=6.0, PVEM=3.0
INITIAL
    PAT= PATM*1332.        $ PVE= PVEM*1332.
END $ 'of Initial'
DYNAMIC
   Cinterval CINT= 0.01
   Constant TF=4.0
 DERIVATIVE
   Algorithm IALG = 5    $ 'Runge Kutta 4'
```

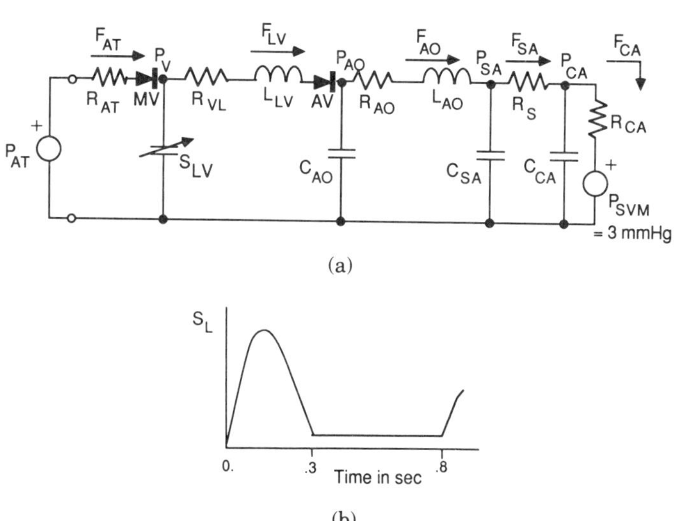

Figure 4.2.5. (a) Lumped-circuit equivalent for model LH-PF-3. (b) Ventricular stiffness, SLV, plotted versus time.

```
     Maxterval MAXT =0.001 $ Nsteps NSTP = 1
     LOGICAL XX
    Constant TH=0.8,TS=0.3,SLD=67.,SLS=2400.0
    Constant PI=3.14159,K1=.9,K2=0.3,B=1.05
     X = T - ZOH(T,0.,0.,TH)
     XX=(X .LE. TS)
     STW= RSW(XX,X,0.0)
     SSW= K1*SIN(PI*STW/TS)-K2*SIN(2.*PI*STW/TS)
     ACT= BOUND(0.,1.0,B*SSW)
     SLV= SLD*(1.-ACT) + SLS*ACT
    Constant RAT=5., QLVIC= 120., QLVU=0.0
     FAT= BOUND(0.0,5000.,(PAT- PLV)/RAT)
     QLV= INTEG((FAT-FLV),QLVIC)
     PLV= (QLV-QLVU)*SLV
    Constant RLV=5.0,LLV=0.5,RAO=5.,LAO=.5, . . .
     CAO=.00015, QAOIC=100., QAOU=85.
     FLV= LIMINT((PLV-PAO)/LLV - RLV *FLV/LLV,0.,0.,5000.)
     QAO= INTEG((FLV-FAO),QAOIC)
     PAO= (QAO=QAOU)/CAO
     FAO= INTEG((PAO-PSA)/LAO - RAO*FAO/LAO,0.0)
    Constant CSA= .0003, RSA= 50.,QSAIC=281.,QSAU=250.
     QSA= INTEG(FAO-FSA,QSAIC)
     PSA= (QSA-QSAU)/CSA
     FSA= (PSA-PCA)/RSA
    Constant CCA=0.0022, QCAIC=1010.,QCAU=810.,RCA=1150.
     QCA= INTEG(FSA-FCA,QCAIC)
     PCA= (QCA-QCAU)/CCA
     FCA= PCA/RCA
   END $ 'of Deriv.'
     PLVM= PLV/1332.
     PAOM= PAO/1332.
     PSAM= PSA/1332.
     PCAM= PCA/1332.
     TERMT (T .GE. TF)
     Q= QLV + QAO + QSA + QCA
   END $ 'of Dynamic'
 END  $ 'of Program'
```

Some runs made with LH-PF-3 are shown in Fig. 4.2.6. It can be seen that the pressure within the ventricle is still somewhat peaked, but that some oscillations appear near the end of systole. The aortic pressure PAO follows PLV during systole, and PCA is much more rounded. During diastole, PAO and PCA nearly coincide. Note, however, that the oscillations in these waves are of a higher frequency than is normally observed, and that no dicrotic notch at the end of systole is observed. The flow pulses, also shown in Fig. 4.2.6b, are improved but are still not very

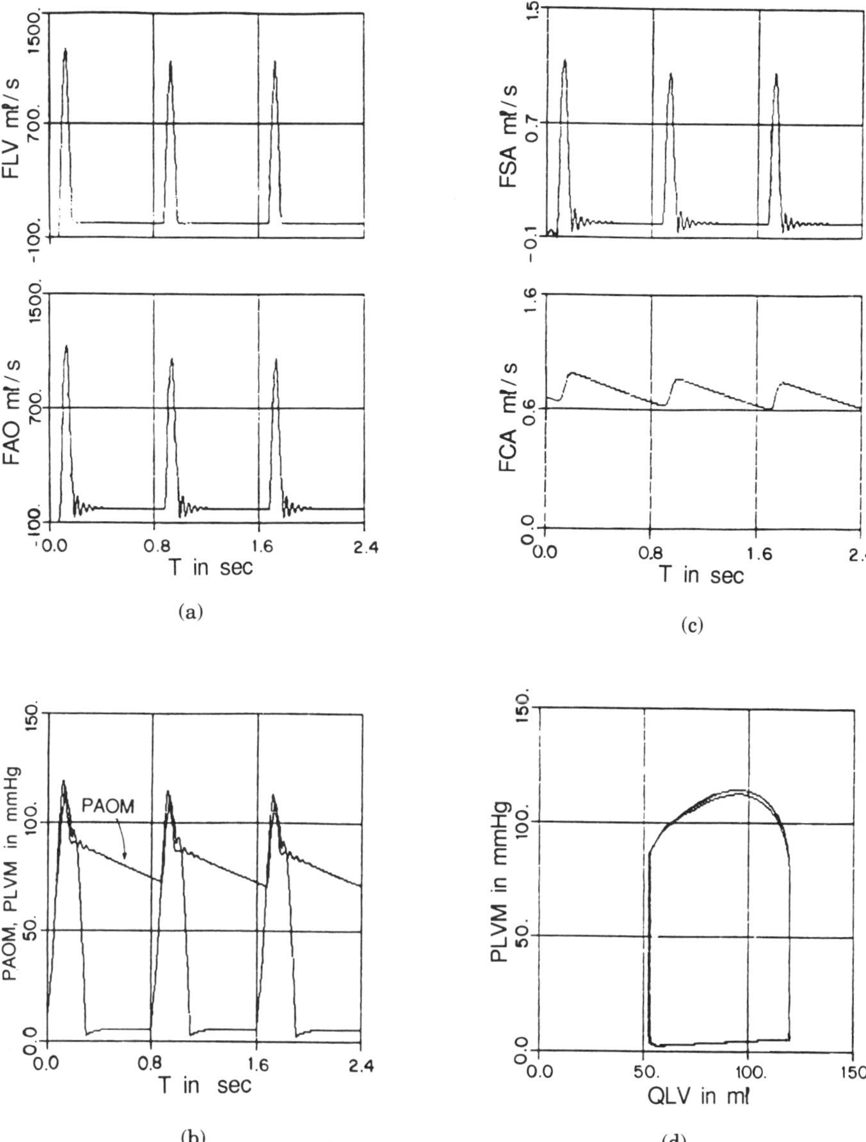

Figure 4.2.6. Pressure and flow waveforms obtained with the left ventricular model LH-PF-3. (a) Left ventricular flow FLV and aortic flow FAO. The latter shows the oscillations which occur in the aorta just after valve closure.
(b) Left ventricular pressure, PLVM, and superimposed aortic pressure PAOM, both in mmHg.
(c) Aortic flow FSA and the much less pulsatile capillary flow FCA.
(d) Left ventricle pressure-versus-volume locus. The height of this loop gives the peak value of PLVM, and the width gives the stroke volume.

realistic. It will be demonstrated later that even a slightly more detailed multisection systemic model will give more satisfactory realism in waveforms.

The slow descent of flow FCA during diastole corresponds approximately to the first part of a decaying exponential of time constant TCA ≈ RCA∗CCA = 2.75 sec (see Fig. 4.2.5a). As an approximate check, note that the peaks of FCA are at about 125 ml/s, and diastolic delay lasts about 0.6 sec. The lowest points in FCA should be given by

$$\begin{aligned} \mathrm{FCA}_{min} &= 125.0*\exp(-T/\mathrm{TCA}) \\ &\approx 125.*(1. - 0.6/2.75) = 98.\ \mathrm{ml/s} \end{aligned}$$

which is fairly close to the value observed. Simple checks of this kind are important to verify that the model is obeying the equations used.

4.3 SIMULATION OF A COMPLETE CARDIOVASCULAR LOOP

A complete cardiovascular loop will now be set up in an uncontrolled form, that is, without the connections to the central nervous system (CNS), which provides much of the control of this system, and without consideration of the membrane connections to the body tissues that permit diffusion of plasma and of substances carried by the blood to and from such tissues. To do this we must devise a right heart model that will be much the same as the left heart model developed in Section 4.2, except that the peak systolic stiffness will need to be less by about a factor of four because of the smaller total capillary bed resistance in the lungs (about 170 CGS units) as compared to the systemic peripheral resistance (about 1300 CGS units). Such a model may be used to study blood volume shifts and other changes in response to parameter changes or defects (e.g., in heart valves).

Figure 4.3.1 shows a simple model of the uncontrolled cardiovascular system with right and left heart and associated arterial pathways much like the partial model of Fig. 4.2.5; the venous segments added to complete the loop are simple resistive segments. This model, which we will call pressure-flow zero (PF-0), is described by the equations in the ACSL program PF-0 below. This model has the following important characteristics:

1. Numerical values of parameters are entered in the equations except for the VSD conductance, GD = $1/R_{40}$, and the four ventricular stiffnesses, LS, LD, RS, and RD. Thus it is not possible to change anything except these five parameters at run time, unless they are introduced into the equations algebraically before compiling, with constants

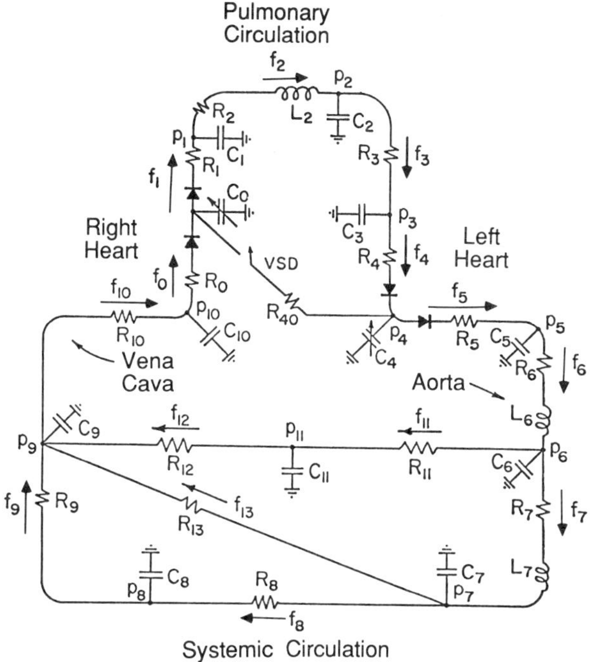

Figure 4.3.1. A simple model of the complete cardiovascular loop shown in lumped circuit form (model PF-0).

shown separately. (Note that the three-letter designation scheme used in Section 4.2 is not used here, in order to be consistent with the first paper in which this model, with parameter values, was described (Rideout-72)).

2. Units are in the CGS system except that pressures are in medical units (mm Hg), requiring that a unit correction factor be included to multiply any pressure appearing in any equation. Thus for the flow f_3 (in ml/s) determined by the pressures across R_3

$$F3 = 1332.*(P2 - P3)/R3 = 8.9*(P2 - P3)$$

If we want to be able to change the pulmonary peripheral resistance R3 in this equation at run time it may be left in algebraic form and the command CONSTANT R3 = 150. added before compiling.

3. Numerical values of equation parameters correspond approximately to an adult male human weighing 70 kg at rest. Some allometric equations are known that enable some of the parameters given here to be roughly estimated for humans of other sizes or for dogs (see Section. 2.6).

4. The heart period TH is constant and corresponds to the radian frequency W of the sinusoid used in generating ventricular stiffness variations:

$$TH = 2.*\pi/W = 2.*3.14159/7.854 = 0.8 \text{ sec} \qquad (4.3.1)$$

5. This model may be used as given to study the effect of a VSD or of changes in the contractility of the ventricles (a myocardial infarction can be simulated by reducing SR and SL). As pointed out in item 2, other parameters can be changed at run time if included wherever they appear in algebraic form. In some cases (leaky or insufficient valves or atrial septal defects) new equations and/or changes in existing equations may be needed.

6. In this model no unstressed volumes need to appear, because no interchange between stressed and unstressed volume is assumed to occur. Thus stressed volumes are used throughout. Volume variables appear only in the ventricle, and here the unstressed volumes are assumed to be zero. (A more general approach to blood volume is used in the next model, PF-1.)

```
PROGRAM PF-0
 DYNAMIC
   CONSTANT TF = 4.0
   TERMT(T .GE. TF)

  DERIVATIVE
     Algorithm IALG = 4  $' 2nd order RK'
     Maxterval MAXT = .001
     Cinterval CINT = .02
     Nsteps NSTP=1
   Constant RD=.044, RS=.30, W=7.854

     F0=133.2*BOUND(0.,2000.,P10-P0)      $'Right Heart'
     Q0=INTEG(F0-F1+F40,154.)
     S0=RS*BOUND(0.,2.,SIN(W*T))+RD
     P0=S0*Q0

     P1=.75*INTEG(F1-F2,23.)              $'Pul. Art. 1'
     F1=133.2*BOUND(0.,2000.,P0-P1)

     F2=1000.*INTEG(P1-P2-F2/50.,.043)   $'Pul. Art. 2'
     P2=.25*INTEG(F2-F3,52.)

     P3=.15*INTEG(F3-F4,41.)              $'Lung Capillaries'
     F3=8.9*(P2-P3)
```

```
    Constant LD=.033, LS=1.5                    $'Left Heart'
      Q4=INTEG(F4-F5-F40,158.)
      S4=LS*BOUND(0.,2.,SIN(W*T))+LD
      P4=S4*Q4
      F4=133.2*BOUND(0.,2000.,P3-P4)

    Constant GD=0.0                             $'VSD'
      F40=1332.*GD*(P4-P0)

      P5=1.5*INTEG(F5-F6,64.)                   $'Ascend. Aorta'
      F5=100.*BOUND(0.,2000.,P4-P5)

      F6=1000.*INTEG(P5-P6-.005*F6.,016)  $'Descend. Aorta'
      P6=.75*INTEG(F6-F11-F7,129.)

      F7=1000.*INTEG(P6-P7-.02*F7,.0024)  $'Abdom. Aorta'
      P7=.562*INTEG(F7-F8-F13,172.)

      P8=.0903*INTEG(F8-F9,97.)                 $'Leg Arteries'
      F8=.25*(P7-P8)

      P9=.075*INTEG(F9-F10+F12+F13,113.) $'Veins'
      F9=100.*(P8-P9)
      P10=.15*INTEG(F10-F0,53.)
      F10=100.*(P9-P10)
      P11=.375*INTEG(F11-F12,145.)

      F11=P6-P11                                $'Upper Body'
      F12=P11-P9
      F13=.25*(P7-P9)                           $'Internal Organs'
      CO=  REALPL(TCO,F12+F13+F8,COIC)          $'Ave. Cardiac Output'
      FP=  REALPL(TFP,F2,FPIC)                  $'Ave. Pul. Flow'
      FVSD=REALPL(TFVSD,F40,FVSDIC)             $'Ave. VSD Flow'
    Constant TCO=4.,TFP=4.,TFVSD=4., . . .
     COIC=70.,FPIC=70.,FVSDIC=50.
  END $ 'of Derivative'

 End $ 'of Dynamic'

End $ 'of Program'
```

If this model is compiled and run, the first variables of interest are the ventricular volumes, Q0 and Q4, shown in Fig. 4.3.2a. Note that the volume pumped out of each ventricle per beat is approximately 90 ml, which means that the cardiac output is 90/0.8 = 112 ml/s. Peak volumes are about the same in each ventricle, approximately 160 ml, and thus the ejection fraction for each ventricle is 90/160 = 0.56.

The model goes into a repetitive steady state at about the second beat. This occurs because the initial conditions are nearly right to start the model at the end of diastole, in steady state. These initial conditions were determined by first guessing at their values and then running the model until it reached steady state and all starting transients had disappeared. The model was stopped at the end of diastole, and the outputs of all variables obtained from integrators were obtained using the DISPLY command. These values were then used as integrator initial conditions.

Figures 4.3.3a shows the right ventricular pressure P0, together with the pulmonary artery pressure, P1; the corresponding pressures for the left ventricle are shown in Fig. 4.3.3c. Figures 4.3.3b and 4.3.3d show the important pressure-volume plots for the right and left ventricles.

Note that in Fig. 4.3.3c the amplitude of the left ventricular pressure is close to an expected peak value of 120 mm Hg, whereas the right ventricle peak in Fig. 4.3.3a is somewhat higher than the normal 18 mm Hg. This might be somewhat corrected by lowering the systolic stiffness, SR. Also, the aortic pressure has a high diastolic value; this might be

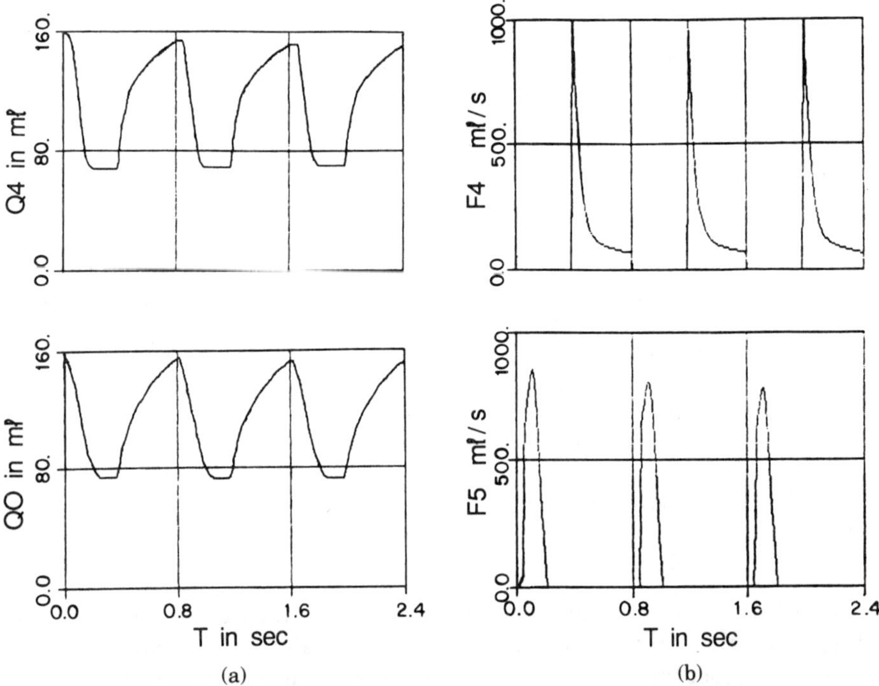

Figure 4.3.2. (a) Ventricular volumes during normal steady-state operation of model PF-0.
(b) Inflow, F_4, and outflow, F_5, for the left ventricle.

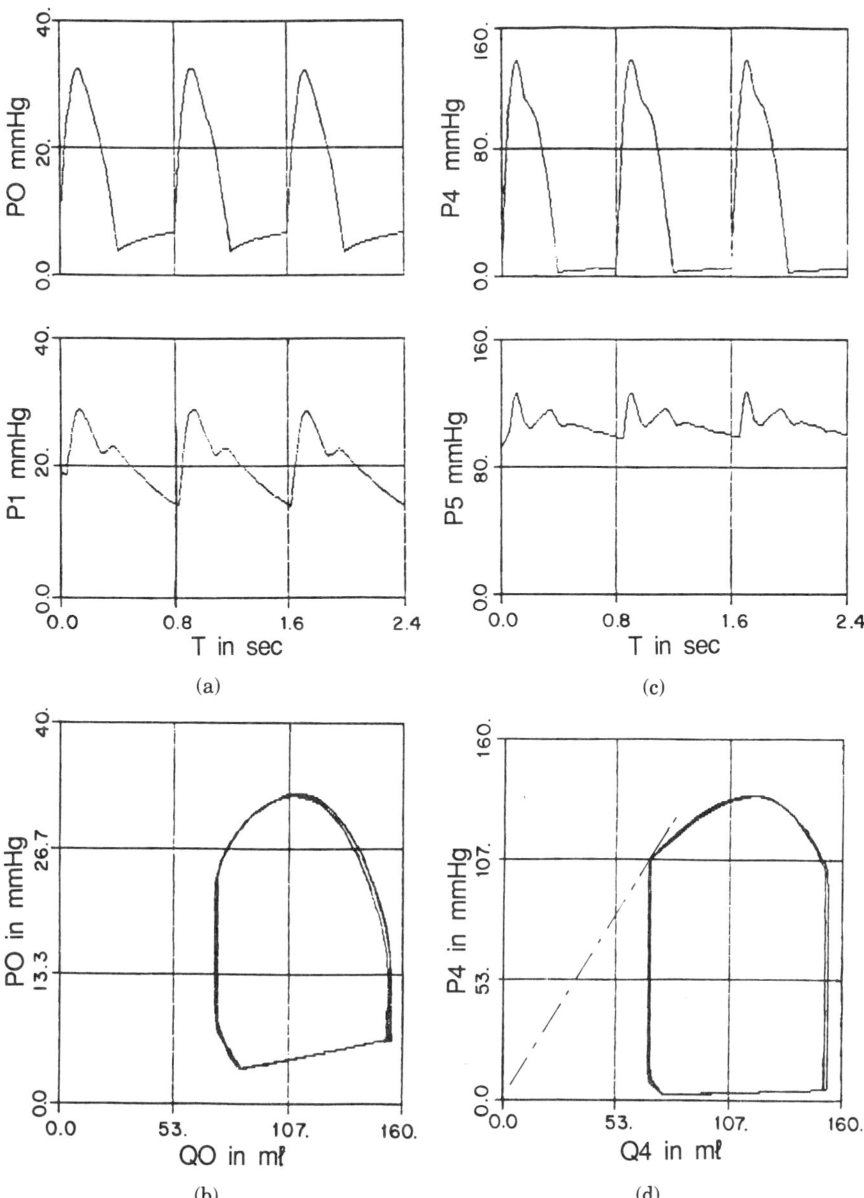

Figure 4.3.3. (a) Right ventricular pressure P0 and pulmonary artery pressure P1.
(b) Pressure versus volume locus for the right ventricle.
(c) Left ventricular and aortic pressures, P4 and P5.
(d) P-V locus for the left ventricle.

corrected by reducing the arterial compliances, C5, C6, and C7, so that the smaller resultant time constants give a faster decay of P5 after the aortic valve closes. Finally, the cardiac output is somewhat high, probably as a result of excess volume; choice of initial volumes will be considered later in model PF-1.

The ventricle pressure-flow loci (see Fig. 4.3.3b) are useful to the modeler in several ways; the stroke volume is easily obtained, as shown, as well as the peak pressure and ejection fraction. The ventricular stiffness slopes have been drawn in for the case of the left ventricle.

If a ventricular septal defect (VSD) is introduced into model PF-0 by setting the ventricle-to-ventricle conductance GD = 0.004, a number of waveforms change, as shown in Fig. 4.3.4, and overall performance is reduced as evidenced by a smaller cardiac output. The flows F5 (aorta) and F40 (VSD) may be seen to be comparable in peak amplitude and more nearly equal in the area under the flow pulses in the two cases. Thus it appears that about half of the left ventricular output is returned to the right ventricle through the defect in this case. (Note that there is a small settling transient after startup in the variables in the VSD case, because the initial conditions are still set for the normal case.)

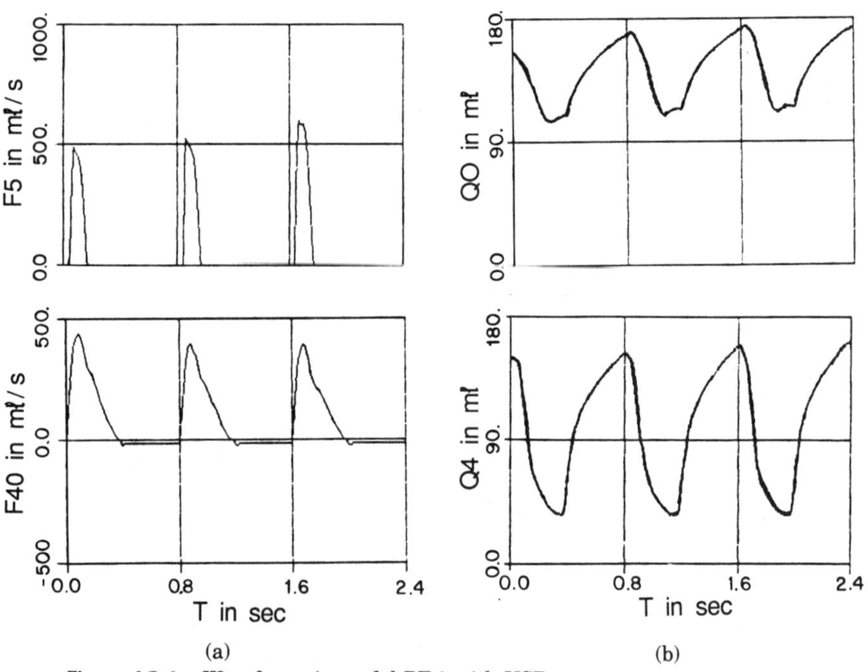

Figure 4.3.4. Waveforms in model PF-0 with VSD.
(a) Top: f_5, aortic flow, and below: f_{40}, VSD flow.
(b) Top: right ventricular average volume Q_0 is increased and volume variation reduced by the effect of the VSD. Below: left ventricular average volume Q_4 is decreased and volume variation increased by the VSD.

When a VSD is present, the cardiac output cannot be determined from the volume variation in either ventricle, because we no longer have a simple blood flow loop. However, it is possible to find the average cardiac output (CO) by filtering F5, or better, by filtering the sum of less pulsatile flows, using the command

```
CO = REALPL(TCO, F8 + F11 + F13, COIC)
```

where TCO = 5.0, (a 5-sec time constant) and COIC = 70.0, (a first guess at cardiac output, in ml/s). This will show that cardiac output is 78 ml/s. It is also possible to filter F40 and show that the average VSD flow is 76 ml/s. If the filtered average pulmonary capillary flow F3 is determined, it may be shown to be 154 ml/s, which is the sum of the other two averaged flows, as would be expected.

Another model, which we will call PF-1, is now introduced. This model has several advantages over PF-0, including the following:

1. PF-1, in its simplest form, is the single-loop model shown in Fig. 4.3.5, but arteriovenous pathways (such as capillary beds in kidneys, skin, fat, brain, muscle, etc.) may easily be included (see Fig. 6.3.1).

2. The venous segments of the model, both pulmonary and systemic, have a structure much like that used in the artery in the left ventricular model (Fig. 4.2.5). This structure has, in very simple form, some tapering of impedance that tends to match the vessels near the heart (of impedance about 120 fluid ohms) to the higher resistive impedance of the capillary beds.

3. PF-1 is set up in algebraic form, so that changes can be made in any parameters at run time. The compliances are regarded as linear but with unstressed volumes (see Fig. 4.1.2). Thus a typical equation at a node in the equivalent lumped circuit model is

$$q_n = \int_0^t (f_{\text{in}} - f_{\text{out}})dt + q_{\text{n}}(0)$$

where $q_n(0) = q_{nu}(0) + q_{ns}(0)$ (the initial volume equals the sum of the initial unstressed and stressed volumes).

Pressure is obtained from stressed volume, using

$$p_n = q_{ns}/c_n = (q_n - q_{nu})/C_n$$

All quantities in this program are in CGS units, so the pressures must be converted to medical units (mm Hg) somewhere in the DYNAMIC part of the program, using PNM = PN / 1332.0.

In the INITIAL part of the program the initial total volumes are determined from initial unstressed volumes and initial end-diastolic pressures, both assumed to be known, using QNIC = QNUIC + PNEDIC*

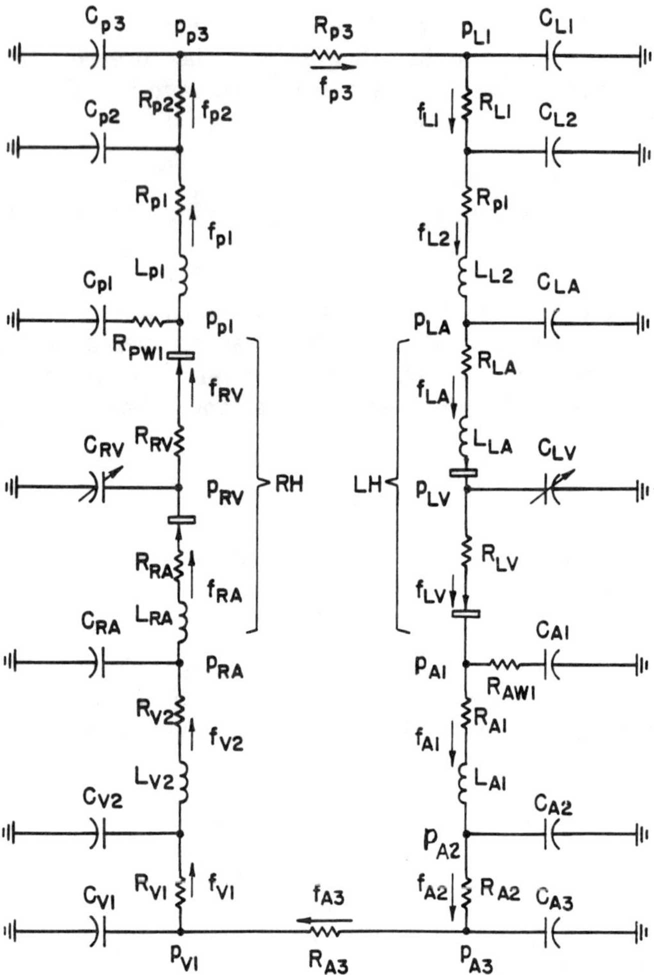

Figure 4.3.5. A single-loop CV model, PF-1. Additional systemic arterial pathways may be added in parallel with R_{A3}.

CN∗1332. for the n-th segment, where the pressure is given in mm Hg, and the model is to start at the beginning of systole.

4. The spaced half-sine wave used to produce the ventricular activity signal is the same as that used in the later ventricular models (see Fig. 4.2.4), but with a second harmonic sine wave added to shape the activity function more realistically (Snyder-68). Note, too, that this program is convenient for including a baroreceptor loop, as will be done in Section 4.4.

The following program for PF-1 contains coding that permits a myocardial infarction (of one or both ventricles) to be introduced at a chosen time. Other defects, such as a VSD, atrial septal defect (ASD), or defective heart valves, may easily be added. The model contains a means for infusing blood or other fluids into the arterial system (flow FIS into QA1 at chosen time TIS). Unstressed volume, QU, is determined in INITIAL, together with initial stressed volume, QS. If infusion or bleeding (FIS negative) is made to occur, the stressed volume QST may be determined as a function of time as given in DYNAMIC. Also, unstressed volumes may be varied with the aid of simple additions to this model, to simulate some aspects of shock, for example.

```
PROGRAM PF-1
 INITIAL
        'Some constants and calculations of initial volumes'
        Constant QP1U=7.8, PP1EDM=7.2,CP1=.0001
       QP1IC= QP1U+ PP1EDM*CP1*1332.        $ 'Pulm. Art. 1'
        Constant QP2U=23.4, PP2EDM = 7.0,CP2=.0003
       QP2IC= QP2U + PP2EDM*CP2*1332.       $ 'Pulm. Art. 2'
        Constant QP3U=210.5,PP3EDM = 6.6,CP3=.0027
       QP3IC= QP3U+ PP3EDM*CP3*1332.        $ 'Pulm. Art. 3'
        Constant QL1U=69.,PL1EDM=4.45,CL1=.001
       QL1IC= QL1U + PL1EDM*CL1*1332.       $ 'Pulm.Veins 1'
        Constant QL2U=69.,PL2EDM=3.62,CL2=.001
       QL2IC= QL2U+ PL2EDM*CL2*1332.        $ 'Pulm.Veins 2'
        Constant QLAU=814.5,PLAEDM=3.45,CLA=.01176
       QLAIC= QLAU + PLAEDM*CLA*1332.       $ 'L. Atrium'
        Constant QLVU=10.,PLVEDM=4.0, LD=45.
       QLVIC= QLVU+ PLVEDM*1332./LD         $ 'L. Ventricle'
        Constant QA1U=35.1,PA1EDM=64.3,CA1=.00018
       QA1IC= QA1U + PA1EDM*CA1*1332.       $ 'Syst. Art. 1'
        Constant QA2U= 85.,PA2EDM=64.,CA2= .00023
       QA2IC= QA2U+ PA2EDM*CA2*1332.        $ 'Syst. Art. 2'
        Constant QA3U=710.,PA3EDM=63.,CA3=.00182
       QA3IC= QA3U + PA3EDM*CA3*1332.       $ 'Syst. Art. 3'
        Constant QV1U=909.,PV1EDM=13.5,CV1=.021
       QV1IC= QV1U+ PV1EDM*CV1*1332.        $ 'Syst. Veins 1'
        Constant QV2U=1948.,PV2EDM=7.2,CV2=.045
       QV2IC= QV2U + PV2EDM*CV2*1332.       $ 'Syst. Veins 2'
        Constant QRAU=1948.,PRAEDM=6.64,CRA=.045
       QRAIC= QRAU+ PRAEDM*CRA*1332.        $ 'Rt. Atrium'
        Constant QRVU=10.,PRVEDM=7.4,RD=72.
       QRVIC= QRVU + PRVEDM*1332./RD        $ 'Rt. Ventricle'

        'Calc. of total initial blood vol. QT, total un- . . .
        stressed volume QU, and stressed volume, QS at T=0.0'
       QT=QP1IC+ QP2IC+ QP3IC+QL1IC+QL2IC+ QLAIC+ QLVIC . . .
        +QA1IC+ QA1IC+ QA3IC+ QV1IC+ QV2IC+ QRAIC+ QRVIC
```

```
        QU=QP1U+ QP2U+ QP3U+ QL1U+ QL2U+ QLAU+ QLVU+ QA1U . . .
         +QA2U+ QA3U+ QV1U+ QV2U+ QRAU+ QRVU
        QS= QT- QU

  END $'of initial'

  DYNAMIC
        CONSTANT TF = 8.
 TERMT(T .GE. TF)
 Cinterval CINT=.02

  DERIVATIVE
        Algorithm IALG = 4    $ '2nd order RK'
        Maxterval MAXT = .002 $ Nsteps NSTP = 1

     Constant THI=800., LSI=2500.,RSI=350.,DLS=0.,DRS=0.
         'DLS and DRS are values of sudden changes in LS, RS at THI'
         'These changes should be negative for an infarct'
        LS= LSI + FCNSW(TI,0.,0.,DLS)
        RS= RSI + FCNSW(TI,0.,0.,DRS)
        TI=T - THI             $' THI is time of infarct'

     Constant TSA=0.1,TS=.3,TH=.8,PI=3.1416,KB=1.,SV1=.9,SV2=.25
        LOGICAL XX
        X=T-ZOH(T,0.0,0.0,TH)
        XX=X .LE. TS
        STW=RSW(XX,X,0.0)
        SSW = SV1*SIN(PI*STW/TS)-SV2*SIN(2.*PI*STW/TS)
        ACTV=KB*BOUND(0.0,1.0,SSW)         $'Ventr. Pumping Activ.'

        'Pressure-Flow Equations start here'
     Constant          RPW1=10.,LP1=1.0,FP1IC=0.0, . . .
        KP1=1.,RP1=10.                     $'Pul. Art. 1'
        PP1= (QP1-QP1U)/CP1 +KP1 *RPW1*(FRV-FP1)
        FP1= INTEG((PP1-PP2-RP1*FP1)/LP1,FP1IC)
        QP1=  INTEG(FRV-FP1,QP1IC)  $'Note:CP1 and QP1IC in INITIAL'
     Constant RP2=40.                      $'Pul. Art. 2'
        PP2= (QP2-QP2U)/CP2
        FP2= (PP2-PP3)/RP2
        QP2= INTEG(FP1-FP2,QP2IC)
     Constant RP3=80.                      $'Pul. Art. 3'
        PP3= (QP3-QP3U)/CP3
        FP3= (PP3-PL1)/RP3
        QP3= INTEG(FP2-FP3,QP3IC)
     Constant    RL1=30.                   $'Pul.    Vein   1'
        PL1= (QL1-QL1U)/CL1
        FL1= (PL1-PL2)/RL1
        QL1= INTEG(FP3-FL1,QL1IC)
```

```
  Constant RL2=10.,LL2=1.0,FL2IC=33.   $'Pul. Vein 2'
     PL2= (QL2-QL2U)/CL2
     FL2= INTEG((PL2-PLA-RL2*FL2)/LL2,FL2IC)
     QL2= INTEG(FL1-FL2,QL2IC)
  Constant RLA=5.,LLA=1.0,FLAIC=0.0    $'Left Atrium'
     PLA= (QLA-QLAU)/CLA
     FLA= LIMINT((PLA-PLV-RLA*FLA)/LLA,FLAIC,0.0,1.E4)
     QLA= INTEG(FL2-FLA,QLAIC)
  Constant RLV=5.,LLV=1.,FLVIC=0.0     $'Left Ventr.'
     SLV= LD*(1.-ACTV) + LS*ACTV
  'LD given in INITIAL, LS in 6-th line of DERIVATIVE'
     PLV= (QLV-QLVU)*SLV
     FLV= LIMINT((PLV-PA1-RLV*FLV)/LLV,FLVIC,0.,1.E5)
     QLV= INTEG(FLA-FLV,QLVIC)
  Constant FA1IC=4.6,RA1=10.,LA1=1.0   $'Aorta 1'
  Constant RPW2=10.,KP2=1.0,FIS=0.0,TIS=3.0
     FI= FCNSW(T-TIS,0.0,0.0,FIS)      $'Infusion FI,T>TIS'
     PA1= (QA1-QA1U)/CA1 +KP2*RPW2*(FLV-FA1)
     FA1= INTEG((PA1-PA2-RA1*FA1)/LA1,FA1IC)
     QA1= INTEG(FLV-FA1+FI,QA1IC)
  Constant RA2=160.                    $'Aorta 2'
     PA2= (QA2-QA2U)/CA2
     FA2= (PA2-PA3)/RA2
     QA2= INTEG(FA1-FA2,QA2IC)
  Constant RA3=1000.                   $'System. Art.'
     PA3= (QA3-QA3U)/CA3
     FA3= (PA3-PV1)/RA3
     QA3= INTEG(FA2-FA3,QA3IC)
  Constant RV1=90.                     $'System. Veins 1'
     PV1= (QV1-QV1U)/CV1
     FV1= (PV1-PV2)/RV1
     QV1= INTEG(FA3-FV1,QV1IC)
  Constant RV2=10.,LV2=1.,FV2IC=95.    $'System. Veins 2'
     PV2= (QV2-QV2U)/CV2
     FV2= INTEG((PV2-PRA-RV2*FV2)/LV2,FV2IC)
     QV2= INTEG(FV1-FV2,QV2IC)
  Constant RRA=5.,LRA=1.0,FRAIC=0.     $'Rt. Atrium'
     PRA= (QRA-QRAU)/CRA
     FRA= LIMINT((PRA-PRV-RRA*FRA)/LRA, FRAIC, 0.,1.E4)
     QRA= INTEG (FV2-FRA,QRAIC)
  Constant RRV=5.,LRV=1.,FRVIC=6.0     $'Rt. Ventr.'
     SRV= RD*(1-ACTV) + RS*ACTV
     PRV= (QRV-QRVU)*SRV
     FRV= LIMINT((PRV-PP1-RRV*FRV)/LRV,FRVIC,0.,1.E5)
     QRV= INTEG(FRA-FRV,QRVIC)

END $'of Deriv.'
```

```
        'Calculate Output Pressures in mmHg'
      PP1M=PP1/1332. $ PP2M=PP2/1332. $ PP3M=PP3/1332.
      PL1M=PL1/1332. $ PL2M=PL2/1332. $ PLAM=PLA/1332.
      PLVM=PLV/1332. $ PA1M=PA1/1332. $ PA2M=PA2/1332.
      PA3M=PA3/1332. $ PV1M=PV1/1332. $ PV2M=PV2/1332.
      PRAM=PRA/1332. $ PRVM=PRV/1332.

  'Find Total Volume and Stressed Volume as Functions of Time'
   QTOT=QP1+QP2+QP3+QL1+QL2+QLA+QLV+QA1+QA2+QA3+QV1+QV2+QRA+QRV
   QST = QTOT - QU   $'Total Stressed Vol. as Fcn. of Time'

  END  $ 'of Dynamic'
 END  $ 'of Program'
```

Running normally, this program has a ventricular activity function and ventricular volumes, as shown in Fig. 4.3.6. The ventricular activity function has a somewhat slower rise and a faster fall as a result of the inclusion of a second harmonic sinusoidal term, but might be improved by clipping its rather sharp peak. The ventricular volume curves are much like those for PF-0 (see Fig. 4.3.2), but stroke volume is small at a value of 64 ml; since the heart period is fixed at 0.8 sec, this corresponds to a cardiac output of 64/0.8 = 80 ml/s, which is slightly low for an adult male. The cardiac output will increase as blood volume is increased. This may be accomplished by including a factor M in all calculations for stressed volumes; M should ordinarily be set to unity but may be set to a larger value at run time to increase blood volume and cardiac output.

Other outputs for PF-1 are shown in Fig. 4.3.7. Here the right ventricular pressure PRVM (in medical units) is shown in part a, together with the pulmonary artery pressure, PP1M; the corresponding left side pressures, PLVM and PA1M, are shown in part b. The flow FLA into the left ventricle is shown in part c, together with the flow FLV into the first segment of aorta; note that FLA has an oscillatory decay after the aortic valve closes. In a better, more detailed model this oscillation may go negative on its downswings. The important left ventricular pressure versus volume locus in Fig. 4.3.7d shows the peak ventricular pressure, stroke volume VS, and ejection fraction (here about 50 percent).

The means for sudden introduction of weakened ventricles (myocardial infarction) are included in model PF-1. This is achieved by modifying the two commands used in the first part of the Derivative section of PF-1 to determine the ventricular systolic stiffnesses, LS and RS. These are normally set equal to the given constants, LSI and RSI, and function switches are included to change these values by DLS and DRS at time THI. Thus, if we set DLS = −625.0 and DRS = −87.5 at run time, a 25 percent weakening of systolic stiffness in each ventricle will occur at

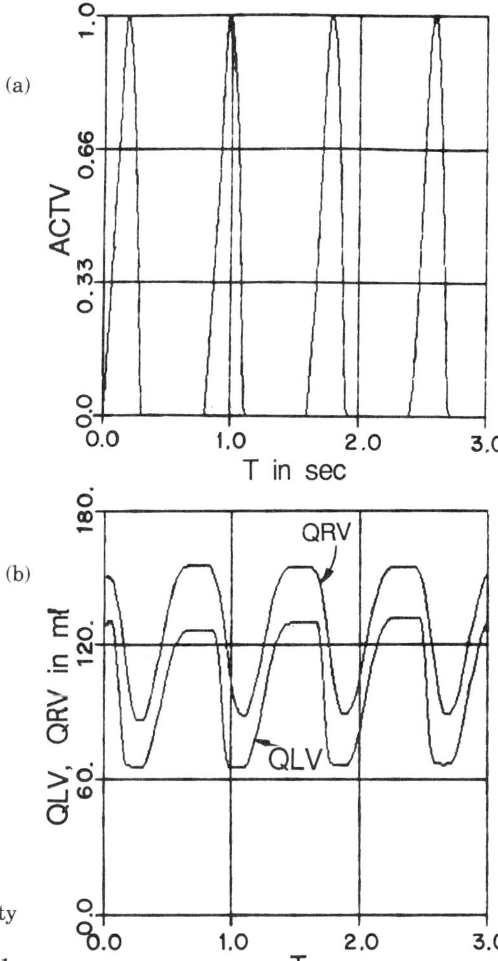

Figure 4.3.6. (a) Ventricular activity function, ACTV, in model PF-1. (b) Ventricular volumes in model PF-1.

time THI—somewhat unrealistically in that the weakening in cardiac muscle will ordinarily tend to occur more slowly.

This model was set to run with DLS and DRS set to the negative values given above, and THI = 2.4; some outputs for this case are shown in Fig. 4.3.8. Here the sudden decrease in ventricular stiffnesses causes a corresponding sudden decrease in stroke volume, as shown in Fig. 4.3.8b, but a slight recovery begins to occur as atrial average volumes and pressures increase, thus causing increased filling, which in turn (by Starling's law) increases ventricular output. Thus the circulatory system has some inherent stability, even without baroreceptor control, which would tend

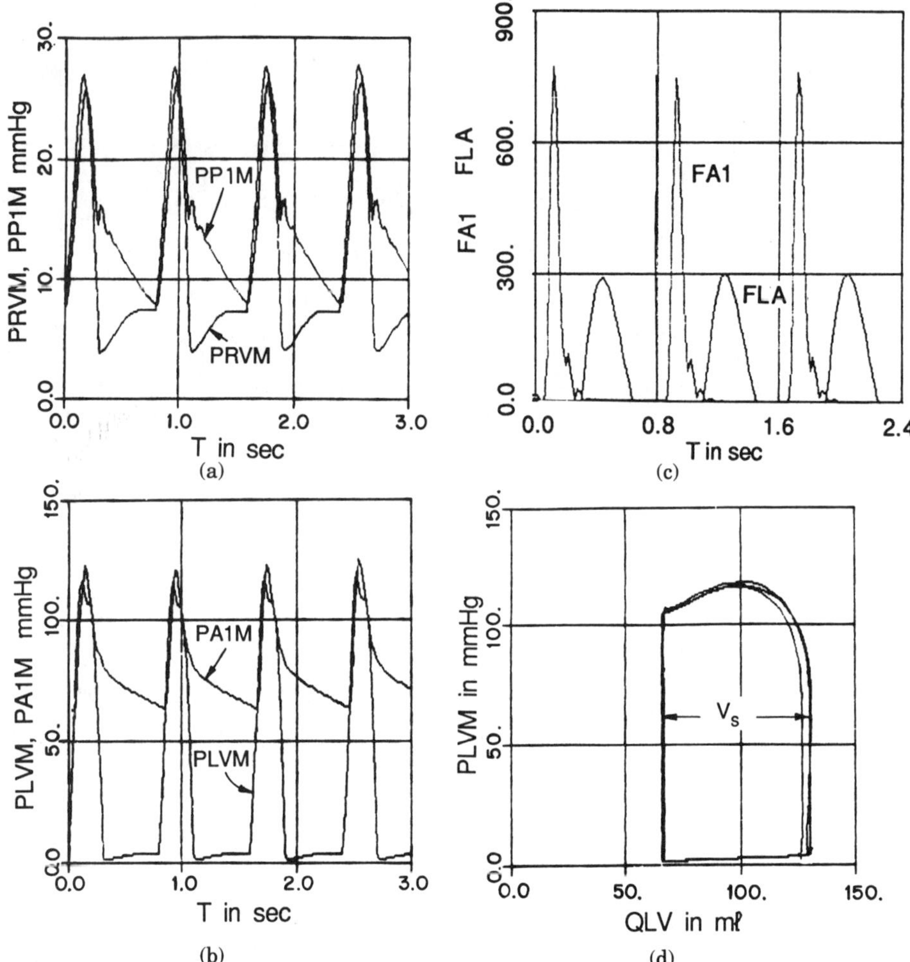

Figure 4.3.7. Model PF-1 in normal operation.
(a) Right ventricular and pulmonary artery pressures.
(b) Left ventricular and aortic pressures.
(c) Aortic flow, FLV and mitral valve inflow FLA, to ventricle.
(d) Pressure-volume plot for the left ventricle.

to give further recovery in case of reduced ventricular strength (see Section 4.5). Note that many other effects not included in this model bear upon the problem being considered; for example, reduced output pressure can reduce coronary flow to the heart muscles, which in turn further reduces pressures and flows.

Program PF-1 also includes means for either fluid infusion or a fixed rate of bleeding from the systemic arteries, as discussed above.

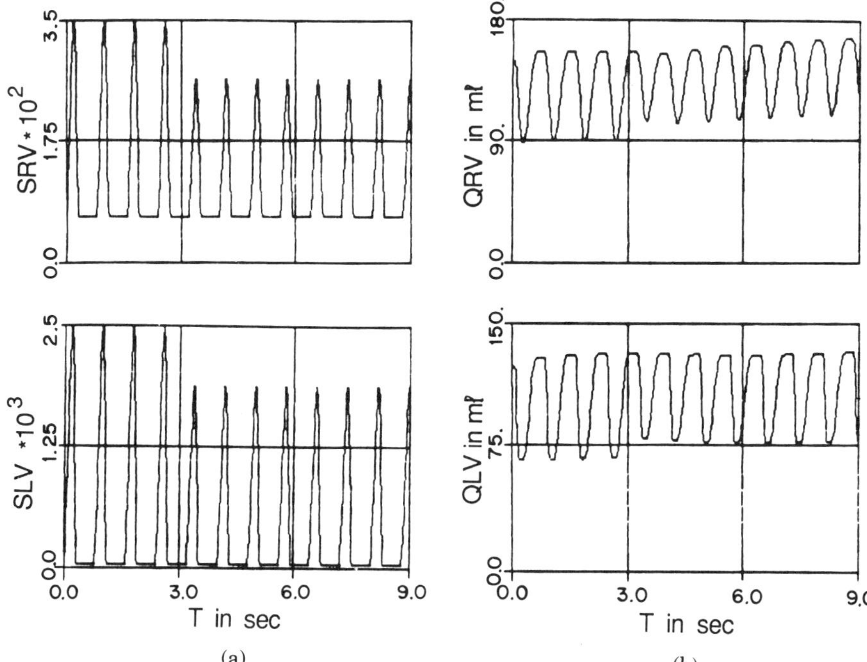

Figure 4.3.8. Model PF-1 with a simulated sudden infarction.
(a) Sudden decreases in SRV and SLV at THI = 2.4 sec.
(b) Ventricular volumes. Note the slow recovery in stroke volume after the infarct.

4.4 PROBLEMS OF DETAIL IN CARDIOVASCULAR MODELS

The cardiovascular system may be modeled in much more detail than in the PF-1 model (see Section 4.3). More commonly, it is only some portion of the whole system that is expanded in detail, such as the systemic arterial model shown in the frontispiece. This model (Snyder-68), whether used by itself or as the arterial part of some more complete system model, will yield very faithful aortic and arterial waveforms that may serve various research purposes. Other successful models of equivalent detail appeared somewhat earlier in Holland (Jager-65, Noordergraaf-63, Beneken-65). A detailed arterial system model of slightly different form with somewhat fewer sections was successfully used by Chang in parameter estimation of the canine systemic arterial system (see Chapter 9), an application in which waveforms are important. Some of the needs in cardiovascular modeling may be found in work on patient management under anesthesia or in intensive care (Ream-82).

To illustrate the progressive addition of detail to a model, we can further examine the kind of changes made in the systemic arterial system in the left heart studies described earlier in this chapter. In the left heart models, a modification of the simple *windkessel* (parallel compliance and capillary resistance) was used with the addition of an added series resistance, as redrawn in Fig. 4.4.1a; this model, called the *westkessel* (Westerhof-69, Noordergraaf-78), has an additional series resistance equal to the characteristic impedance Z_0 of the aorta, as given by transmission line theory. This impedance, using expressions for L and C from (4.1.8) and (4.1.9), and assuming a low-loss distortionless line (Rideout-67), is

$$Z_0 = \sqrt{L/C} = \sqrt{3\rho E h / 2\pi^2 r^5} \tag{4.4.1}$$

The terms in this expression may be fairly well known, with the important exception of E, the bulk modulus of elasticity. E is so difficult to measure that it may be easier to use (4.4.1) to find E from a measured Z_0! (Note that Z_0 may be determined by taking the quotient of the change in pressure during the initial part of systole and the resultant change in flow.)

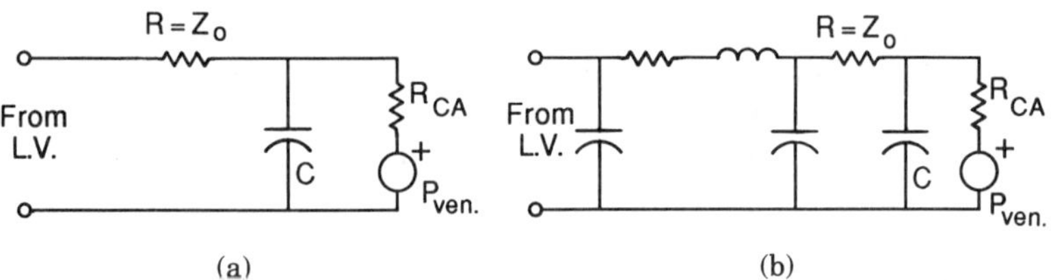

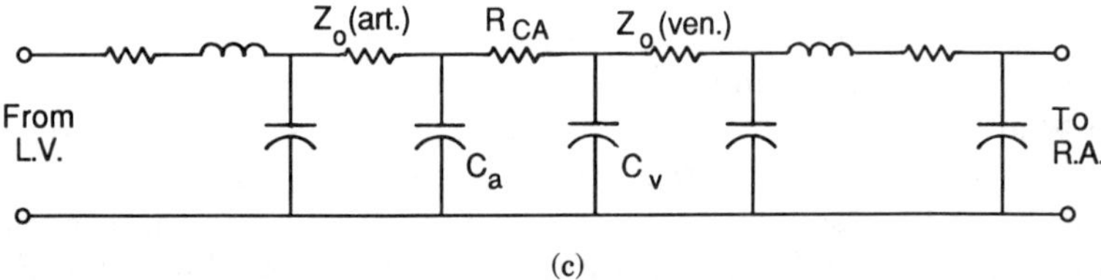

Figure 4.4.1. (a) Westkessel model, the simplest arterial system model for pulsatile system modeling.
(b) Modified westkessel model, with one added RLC pi-section.
(c) Use of two models of the form shown in (b), used back-to-back to represent the systemic arterial and venous system rather simply. Here the impedance can taper up from the arterial characteristic impedance (of 100 to 150 cgs ohms) to the major part of the peripheral impedance ($R_{CA} \approx 1300$) in the capillary beds, and then taper back down to the characteristic impedance of the large veins.

The westkessel model may be improved by adding one (or more) pi sections of RLC models, as shown in Fig. 4.4.1b. These simple model forms may be combined in other ways and can more accurately represent the cardiovascular system if a branching out is used in the arterial tree and a recombining in the venous (Fig. 4.4.1c).

Beneken devised a highly detailed heart model, involving muscle models and concerned with the structural form of the heart (Beneken-65), a model form also used later in a study of the canine heart and circulation (Dick-68). At the other end of the spectrum is the nonpulsatile cardiovascular model (see Section 4.6), which has many possible applications in pharmacokinetics.

The left heart is shaped as shown in Fig. 4.4.2a, with the input

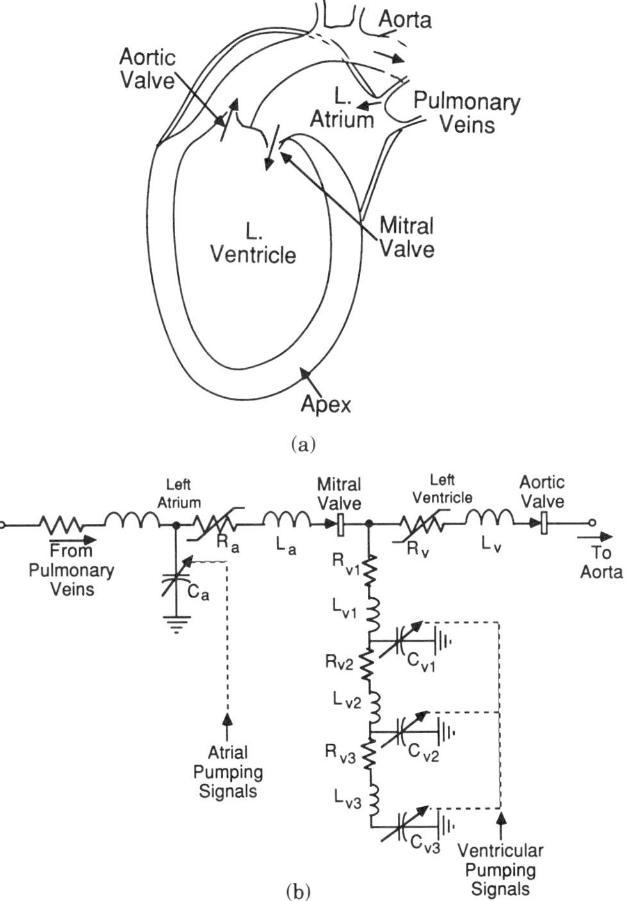

Figure 4.4.2. (a) An approximate cross-sectional view of the left heart. (b) Model of the left heart, with a multi-segment representation of the ventricle, and atrial pumping.

(mitral) valve and output (aortic) valve close to one another. Thus these valves may be considered to be at one end of a fluid-flow transmission line running down from the valves to the apex of the heart, as shown in Fig. 4.4.2b, where a three-segment lumped model represents this transmission line. Note that if the resistances R_{vi} and inertances L_{vi} (for $i = 1, 2$, and 3) are assumed to be zero, this model closely resembles the ventricular model in Fig. 4.2.5, with the variable compliance $C_v = C_{v1} + C_{v2} + C_{v3}$. The number of segments used may be larger than three (Gianunzio-67), just as more may be used in an aortic or systemic arterial model (Snyder-68). In addition to the inclusion of multiple segments within the ventricle, the model shown indicates that atrial pumping (of compliance C_a) may also be used (Katra-66 and Lau-79), as well as square-law nonlinear valve resistances (Blackstone-77). Models of this kind should have the contractions of the individual ventricular compliances begin with the compliance nearest the apex of the heart, corresponding to the timing of the spread of excitation in the heart.

Adequate treatment of the venous system is important in models of the entire cardiovascular system. Veins and the venous system have also been studied (Moreno-78 and Brower-78). In a model of the venous system that was general enough to study the effects of changes in gravitational force, Snyder included the venous valves in the limbs and the possibilities of collapse in the large veins within the chest in certain circumstances (Snyder-72); a diagram that appeared in this study and elsewhere in his work is shown in Fig. 4.0.1b.

Physiological control of the cardiovascular system is achieved with the aid of many control loops; perhaps of most importance among these is the baroreceptor loop (Katona-62, Sagawa-80, Tham-88) which is modeled in a simplified form in Section 4.5.

Enough has been said to indicate that a major problem in simulation is the inclusion of enough detail in the model to serve the needs of the modeler without overloading the computer—or the modeler. Note that there are three major ways in which detail may have to be added to cardiovascular models. These are, with their advantages:

1. Use more segments to represent any given part of the system, and thus increase bandwidth.
2. Add subsystems such as baroreceptor control of the heart and vasculature, and thus represent more aspects of the system.
3. Include nonlinearities, such as nonlinear elastance of vessel walls or valves in leg veins, and thus represent system dynamics more accurately.

There has been some tendency to philosophize about problems of model size, with investigators finding that as more and more details are added to models, they tend to become slow and unwieldy, and thus only isolated subsystems can be properly studied by computer model methods (Noordergraaf-78). But as more powerful computers (particularly parallel digital machines) become available, and with the aid of modular approaches (discussed in Chapters 1 and 6 of this book), it may become possible to work with more useful and meaningful simulations. Nevertheless, it should be noted that the typical modeler always tends to push model size to the limits of the computer equipment available.

4.5 BARORECEPTOR CONTROL OF THE CIRCULATORY SYSTEM

Pressures and flows in the uncontrolled circulation tend to be stabilized by the Frank-Starling mechanism (Noordergraaf-78); this may be shown by the partial recovery of cardiac output after a left ventricular infarction in model PF-0 of Section 4.3. However, the normal cardiovascular system has a more important stabilization mechanism as a result of feedback control acting through the central nervous system. This control depends on pressure signals that are converted to efferent nerve signals by the baroreceptors in the carotid arch. These nerve pathways are shown in Fig. 4.5.1, together with the afferent nerves, which carry signals from the baroreceptors to the central nervous system.

Studies of the baroreceptor control system (Katona-70 and 80;

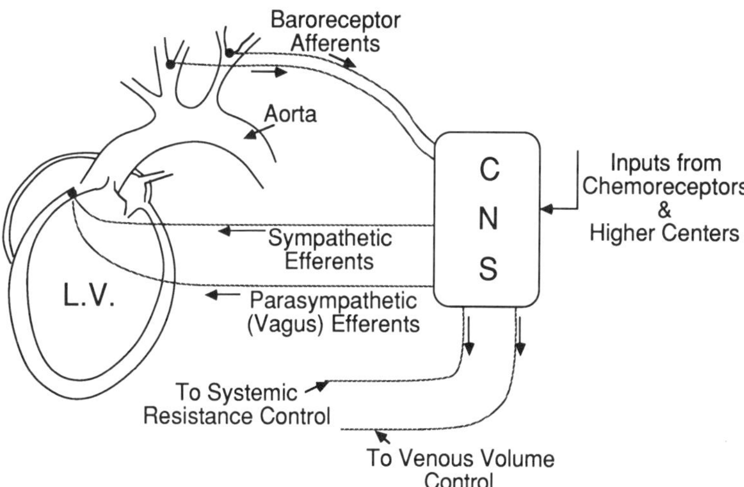

Figure 4.5.1. The activity of the heart is affected by two sets of efferent nerves carrying signals from the CNS to the heart, the sympathetic and the parasympathetic (or vagus) nerves. These signals, in turn depend upon the afferent messages carried to the CNS from the baroreceptors.

Dick-68) have shown that the signals returned to the heart tend to reduce both heart rate and strength of contraction in response to increased pressure in the carotid arteries and to increase both if there is decreased pressure in the carotids. In addition, other signals lead to an increase in peripheral systemic resistance and decreased venous volume with decreasing carotid pressure, and vice versa.

It is interesting to add elementary negative feedback regulation, corresponding to the baroreceptor system, to the cardiovascular model PF-1; the new program will be called PF-1-REG. In this program, the pressure PA3M, corresponding approximately to the carotid pressure, is filtered by a simple lag with time constant TFIL = 3.2

```
PA3MF = REALPL(TFIL, PA3M, PA3MIC)                    (4.5.1)
```

where DPA3MF = PA3MF − PREF is the error in pressure. Here pressures are in mm Hg, and both PREF and PA3MIC are set at 72 mm Hg for normal startup of PF-1-REG.

We now define

```
Z3 = KX * DPA3MF                                      (4.5.2)
```

where KX, a gain constant, is normally set to 0.2, and Z3 is a feedback quantity that may be positive or negative, according to whether the average carotid pressure is greater or less than PREF. We want a feedback quantity Y that is normally unity and bounded between the limits 0.1 and 1.9,

```
Y - BOUND(LLT, ULT, (1.0 + Z3))
where LLT = 0.1, ULT = 1.9 .                          (4.5.3)
```

The feedback signal Y is now used to control automatically the heart period TH, as well as the systolic period TS and the strength of contraction of both ventricles, according to the equations:

```
TH = 0.2 + 0.6*Y
TS = 0.14 + 0.2*TH
LS = LSI/(0.5*Y+0.5) + FCNSW(TI,0.0,0.0,DLS)
RS = RSI/(0.5*Y+0.5) + FCNSW(TI,0.0,0.0,DRS)          (4.5.4)
```

Note that an increase in Y, which might result from an increase in carotid pressure, will tend to increase heart period (decrease heart rate) and also will decrease strengths of contraction of the ventricles. The result of these changes will tend to return arterial pressures, and thus cardiac output, back to their original levels.

The program PF-1-REG is shown next. Here the same scheme has been used in INITIAL to find integrator initial conditions (chiefly for volumes) as in its predecessor, PF-1, although simpler methods could have been used to find initial conditions in this program.

```
PROGRAM PF-1-REG
 INITIAL
      'Some constants and calculations of initial volumes'
      Constant QP1U=7.8, PP1EDM=7.2,CP1=.0002
     QP1IC= QP1U+ PP1EDM*CP1*1332.         $ 'Pulm. Art. 1'
      Constant QP2U=23.4, PP2EDM=7.0,CP2=.0004
     QP2IC= QP2U + PP2EDM*CP2*1332.        $ 'Pulm. Art. 2'
      Constant QP3U=210.5,PP3EDM=6.6,CP3=.0027
     QP3IC= QP3U + PP3EDM*CP3*1332.        $ 'Pulm. Art. 3'
      Constant QL1U=69.,PL1EDM=4.45,CL1=.001
     QL1IC= QL1U + PL1EDM*CL1*1332.        $ 'Pulm.Veins 1'
      Constant QL2U=69.,PL2EDM=3.62,CL2=.001
     QL2IC= QL2U+ PL2EDM*CL2*1332.         $ 'Pulm.veins 2'
      Constant QLAU=814.5,PLAEDM=3.45,CLA=.01176
     QLAIC= QLAU + PLAEDM*CLA*1332.        $ 'L. Atrium'
      Constant QLVU=10.,PLVEDM=4.0, LD=45.
     QLVIC= QLVU+ PLVEDM*1332./LD          $ 'L. Ventricle'
      Constant QA1U=35.1,PA1EDM=64.3,CA1=.00018
     QA1IC= QA1U + PA1EDM*CA1*1332.        $ 'Syst. Art. 1'
      Constant QA2U= .85.,PA2EDM=64.,CA2= .00023
     QA2IC= QA2U+ PA2EDM*CA2*1332.         $ 'Syst. Art. 2'
      Constant QA3U=710.,PA3EDM=63.,CA3=.00182
     QA3IC= QA3U + PA3EDM*CA3*1332.        $ 'Syst. Art. 3'
      Constant QV1U=909.,PV1EDM=13.5,CV1=.021
     QV1IC= QV1U+ PV1EDM*CV1*1332.         $ 'Syst. Veins 1'
      Constant QV2U=1948.,PV2EDM=7.2,CV2=.045
     QV2IC= QV2U + PV2EDM*CV2*1332.        $ 'Syst. Veins 2'
      Constant QRAU=1948.,PRAEDM=6.64,CRA=.045
     QRAIC= QRAU+ PRAEDM*CRA*1332.         $ 'Rt. Atrium'
      Constant QRVU=10.,PRVEDM=7.4,RD=68.
     QRVIC= QRVU + PRVEDM*1332./RD         $ 'Rt. Ventricle'

      'Calc. of total blood vol. QT, total unstressed . . .
       volume QU, and initial stressed volume, QS, at T=0.0'
     QT=QP1IC+ QP2IC+ QP3IC+QL1IC+QL2IC+ QLAIC+ QLVIC . . .
       +QA1IC+ QA2IC+ QA3IC+ QV1IC+ QV2IC+ QRAIC+ QRVIC
     QU=QP1U+ QP2U+ QP3U+ QL1U+ QL2U+ QLAU+ QLVU+ QA1U . . .
       +QA2U+ QA3U+ QV1U+ QV2U+ QRAU+ QRVU
     QS= QT- QU

 END $'of initial'

 DYNAMIC
     Constant TF = 8.
```

```
    TERMT(T .GE. TF)
    Cinterval CINT=.02
 DERIVATIVE
    Algorithm IALG = 4    $ '2nd order RK'
    Maxterval MAXT = .002 $ Nsteps NSTP = 1

   Constant THI=800., LSI=2500.,RSI=350.,DLS=0.,DRS=0.
     'DLS and DRS are values of changes in LS, RS at THI'
     'These changes will be negative for an infarct'
    LS= LSI/(0.5*Y + 0.5) + FCNSW(TI,0.,0.,DLS)
    RS= RSI/(0.5*Y = 0.5) + FCNSW(TI,0.,0.,DRS)
    TI=T - THI                   $'Infarct at THI'

   Constant PI=3.1416,KB=1.,SV1=.9,SV2=.25
   Constant TFIL=3.2,PA3MIC=72., LLT=0.1,ULT=1.9,PREF=72.
    PA3M=PA3/1332.
    PA3MF= REALPL(TFIL,PA3M,PA3MIC)      $'Filter Carotid Press.'
    DPA3MF=PA3MF -PREF
    Z3 = KX * DPA3MF
   Constant KX = .02                     $'Use KX=0.0 for no Reg.'
    Y = BOUND(LLT,ULT,(1.0 + Z3))        $'Y appears above in LS, RS'
    TH = 0.2 + 0.6*Y                     $ TS= 0.14 + 0.2 *TH


   LOGICAL XX
   X=T-ZOH(T,0.0,0.0,TH)
   XX=X .LE. TS
   STW=RSW(XX,X,0.0)
   SSW=SV1*SIN(PI*STW/TS)-SV2*SIN(2.*PI*STW/TS)
   ACTV=KB* BOUND(0.0,1.0,SSW)           $'Ventr. Pumping Activ.'


    'Note, TH appears in Eqn. for X, TS in XX and SSW'
    'Pressure-Flow Equations start here'
   Constant RPW1=10.,LP1=1.0,FP1IC=0.0, . . .
      KP1=1.,RP1=10.                     $'Pul. Art. 1'
    PP1= (QP1-QP1U)/CP1 +KP1 *RPW1*(FRV-FP1)
    FP1= INTEG((PP1-PP2-RP1*FP1)/LP1,FP1IC)
    QP1= INTEG(FRV-FP1,QP1IC)        $'CP1 AND QP1IC in INITIAL'
   Constant RP2=40.                      $'Pul. Art. 2'
    PP2= (QP2-QP2U)/CP2
    FP2= (PP2-PP3)/RP2
    QP2= INTEG(FP1-FP2,QP2IC)
   Constant RP3=80.                      $'Pul. Art. 3'
    PP3= (QP3-QP3U)/CP3
    FP3= (PP3-PL1)/RP3
    QP3= INTEG(FP2-FP3,QP3IC)
   Constant   RL1=30.                    $'Pul. Vein 1'
    PL1= (QL1-QL1U)/CL1
```

```
  FL1= (PL1-PL2)/RL1
  QL1= INTEG(FP3-FL1,QL1IC)
 Constant RL2=10.,LL2=1.0,FL2IC=33. $'Pul. Vein 2'
  PL2= (QL2-QL2U)/CL2
  FL2= INTEG((PL2-PLA-RL2*FL2)/LL2,FL2IC)
  QL2= INTEG(FL1-FL2,QL2IC)
 Constant RLA=5.,LLA=1.0,FLAIC=0.0  $'Left Atrium'
  PLA= (QLA-QLAU)/CLA
  FLA= LIMINT((PLA-PLV-RLA*FLA)/LLA,FLAIC,0.0,1.E4)
  QLA= INTEG(FL2-FLA,QLAIC)
 Constant RLV=5.,LLV=1.,FLVIC=0.0   $'Left Ventr.'
  SLV= D*(1.-ACTV) + LS*ACTV
'LD given in INITIAL, LS in 4-th line of DERIVATIVE'
  PLV= (QLV-QLVU)*SLV
  FLV= LIMINT((PLV-PA1-RLV*FLV)/LLV,FLVIC,0.,1.E5)
  QLV= INTEG(FLA-FLV,QLVIC)
 Constant FA1IC=4.6,RA1=10.,LA1=1.0,FI=0.$'Aorta 1'
   'Note:RPW1, KP1 given above PP1'
  PA1= (QA1-QA1U)/CA1 +KP1*RPW1*(FLV-FA1)
  FA1= INTEG((PA1-PA2-RA1*FA1)/LA1,FA1IC)
  QA1= INTEG(FLV-FA1+FI,QA1IC)
 Constant RA2=160.                  $'Aorta 2'
  PA2= (QA2-QA2U)/CA2
  FA2= (PA2-PA3)/RA2
  QA2= INTEG(FA1-FA2,QA2IC)
 Constant RA3=1000.                 $'System. Art.'
  PA3= (QA3-QA3U)/CA3
  FA3= (PA3-PV1)/RA3
  QA3= INTEG(FA2-FA3,QA3IC)
 Constant RV1=90.                   $'System. Veins 1'
  PV1= (QV1-QV1U)/CV1
  FV1= (PV1-PV2)/RV1
  QV1= INTEG(FA3-FV1,QV1IC)
 Constant RV2=10.,LV2=1.,FV2IC=95. $'System. Veins 2'
  PV2= (QV2-QV2U)/CV2
  FV2= INTEG((PV2-PRA-RV2*FV2)/LV2,FV2IC)
  FV2F=REALPL(3.2,FV2,FV2FIC)       $'Use for Cardiac Output'
  Constant FV2FIC=78.
  Constant GBS=0.0,TB=3.0
  GB = FCNSW(T-TB,0.,0.,GBS)
  FB= PV2*GBS          $'Venous bleeding at TB if GBS > 0.0'
  QV2= INTEG(FV1-FV2-FB,QV2IC)
 Constant RRA=5.,LRA=1.0,FRAIC=0.  $'Rt. Atrium'
  PRA= (QRA-QRAU)/CRA
  FRA= LIMINT((PRA-PRV-RRA*FRA)/LRA, FRAIC, 0.,1.E4)
  QRA= INTEG (FV2-FRA,QRAIC)
 Constant RRV=5.,LRV=1.,FRVIC=6.0  $'Rt. Ventr.'
  SRV= RD*(1-ACTV) + RS*ACTV
```

```
        PRV= (QRV-QRVU)*SRV
        FRV= LIMINT((PRV-PP1-RRV*FRV)/LRV,FRVIC,0.,1.E5)
        QRV= INTEG(FRA-FRV,QRVIC)

     END $'of Deriv.'

          'Calculate Output Pressures in mmHg'
        PP1M=PP1/1332. $ PP2M=PP2/1332. $ PP3M=PP3/1332.
        PL1M=PL1/1332. $ PL2M=PL2/1332. $ PLAM=PLA/1332.
        PLVM=PLV/1332. $ PA1M=PA1/1332. $ PA2M=PA2/1332.
        PA3M=PA3/1332. $ PV1M=PV1/1332. $ PV2M=PV2/1332.
        PRAM=PRA/1332. $ PRVM=PRV/1332.
       QTOT=QP1+QP2+QP3+QL1+QL2+QLA+QLV+QA1+QA2 . . .
            +QA3+QV1+QV2+QRA+QRV       $'Total blood'
       QSTOT=QTOT-QU                           $'Total blood,
  stressed'
   END $ 'of Dynamic'
  END  $ 'of Program'
```

Some open-loop outputs obtained with this model are shown in Fig. 4.5.2; here feedback was removed by setting KX = 0.0, so that Y remains at unity, giving normal steady-state operation. At $T = 11.0$ the left ventricle stiffness was reduced by 650.0, giving responses to a sudden infarction. The filtered carotid pressure PA3MF for this open-loop case is shown.

Closed-loop response, with KX set at 0.2, appears in Fig. 4.5.3; note that at the time of infarction (of the left ventricle, as in the open-loop responses of Fig. 4.5.2), the arrows in (4.5.5) show the expected sequence of responses,

$$\begin{gathered}\mathrm{SL}\downarrow,\ \mathrm{PLVM}\downarrow,\ \mathrm{QLVM(peak\text{-}to\text{-}peak)}\downarrow,\ \mathrm{PA3M}\downarrow,\\ \mathrm{Y}\downarrow,\ \mathrm{TH}\downarrow,\ \mathrm{SL}\uparrow\end{gathered} \tag{4.5.5}$$

The resulting increased heart rate and strength of both ventricles tend to counter the effect of the original system parameter disturbance.

The effectiveness of the control system may also be studied by comparing open- and closed-loop plots of system response to other sudden disturbances, such as valve failure, opening of an anastomosis, hemorrhage, or opening (or closing) of a ventricular or atrial septal defect. Note that in PF-1-REG the arterial infusion FI is simpler than in PF-1, in that it can only start at $T = 0.0$; however, venous bleeding is now possible, starting at time TB, as determined by the choice of bleeding conductance GBS, according to

$$\mathrm{FB = PV2 * GBS} \tag{4.5.6}$$

In case of bleeding it may be interesting to determine changes in blood volume using the commands at the end of Dynamic (See Prob.4.7e).

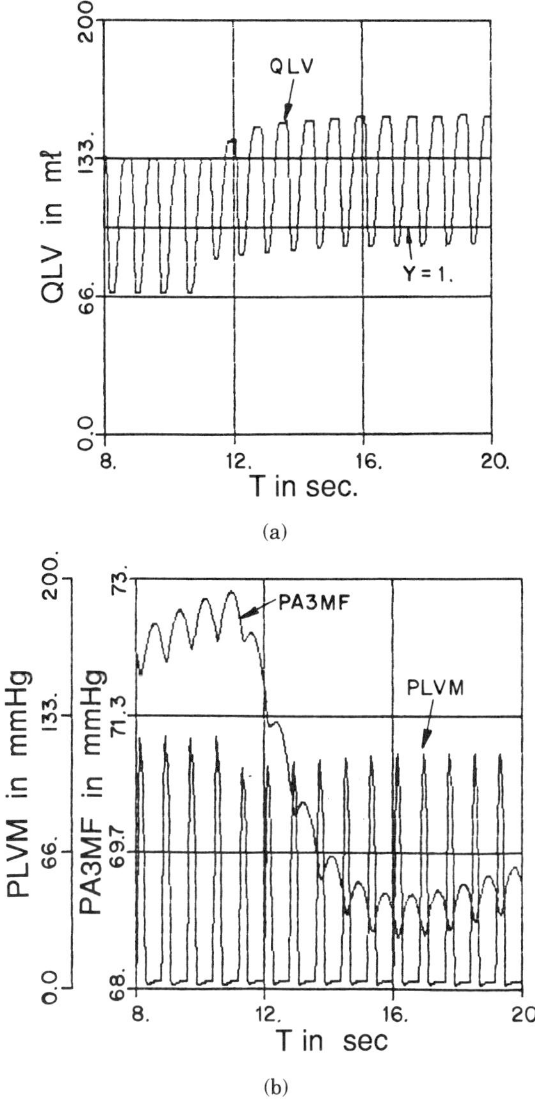

Figure 4.5.2. Open loop response of the system PF-1-REG with no baroreceptor feedback (Y held at 1.0), showing normal operation followed by an infarct at T = 11.
(Note that plots begin at T = 8.0).
(a) Left ventricular volume.
(b) Left ventricular pressure, PLVM, and carotid pressure, PA3MF (after filtering).

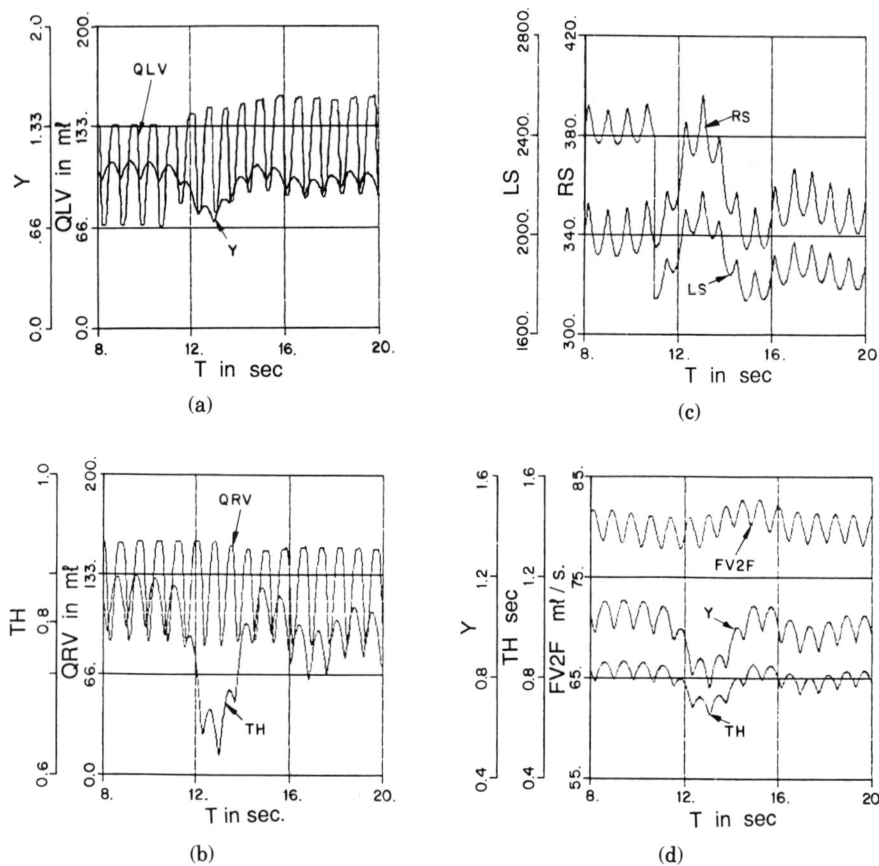

Figure 4.5.3. Closed-loop response of the cardiovascular system (program PF-1-REG, with KX = 0.2), to a left ventricle infarct at T = 11.0 sec.
(a) Feedback signal, Y, and left ventricular volume QLV.
(b) Heart period TH and right ventricular volume QRV.
(c) Ventricle muscle stiffnesses LS and RS.
(Note that LS drops suddenly at T = 11., but after one oscillation, LS partially recovers, and RS shows a slight increase.
(d) The feedback Y and heart period TH respond to the infarct with lower values and some oscillation, but final TH and Y tend to recover after T = 11.

A more detailed and realistic model of the baroreceptor control system (Tham-88) will include a better representation of the responses of the central nervous system, as well as feedback effects which change the flow resistances and compliances. This model is based on one introduced by Katona, and used by Dick and Tham (Katona-80, Dick-68, Tham-88). It is

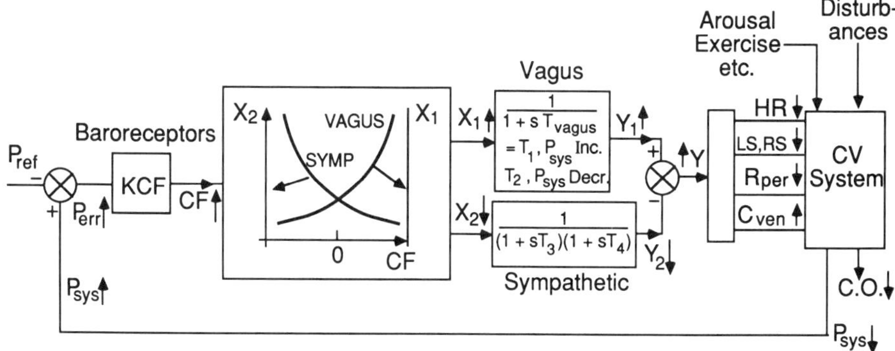

Figure 4.5.4. Baroreceptor Feedback Control Loop

shown in block form in Fig. 4.5.4, depicting the neural feedback system for control of blood pressure. Note the "push-pull" action provided by the opposing sympathetic and vagus channels. The vertical arrows on variables indicate the results if the loop is opened in the feedback line and P_{sys} is applied at the lower left; the "returned" P_{sys} at the right of the diagram is of the opposite sign to that first applied, indicating that the system would serve to correct the pressure P_{sys} toward P_{ref} if the loop were closed.

4.6 NONPULSATILE CARDIOVASCULAR MODELS

The frequencies in human cardiovascular pulsations tend to be harmonics of a fundamental heart rate of approximately 1.2 beats per second; healthy adults at rest may have rates ranging from about 0.8 to 1.5 beats per second, and harmonics up to the tenth are important if waveforms near the ventricular outputs are of interest. Exercise or illness may increase the heart rate significantly, and sometimes modelers may have to consider bandwidths of 40 or 50 Hz. These frequencies are much higher than those of concern in the kinetics of most pharmaceutical substances. Thus, for example, most anesthetic agents and muscle relaxants function in the body with their fastest time constants in minutes. Since the pulsatility seems to be added to the slower changes in blood flow, schemes for nonpulsatile cardiovascular modeling have been developed (Rideout-83b, Möller-83, Peskin-79). These methods appear to be particularly useful in multiple models for pharmacokinetic studies, especially in anesthesiology. The dynamic model described here is based on a fourth-order nonpulsatile model (Rideout-83b, pp. 156–157).

Figure 4.6.1a shows the ventricular compliance curves of maximum (systolic) slope and minimum (diastolic) slope; a typical pressure-flow locus is also shown. This diagram is of key importance in setting up a nonpulsatile cardiovascular model, because it shows that the stroke volume for a ventricle is

$$Q_{SV} = P_{ED}*C_D - P_{ES}*C_S \tag{4.6.1}$$

where C_D and C_S are the diastolic and maximum systolic compliance of the myocardium and P_{ED} is the end-diastolic and P_{ES} the end-systolic pressure, ignoring some nonlinearities which will be given some consideration later (Sunagawa-81, Tham-88). This equation, if multiplied by heart rate H, gives the average outflow of either ventricle:

$$F = (C_D*H)*P_{ED} - (C_S*H)*P_{ES} \tag{4.6.2}$$

Factors K_d and K_s may be introduced, which are such that average atrial pressure is related to end-diastolic pressure by

$$P_{at} = P_{ED}/K_d \tag{4.6.3}$$

and average arterial pressure is similarly related to end-systolic pressure by

$$P_{art} = P_{ES}/K_s \tag{4.6.4}$$

The ventricular outflow, from (4.6.2), (4.6.3), and (4.6.4), is

$$F = G_{pre}*P_{at} - G_{after}*P_{art} \tag{4.6.5}$$

where the preload and afterload conductances are given by

$$\begin{aligned} G_{pre} &= C_D*H*K_d \\ G_{after} &= C_S*H*K_s \end{aligned} \tag{4.6.6}$$

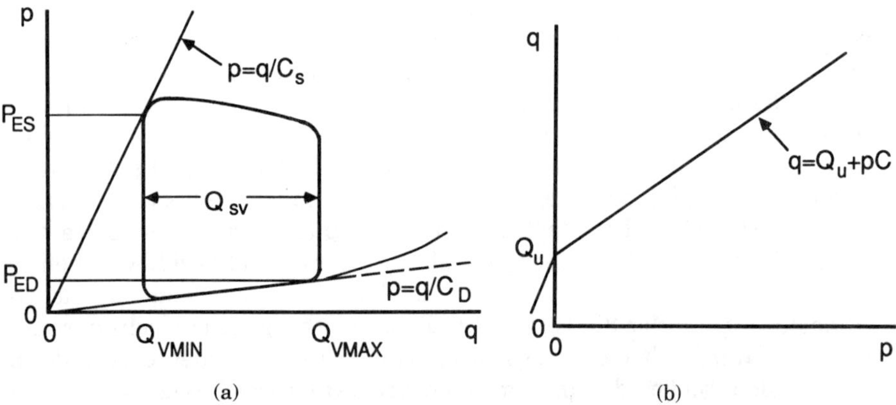

Figure 4.6.1. (a) Ventricular pressure-volume locus, related to minimum and maximum ventricular stiffness (or reciprocal compliance).
(b) Venous and arterial pressure-volume relationships.

Figure 4.6.1b shows that the arterial or venous segmental compliance C, together with unstressed volume Q_U, gives total average volume in a segment as

$$q = q_U + p*C \tag{4.6.7}$$

where P is the average pressure. Here q may vary as a result of changes in any of the quantities q_U, p, and/or C. Note that a nonlinear relationship may be used in place of (4.6.7).

If the preload and afterload conductances for the left ventricle are called G_1 and G_2, and those for the right ventricle G_3 and G_4, then the ventricular nonpulsatile flow equations may be written as

$$\begin{aligned} G_1*p_L - G_2*p_S &= f_L \\ G_3*p_R - G_4*p_P &= f_R \end{aligned} \tag{4.6.8}$$

where lowercase letters (p and f) indicate the variables, and uppercase letters the quantities that are ordinarily constant. Also, subscripts L and R have been chosen to indicate the left and right atria, and S and P the systemic and pulmonary arteries.

The systemic and pulmonary equations expressing the pressure drops (principally in capillary beds) are

$$\begin{aligned} p_S - p_R &= R_S*f_S \\ p_P - p_L &= R_P*f_P \end{aligned} \tag{4.6.9}$$

where R_P is the pulmonary peripheral resistance and f_P the total pulmonary flow; R_S and f_S are the corresponding systemic quantities, but may need to be modified if a number of parallel paths are to be considered, as will be shown below.

The volumes q_S, q_R, q_P, and q_L associated with each compliance are given by the integrals of inflow and outflow as shown in (4.6.10). Also, the compliances C_S (total arterial), C_R (total systemic venous), and corresponding pulmonary compliances C_P and C_L may be used with the four volumes (see (4.6.7)) to obtain pressures, as shown below:

$$\begin{aligned} q_S &= \int_0^t (f_L - f_S)dt & p_S &= (q_S - Q_{SU})/C_S \\ q_R &= \int_0^t (f_S - f_R + f_I)dt & p_R &= (q_R - Q_{RU})/C_R \\ q_P &= \int_0^t (f_R - f_P)dt & p_P &= (q_P - Q_{PU})/C_P \\ q_L &= \int_0^t (f_P - f_L)dt & p_L &= (q_L - Q_{LU})/C_P \end{aligned} \tag{4.6.10}$$

where an infusion flow of blood or plasma, f_I, into the systemic veins is assumed. The 12 equations—(4.6.8), (4.6.9), and (4.6.10)—serve to define a nonpulsatile model, shown in Fig. 4.6.2.

Several parallel systemic paths may need to be included in Fig. 4.6.2, corresponding to capillary beds that run through different kinds of tissue (Tham-90). If there are three such paths, for example, with flow resistances R_{S1}, R_{S2}, and R_{S3}, then the total peripheral systemic resistance used in the first equation of (4.6.9) will be

$$R_S = 1/(1/R_{S1} + 1/R_{S2} + 1/R_{S3}) \tag{4.6.11}$$

The individual flows are given by equations of the form

$$f_{S1} = f_S * R_S/R_{S1} \tag{4.6.12}$$

It should also be noted that if the total volume q_T of the system in Fig. 4.6.2,

$$q_T = q_S + q_R + q_P + q_L \tag{4.6.13}$$

is fixed, with no flow paths to "ground" or to some other system, then there is an "excess integration" in the equations of (4.6.10). This extra integration can be shown to be present because only three integrator commands are needed (to find, for example, q_R, q_P, and q_L), with the remaining blood volume determined from (4.6.13), using

$$q_S = q_T - q_R - q_P - q_L \tag{4.6.14}$$

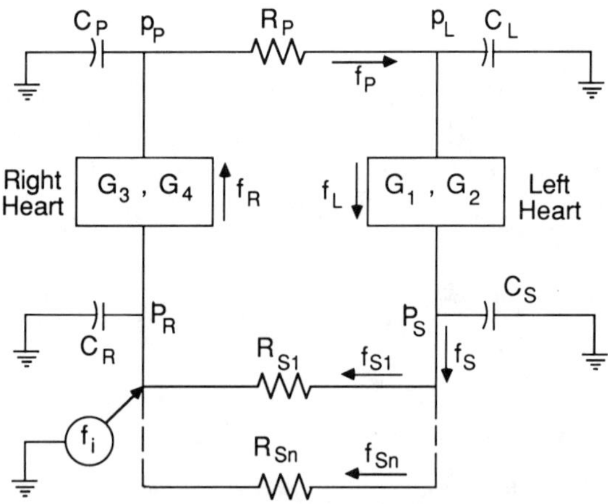

Figure 4.6.2. Basic non-pulsatile model, with two parallel systemic paths shown.

If four integrations are used, a drift problem may result, with Q_T gradually increasing or decreasing, because of slight inaccuracies in the integrations. However, note that in the following program an excess integration was used without errors appearing; this will usually be possible when digital computation is used. Also, in real physiological systems, blood volume or fluid balance is maintained by the thirst reflex, which governs water intake, and the kidneys, which tend to remove more water when increased volume causes increased system pressure. If such fluid balance equations are included in this model, then they will control Q_T, and four integrations must then be used or the four volumes associated with the four compliances.

The system described by (4.6.8), (4.6.9), and (4.6.10) may be set up in the ACSL program PF-NP. This program includes a means for changing the left ventricular stiffness; here an increase of a factor of two (obtained by decreasing G_2) is shown, and may be moved into the time range of the program by changing TCH to a value such as TCH = 1.

An infusion flow f_I is provided here, in the form of a pulse of amplitude A = 25.0 ml, starting at TSTT = 1.0 sec, and lasting for WID = 2.0 sec; it is not set to repeat within the time range of the problem, but could be by reducing PER.

```
PROGRAM PF-NP
 DYNAMIC
   Cinterval CINT= 0.1
   Constant TF=10.
  DERIVATIVE
   Algorithm IALG = 4  $ 'Runge Kutta 2'
   Maxterval MAXT =.05
   Nsteps NSTP = 1

   'Generate LV afterload stiffness G2'
  Constant G2IC=.821, G2NEW=.4105,TCH=1.E6
   Z= T - TCH
   G2= FCNSW(Z,G2IC,G2IC,G2NEW)

   'Flow equations'
  Constant G1=24.,G3=40.,G4=3.889
   FL= G1*PL-G2*PS
   FR= G3*PR-G4*PP
  Constant RS=1.0111,RP=.12222
   FS= (PS-PR)/RS
   FR= (PP-PL)/RP

   'Generate infusion flow FI at STT with period . . .
   PER, width WID, and amplitude A'
```

```
    Constant A=25.,TSTT=1., PER=1.E6, WID=2.
     FI=A*PULSE(TSTT, PER, WID)

     'Differential Equations'
    Constant QSIC=1000.,QRIC=5400., . . .
     QPIC=500.,QLIC=1800.
     QS= INTEG (FL-FS,   QSIC)
     QR= INTEG (FS-FR+FI,QRIC)
     QP= INTEG (FR -FP,  QPIC)
     QL= INTEG (FP-FL,   QLIC)

     'Check total volume'
     QT= QS + QR + QP + QL

     'Find Pressures'
    Constant CS=2.6316,CR=225.0,CP=6.9444,CL=42.857
    Constant QSU=750.,QRU=4500.,QPU=375.,QLU=1500.
     PS= (QS-QSU)/CS
     PR= (QR-QRU)/CR
     PP= (QP-QPU)/CP
     PL= (QL-QLU)/CL
     END $ 'of Deriv.'
      TERMT (T .GE. TF)
    END $ 'Of Dynamic'
   END $ 'Of Program'
```

The units used in this example are the so-called "medical" units, with Q in ml, F in ml/s, and P in mmHg. In these units resistances are in mmHg* sec/ml, and compliances in ml/mmHg.

This program was first run as shown (with infusion FI, but with no change in G2) for TF = 10 sec (see Fig. 4.6.3). The total infusion (25 ml/s for 2 s) was 60 ml, and this amount of change in QT would be expected during the period from T = 1 to T = 3 sec.

The program was also run with FI zero during the operating period, but with G2 decreased (corresponding to an increase in left ventricular stiffness) at T = 1 sec (see Fig. 4.6.4). This results in increased PS and QS; PR and QR also increase, but somewhat more slowly. As a result of these increases, the variables PP, QP, PL, and QL decrease. The flow, after transients settle out, will again be equal, but will be larger because of the stronger left heart. Total volume QT will be constant.

Many changes may be made in the model in addition to the introduction of a number of parallel paths in the systemic circulation (See Eqns. 4.6.11 and 4.6.12) and similar introduction of parallel paths in the pulmonary circulation. Some of these are nonlinear changes, such as the introduction of a square-law term in the diastolic compliance, and nonlinearities in the peripheral resistances.

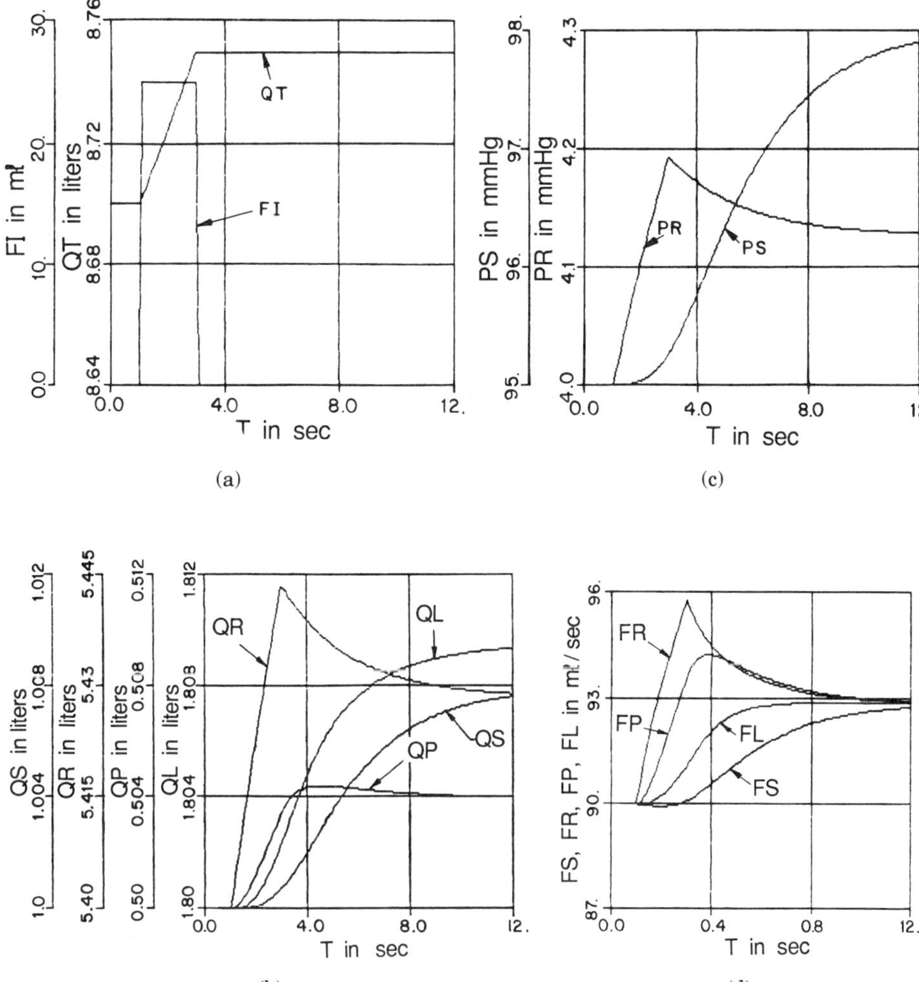

Figure 4.6.3. Response of the non-pulsatile model of Fig. 4.6.2 to an infusion pulse, FI.
(a) Input FI and total volume QT. Note that the change in QT is linear and occurs only during the infusion.
(b) Volumes associated with the four compliances. All volumes tend to increase with a total which equals 50 ml. Volume QR shows the fastest response, and has the most overshoot.
(c) The varying parts of pressures PR and PS have the same forms as QR and QS, as would be expected.
(d) The flows all tend to be equal, initially, and after transient excursions which are slower as we go from FR through FP, FL and FS, they are again equal.

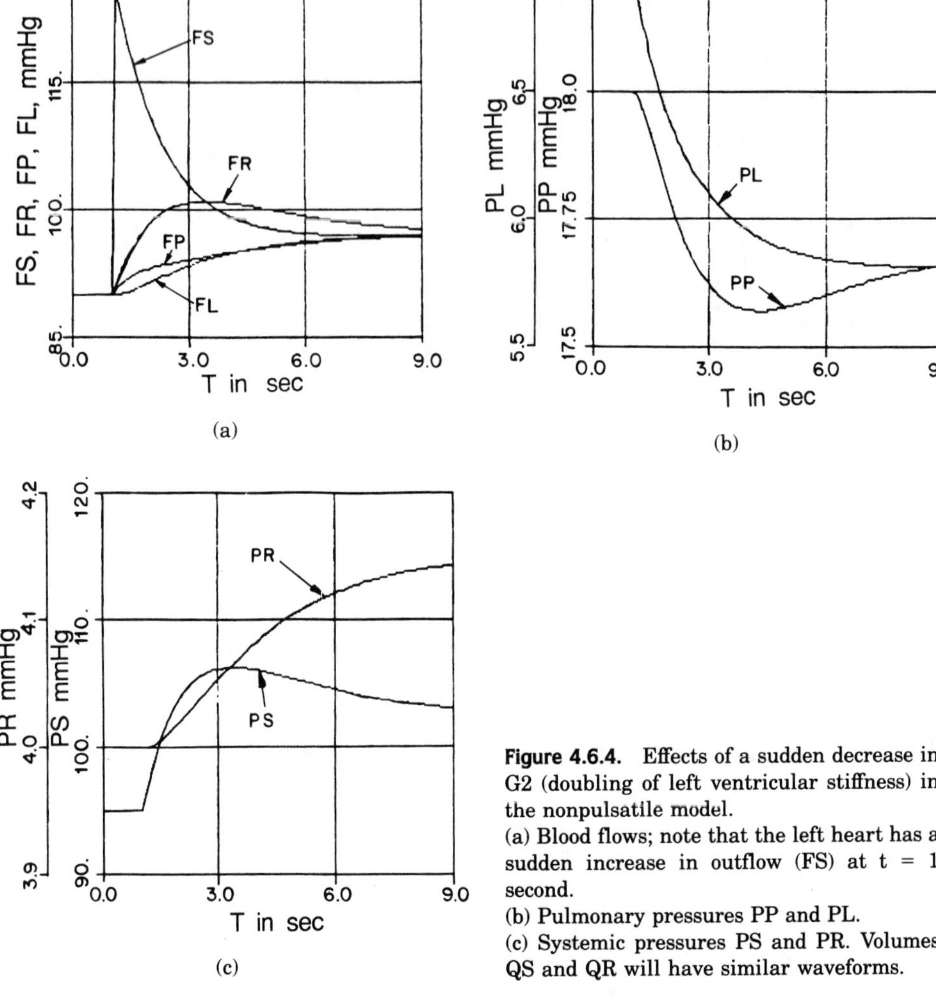

Figure 4.6.4. Effects of a sudden decrease in G2 (doubling of left ventricular stiffness) in the nonpulsatile model.
(a) Blood flows; note that the left heart has a sudden increase in outflow (FS) at t = 1 second.
(b) Pulmonary pressures PP and PL.
(c) Systemic pressures PS and PR. Volumes QS and QR will have similar waveforms.

The transients shown in the nonpulsatile model solutions indicate that the human CV system has time constants that are not much greater than a typical pulse period (of about 0.8 sec). It was deemed important, therefore, that comparisons be made to check the nonpulsatile model against the corresponding responses for a pulsatile model. This was done, and the nonpulsatile model outputs were found to follow closely the pulsatile outputs, when the latter were averaged over each pulse (Rideout-88).

It is possible to find some closed-form expressions that give the changes in the steady-state conditions in the linear nonpulsatile model, by solving the set of algebraic equations for this system that results when derivative terms are set to zero (Rideout-83b). This may be done using a nonnumeric language such as REDUCE (Hearn-73) or MAXSYMA. Some interesting results are as follows:

1. For a change Δq in total blood volume, the change Δf in cardiac output will be

$$\Delta f = (G_1 * G_3 - G_2 * G_4) * \Delta q / (-\mathrm{det}) \qquad (4.6.15)$$

where

$$\begin{aligned} -\mathrm{det} = {} & (C_L + C_P) * [G_3 * (1 + G_2 * R_S) + G_2] \\ & + (C_R + C_S) * [G_1 (1 + G_4 * R_P) + G_4] \\ & + G_1 * G_3 * (R_P + R_S * C_S) + G_2 * G_4 * (R_P * C_L \\ & + R_S * C_R) \end{aligned} \qquad (4.6.16)$$

2. For a change ΔR_S in total systemic peripheral resistance, the change in cardiac output will be

$$\begin{aligned} \Delta f = {} & -F * [G_1 * G_3 * C_S + G_2 * G_4 * C_R \\ & + G_2 * G_3 * (C_L + C_P)] * \Delta R_S / (-\mathrm{det}) \end{aligned} \qquad (4.6.17)$$

PROBLEMS

4.1 **(a)** Using a parameter sweep program with the left ventricular model, LH-PF-1, plot a set of curves of the ventricular outflow, FCA, versus time as PATM is swept from 3.0 to 9.0 mmHg in increments of 1.5 mmHg. Repeat this for QLV and FLV, and be sure to indicate the direction of increasing PATM on each family of curves. (Check your curves for PATM = 6.0 mmHg in each plot against those shown in Fig. 4.2.3b)

(b) Cardiac output (CO) may be determined by taking the product of stroke volume and heart rate. Find stroke volumes from (a), and determine CO for PATM equal to 3.0, 6.0 and 9.0 mmHg. Sketch a plot of CO versus PATM.

4.2 **(a)** Repeat P4-1(a) for model LH-PF-2, which incorporates an improved heart activity generator, and again plot FCA, QLV and FLV as PATM is swept from 3.0 to 9.0 mmHg.

(b) Discuss the agreement of the results in (a) with Starling's Law.

(c) Are the waveforms in (a) more realistic than those in Problem 4.1(a), and in what way?

4.3 Using the left ventricular model LH-PF-2, plot the locus of the pressure PLVM versus volume QLV using MAXT = .001, CINT = .001, and TF = 2.4 sec, for PATM = 4.5 mmHg; repeat for PATM = 7.5 mmHg. Note and explain the changes in the locus during the 3 heart cycles in each case.

4.4 **(a)** Using the left ventricular model, LH-PF-2, sweep the maximum systolic stiffness, SLS, from 1500 to 2500 in increments of 250.0 gm/(cm^4*sec^2), and make plots of the resultant families of curves for QLV and PLVM. Explain the observed results, particularly in stroke volume; (here it may help to sketch the pressure-volume loci for the extreme values of SLS).

(b) Make pressure-volume loci plots as in Problem 4.3, but with PATM fixed at 6.0 and using SLS = 1750 and then SLS = 2250. Do the results (after settling) agree with your sketches in the (a) part of the problem?

4.5 In response to exercise the heart may have an increase in maximum systolic stiffness that accompanies any increase in heart rate, as discussed in Section 4.5. However, a change in heart rate only may occur in response to the signal from an electronic heart pacer. To study this in a model, assume that the total period TH equals EH, the signal from a pacer, and let the systolic period be TS = EH*0.3/0.8, in LH-PF-2. Examine the cardiac output obtained by filtering FCA, using a simple low-pass filter with a 2-second time constant and an initial flow assumed to be 90.0 ml/sec,

```
CO = REALPL(2.0,FCA,90.).
```

Sweep EH from 0.4 to 1.6 sec. in steps of 0.2 sec, using TF = 16.0 to give the system more time to settle during each run, and observe the changes in final FCA as period increases (or heart rate decreases) and explain.

4.6 Use the single-loop cardiovascular model PF-1 to simulate and study the effects of disturbances or changes in CV system parameters in an unregulated system as follows:

(a) Program PF-1 is set up to permit the left and right maximum systolic stiffnesses, LS and RS, to be changed as in a myocardial infarction. Figure 4.3.8 shows the effect of a simulated sudden infarction at THI = 2.4 affecting both ventricles (DLS = −625.0 and DRS = −87.5). Repeat this and compare your results with the plots in Fig. 4.3.8; then introduce only a right side infarct (DLS = 0.0, DRS = −87.5) and explain the transient and steady state responses.

(b) Increase the systemic peripheral resistance in PF-1 by nearly 50% at T = 3.0 sec., by doubling the value of RA3. Make a run of TF = 12 sec. and show FA2 and FP2 on one plot, and the volumes QLV and QRV on another. Explain the initial response, and the final response that is being approached at time TF.

(c) A command for a flow FI into the aorta at QA1 is given in PF-1; find the effect of such infusion if the level of FI is 10.0 after T = TIS = 3., by setting FIS = 10., and observe and explain the effects on cardiac output and ventricular volumes.

(d) Improve the command for infusion by changing the command for FI to FI = FCNSW((T−TIS)*TES−T), 0.0, 0.0, FIS) to permit infusion into the aorta from time TIS to TES if FIS is positive, or fixed-rate bleeding during the same period if FIS is negative. Observe the effect if FIS is set at 10.0 (use TF = 20.). Repeat for the case of a hemorrhage by setting FIS at −10.0. Observe and compare results in CO and in QLV and QRV for these two disturbances.

(e) A more correct way to simulate bleeding is to introduce a conductance GB as shown in program PF-1-REG in Section 4.5, for venous bleeding from QV2. Use this method to simulate venous bleeding in PF-1, setting GBS = .002; then use the same scheme for arterial bleeding from QA2, setting GBS at a value to give an approximate average outflow of 10.0 ml/s. In both cases plot PA2M, PP2M, FA3 and QS and explain your results.

4.7 In Section 4.5 baroreceptor feedback has been added to PF-1 to give the pressure-regulated model PF-1-REG.

(a) Repeat Problem 4.6(a) using PF-1-REG, and compare results with and without baroreceptor regulation.

(b) Repeat Problem 4.6(b) using PF-1-REG, and compare.

(c) Repeat Problem 4.6(e) for venous bleeding, using PR-1-REG and compare the same plotted variables.

4.8 A non-pulsatile CV model program, PF-NP, is shown in Section 4.6, and corresponds approximately to the pulsatile program PF-1. Compare the transients in aortic flow for these two programs, if the left ventricle is weakened by 30% in each case, in a simulated infarction.

4.9 The final change in flow after blood infusion may be determined by using algebraic solutions of the equations that result if the derivatives in the differential equations describing the system in Fig. 4.6.2 are set to zero. If the system compliances, resistances and heart constants (use G2 = G2IC) are as given in program PF-NP, use equations (4.6.15) and (4.6.16) to find the change in flow, Δf, for an infusion $\Delta q = 60$ ml, and check this against final values in the transient solutions plotted in Fig. 4.6.3d.

REFERENCES

BENEKEN, JAN E. W. "A Mathematical Approach to Cardiovascular Function," (Ph.D. thesis, University of Utrecht); 1965.

______. "Some computer models in cardiovascular research," Chap. 5 in *Cardiovascular Fluid Dynamics,* D. H. Bergel, (Ed.); New York: Academic Press; 1972.

BLACKSTONE, E. H., A. K. GUPTA AND V. C. RIDEOUT, "Cardiovascular simulation study of infants with transposition of the great arteries after surgical correction," *Math. Computers in Simulation,* Vol. 19, pp. 39–50; 1977.

BLACKSTONE, E. H., V. C. RIDEOUT AND D. L. BEDUHN, "Simulation analysis of interatrial transposition of venous return (Mustard's operation)," *Ann. BME,* Vol. 10, No. 5, pp. 193–218; 1982.

BROWER, R. W. AND A. NOORDERGRAAF, "Theory of steady flow in collapsible tubes and veins," in *Cardiovascular System Dynamics,* J. Baan *et al* (Eds.); Cambridge, Mass.: MIT Press; 1978.

BRUBAKK, A. O. AND R. AASLID, "Use of a model for simulating individual aortic dynamics in man," *Med. Biol. Eng. Comput.,* Vol. 16: pp. 231–242; 1978.

CHARM, S. E. AND G. S. KURLAND, "Blood Rheology," Chap. 15 in *Cardiovascular Fluid Dynamics,* Vol. 2, D. H. Bergel, (Ed.); New York: Academic Press; 1972.

COX, ROBERT H. "Wave propagation through a Newtonian fluid contained within a thick-walled visoelastic tube," *Biophys. J.,* Vol. 8, No. 6, pp. 691–709; 1968.

DICK, D. E. "A Hybrid Computer Study of Major Transients in the Canine Cardiovascular System," (Ph.D. thesis, University of Wisconsin); 1968.

DICKINSON, C. J. ET AL, "MACMAN: A digital computer model for teaching some basic principles of hemodynamics," *J. Clin. Comp.,* 2: pp. 42–50; 1973.

FRY, D. L. AND J. C. GREENFIELD, JR., "The mathematical approach to hemodynamics with particular reference to Wormersley's theory," pp. 85–99 in *Pulsatile Blood Flow,* E. O. Attinger, (Ed.), New York: McGraw-Hill Book Co.; 1964.

FUKUI, YASUHIRO, "A Study of the Human Cardiovascular-Respiratory System using Hybrid Computer Modeling," (Ph.D. thesis, University of Wisconsin); 1971.

FUNG, Y. C., ET AL. "Pseudoelasticity of arteries and the choice of its mathematical expression," *Am. J. Physiol.* 237(5), pp. H620–H631; 1979.

GIANUNZIO, J. W., "Hybrid Computer Simulation of Cardiac Dynamics," (M.S. thesis, University of Wisconsin); 1967.

GOW, B. S., "The influence of vascular smooth muscle on viscoelastic properties of blood vessels," Chapter 12 in *Cardiovascular Fluid Dynamics,* D. H. Bergel (Ed.); New York: Academic Press; 1972.

GRODINS, F. S., "Integrative cardiovascular physiology: a mathematical synthesis of cardiac and blood vessel hemodynamics," *Q. Rev. Biol.,* 34: pp. 93–116; 1959.

HEARN, A. C. "REDUCE-2 User's Manual," Department of Computer Science, University of Utah; 1973.

HILLESTAD, R. J., "Hybrid computer studies of the cardiovascular systemic circuit," (M.S. thesis, University of Wisconsin); 1966.

HUNG, TIN-KAN, "A computation of pulsatile flows in rigid and deformable coiled tubes," *Proc. 3rd Intl. Conf. on Mechanics in Medicine and Biology,* Paris; 1982.

JAGER, G. N., "Electrical Model of the Human Arterial Tree," (Ph.D. thesis, University of Utrecht); 1965.

KATONA, PETER G., "Automated control of physiological variables and clinical therapy," *CRC Crit. Revs. Biomed. Eng.,* Vol. 8, Issue 4, pp. 281–310; 1980.

——— ET AL, "An analysis of heart rate control," *Fed. Am. Soc. Exp. Biol. Proc.;* Vol. 22, p. 182; 1962.

———, "Cardiac vagal efferent activity and heart period in the carotid sinus reflex," *Am. J. Physiol.,* Vol. 218, p. 1030; 1970.

KATRA, J. A., "Hybrid computer studies of the cardiovascular pulmonary circuit," (M.S. thesis, University of Wisconsin); 1966.

LAU, VENG-KIN AND KIICHI SAGAWA, "Model analysis of the contribution of atrial contraction to ventricular filling," *Ann. Biomed. Eng.,* Vol. 7, pp. 167–201; 1979.

MILNOR, W. R., *Hemodynamics,* Baltimore: Williams & Wilkins; 1982.

MÖLLER, DIETMAR, D. POPOVIC AND G. THIELE, *Modeling, Simulation and Parameter Estimation of the Human Cardiovascular System,* Braunschweig: Friedr. Vieweg & Sohn; 1983.

MORENO, A. H., "Dynamics of Pressure in the Central Veins," in *Cardiovascular System Dynamics,* J. Baan et al (Eds.); Cambridge, Mass.: MIT Press; 1978.

NOORDERGRAAF, A., "Development of an analog computer for the human systemic circulatory system," A. Noordergraaf (Ed.); *Circulatory Analog Computers,* Amsterdam: North-Holland Publ. Co.; 1963.

______, *Circulatory System Dynamics,* New York: Academic Press; 1978.

PESKIN, C. S., "Lectures on mathematical aspects of physiology," New York: Courant Institute of Mathematical Sciences; 1979.

REAM, A. K. AND R. P. FOGDALL, "Cardiovascular Management in Anesthesia and Intensive Care," Philadelphia: Lippincott; 1982.

RIDEOUT, V. C., "Cardiovascular system simulation in biomedical engineering education," *IEEE Trans. Biomed. Eng.,* Vol. BME-21, pp. 101–07; March 1972.

______, "The importance of nonlinear effects in arterial system dynamics," pp. 79–82 in *Modelling and data analysis in biotechnology and Medical Engineering,* G. C. Vansteenkiste and P. C. Young, (Eds.); Amsterdam: North-Holland Pub. Co.; 1983.

______, "Linear analysis of the cardiovascular system," Ch. 11 in *Integrated Approaches to Monitoring,* J. S. Gravenstein, et al (Eds.); Boston: Butterworths; 1983.

______, AND D. E. DICK, "Difference-differential equations for fluid flow in distensible tubes," *IEEE Trans. Biomed. Eng.,* Vol. BME-14, No. 3, pp. 171–77; July 1967.

______, AND J. A. KATRA, "Computer simulation study of the pulmonary circulation," *Simulation,* Vol. 14, No. 11, pp. 239–45; May, 1969.

______, AND R. Q. Y. THAM, "A non-pulsatile multiple model for pharmacokinetic simulation," *Proc. 25th Annual Rocky Mountain Bioengineering Symposium;* 1988.

RUSHMER, R. F., *Organ Physiology: Structure and Function of the Cardiovascular System,* Philadelphia, PA: W. B. Saunders Co.; 1976.

SAGAWA, KIICHI, "Closed-loop physiological control of the heart," *Annals of Biomedical Eng.,* Vol. 8, pp. 415–29; 1980.

______, "The ventricular pressure-volume diagram revisited," *Circ. Res.* Vol. 43, No. 5, pp. 677–687; Nov. 1978.

SKALAK, RICHARD, "Synthesis of a complete circulation," Chap. 19, pp. 341–376 in *Cardiovascular Fluid Dynamics,* Vol. 2, D. H. Bergel, (Ed.), New York: Academic Press; 1972.

SNYDER, M. F. AND V. C. RIDEOUT, "Computer model studies of blood flow in the venous system," *IEEE Trans. Biomed. Eng.,* Vol. BME-16, No. 4, pp. 325–34; Oct. 1969.

______. "The study of human venous system dynamics using hybrid computer modeling," NASA Contractor Report, NASA CR-2084; July, 1972.

_____ AND R. J. HILLESTAD, "Computer modeling of the human systemic arterial tree," *J. Biomechanics,* Vol. 2, No. 4, pp. 341–53; 1968.

SUNAGAWA, K., AND K. SAGAWA, "Models of ventricular contraction based on time-varying elastance," *CRC Crit. Revs. Biomed. Eng.;* Vol. 9, pp. 193–228; 1982.

THAM, R. Q. Y., "A Study of the effects of Halothane on the Canine Cardiovascular System and Baroreceptor Control," (Ph.D. thesis, University of Wisconsin); 1988.

THAM, R. Q. Y., F. J. SASSE AND V. C. RIDEOUT, "Large-scale multiple model for the simulation of anesthesia," *Advanced Simulation in Biomedicine,* pp. 173–95, D. P. F. Moller, (Ed.); New York: Springer Verlag; 1990.

WARNER, HOMER R., "Use of analog computers in the study of the control mechanism in the circulation," *Fed. Proc.,* Vol. 21, pp. 87–96; 1962.

WESTERHOF, N. AND A. NOORDERGRAAF, "Reduced models of the systemic arteries," *Proc. 8th Intl. Conf. Med. Biol. Eng.:* Chicago; 1969.

WOMERSLEY, J. R., "An elastic tube theory of pulse transmission and oscillatory flow in mammalian arteries," Wright Air Dev. Rpt., WADC-TR 56-614; 1957.

5 Respiratory System Modeling

5.0 INTRODUCTION: THE GAS LAWS

The respiratory system is important principally as a means of oxygen uptake and carbon dioxide elimination. It may be compared with the cardiovascular system because gases are carried in it by pulsatile fluid flow somewhat as gases and many other substances are carried by pulsatile blood flow in the CV system. The respiratory system is simpler in that it has but one branching out of the air-flow passages (Weibel-84, West-74, Grodins-78), whereas the CV system fans out to the many body capillaries from the aorta, then fans in to the vena cavae, and finally repeats this pattern in the pulmonary circulation. However, analysis and modeling are more complex for the respiratory system because air is a compressible fluid and because the flow of air in the lungs is a tidal, or back-and-forth, flow, in contrast to the one-way flow with superimposed pulsatility in the CV system. Also, although the respiratory system does not have valves as the CV system does, there are some important and rather difficult nonlinearities.

Ventilation rate is controlled by nervous and endocrine means (Yamamoto-80), as are the blood pressure and cardiac output. The respiratory control system serves as a regulator that maintains approximately constant levels of oxygen and carbon dioxide in the blood, and, like the CV control system, it responds to disturbances such as the onset of exercise (Comroe-65, Brown-73, Grodins-78, and Jacquez-79).

The physical units used in studies of the respiratory system are

TABLE 5.0.1

T,°C	P_{H_2O} mm Hg
0	4.6
20	17.4
36	44.2
37	46.6
38	49.3

much the same as those for the CV system; metric SI units are used (see Section 2.6), but in the United States, mm Hg may be used as pressure units. In the case of measurements of respiratory pressure, however, water rather than mercury is commonly used, with pressures expressed in terms of cm H_2O. Note that 1 cm H_2O is equal to 0.735 mm Hg, or to 98.1 n/m^2 (pascals); thus, conveniently, 1 cm $H_2O \approx 0.1$ kilopascal.

Some simple basic gas laws (Duffin-76, Cooney-76, Grodins-78) are useful in setting up models of respiration. Thus *Charles' Law,* also called the *ideal gas law,* is expressed as

$$p*v = n*R*T \tag{5.0.1}$$

where p is pressure in millimeters of mercury, v is volume in liters, T is temperature in degrees Kelvin, and n is the quantity of gas in moles (n = mass of gas/molecular weight); in these units the constant $R = 62.37$.

Two important abbreviations describe conditions used in discussing gases. One is standard temperature and pressure, or STPD (standard temperature 0°C = 273 K, dry and at a sea-level pressure of 760 mm Hg); the other is body temperature and pressure, BTPS (body temperature 37°C or 310°K, 760 mm Hg pressure, and saturated with water vapor, 47 mm Hg partial pressure at body temperature).

Dalton's Law for gas mixtures expresses the fact that gas mixtures have a total pressure equal to the sum of the partial pressures of components. Thus normal dry air at sea level is made up of oxygen (O_2), nitrogen (N_2), carbon dioxide (CO_2), and water vapor (H_2O), with

$$\begin{aligned} P &= P_{O_2} + P_{N_2} + P_{CO_2} + P_{H_2O} \\ &= 159 + 597 + 0.3 + 3.7 = 760 \text{ mm Hg} \end{aligned} \tag{5.0.2}$$

Note that water vapor pressure changes rapidly with temperature, as shown in Table 5.0.1. Normally, body core temperature is slightly higher than 37°C, and a rounded-off figure of 47.0 mm Hg is ordinarily used for water pressure in the alveoli, where saturation is assumed to occur.

Some typical figures for partial pressures of air (in mm Hg) in a normal adult at sea level as air enters and leaves the lungs are listed in Table 5.0.2 (Guyton-76, Chap. 40):

TABLE 5.0.2

Gas	"Normal" Atmosphere	Humidified and Warmed	Alveolar Partial Pressure	Expired Partial Pressure
N_2	597	563.4	569	566
O_2	159	149.3	104	120
CO_2	0.3	0.3	40	27
H_2O	3.7	47.0	47	47
Total	760	760	760	760

Note that when normal dry air is humidified at body temperature (second column), the appearance of water vapor at 47 mm Hg results in reduced partial pressures of other gases, with total pressure remaining unchanged. (Here the total pressure of oxygen, nitrogen, and carbon dioxide changes from 760 − 3.7 = 756.3 to 760 − 47 = 713, and individual partial pressures of these gases change by 713/756.3 = 0.94 times. Alveolar pressures are further changed by oxygen uptake and carbon dioxide release; expired air is a mixture of alveolar air and inspired air that does not reach the alveoli.

The *Ostwald solubility coefficients* (Papper-63, Duffin-76), for a given fluid (usually blood) and a given gas is the volume of gas at body temperature that dissolves in a liter of the fluid. Thus 2.3 liters of halothane anesthetic dissolve in 1 liter of blood at BTPS, and the Ostwald coefficient is $\lambda_{bg} = 2.3$. (Note that in chemistry the Bunsen solubility coefficient, α, is used; it is defined in the same way as the Ostwald coefficient, except that the temperature used is 0°C.) Some Ostwald solubility coefficients are shown in Table 5.0.3 (Steward-73, Papper-63).

Note that the relatively safe and useful anesthetic gases halothane and enflurane have very high solubility in fat; this causes very long time constants to occur in the elimination of these gases in obese patients.

The *partition coefficient* for inert gases is equal to the Ostwald coefficient, but is defined as the volume of gas (at body temperature) dissolved in a unit volume of the fluid solute when the partial pressure of the dissolved gas is 760 mm Hg. The effective solubility (or partition) is

TABLE 5.0.3

Gas	λ_{bg} (blood gas)	λ_{tb} (tissue blood, muscle)	λ_{tb} (tissue blood, fat)
N_2	0.014	1.0	5.2
N_2O	0.47	1.15	2.3
Halothane	2.3	3.5	60.0
Enflurane	1.78	1.7	36.2

quite different for an active gas such as oxygen, which combines readily with the hemoglobin in red blood cells. The amount of oxygen thus taken up is much larger than what is dissolved in plasma and is nonlinearly related to its partial pressure. The important partition curves for oxygen and carbon dioxide in blood are discussed in section 5.3 and used in model RESP-OX.

Henry's law states that gases that do not react with the solvent, or ionize, but go into solution in proportion to their partial pressure. Thus, in BTPS, for 2 percent halothane (dry gas ratio) in equilibrium with blood of volume $V_B = 0.5$ liter, the partial pressure of halothane is $P_{Ha} = 0.02*(760 - 47) = 14.26$ mm Hg, and the volume of dissolved halothane in this case is

$$V_{Ha} = V_B * \lambda_{bg} * P_{Ha}/P_{At} = 0.5*2.3*14.26/760$$
$$= 0.022 \text{ liter}$$

(Note that this is its volume at body temperature.)

5.1 STEADY-STATE QUANTITIES IN THE RESPIRATORY SYSTEM

It is helpful to begin the modeling of the respiratory system by finding the normal steady-state values of variables relating to oxygen and carbon dioxide, initially ignoring the pulsatility of breathing (Grodins-78, West-74). Unless otherwise indicated, the system considered will be that of a normal human male adult, at rest but awake. In this case, the rate of oxygen consumption is given approximately by an allometric equation (see Section 2.7):

$$F_{VO_2} = 10 * B^{0.75} \text{ ml/min} \quad (5.1.1)$$

where B is the body mass in kilograms. Thus, for a 70-kg normal human adult, oxygen uptake should be

$$F_{VO_2} = 10*(70)^{0.75} = 242 \text{ ml/min} \quad (5.1.2)$$

The air ventilation rate, F_V, for the normal human adult is about 6.6 l/min, given by the product of a tidal volume (see Fig. 5.1.1) of 0.6 liter and a breathing rate of eleven/min. Some air moves back and forth within the respiratory system in the so-called "dead space" without reaching the alveoli or leaving the body, causing the effective ventilation to be less than F_{VA}. Thus the *alveolar* ventilation is approximately

$$F_{VA} = 5 \text{ l/min} \quad (5.1.3)$$

Air is normally 21 percent oxygen, and thus dry air breathed in would (by Dalton's law) have a partial pressure of

$$P_{O_2} \text{(dry air)} = 0.21 * 760 = 160 \text{ mm Hg} \quad (5.1.4)$$

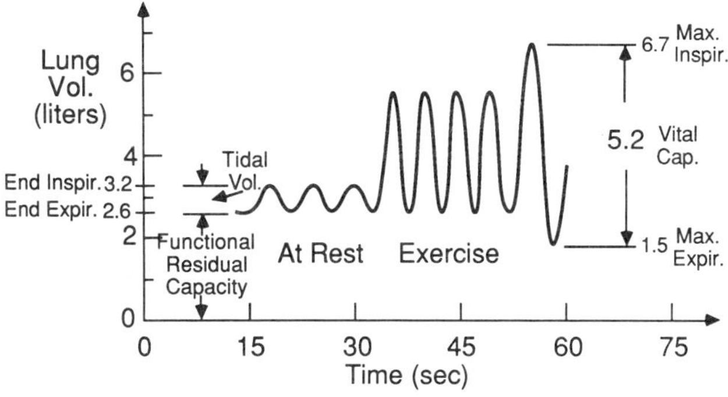

Figure 5.1.1. Breathing pulsatility during rest and exercise for a normal human adult, with typical values of some important respiratory quantities shown. (From Grodins-78, with permission).

for a sea-level air pressure of 760 mm Hg. However, air normally has some moisture, and in the lungs it tends to become saturated with water vapor at 47 mm Hg. Thus the partial pressure of oxygen in the lungs at 37°C and sea level would be, if no oxygen were taken up (or CO_2 released)

$$P_{O_2in} = 0.21 * (760 - 47) = 150 \text{ mm Hg} \tag{5.1.5}$$

These and other steady-state average values of partial pressures and flows, given below, arc shown in Fig. 5.1.2.

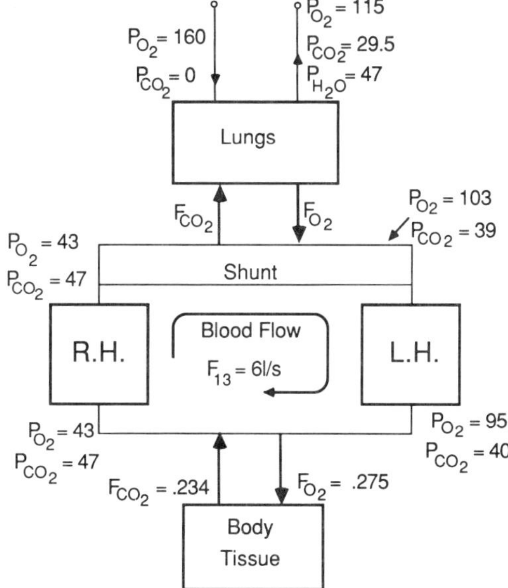

Figure 5.1.2. Average O_2 and CO_2 partial pressures in the respiratory and CV systems for a normal human male, at rest. Some flows are also shown (from Grodins-78, with permission).

The partial pressure of oxygen in the alveoli will be somewhat less than 150 mm Hg because of the effects of dead space and admixture with the water vapor and carbon dioxide given off by the blood, so that, approximately

$$P_{AO_2} = 103 \text{ mm Hg} \tag{5.1.6}$$

The oxygen partial pressure in the air breathed out will be higher because of mixing in the dead space with the most recently inspired air, and may be shown to be

$$P_{O_2out} = 113 \text{ mm Hg} \tag{5.1.7}$$

The relationship between alveolar ventilation, or effective alveolar airflow, F_{VA}, and the alveolar oxygen ventilation, F_{VAO_2}, is

$$F_{VAO_2} = F_{VA} * (P_{O_2in} - P_{O_2out})/760 \tag{5.1.8}$$

Use of values from (5.1.3), (5.1.5), and (5.1.7) in (5.1.8) gives F_{VAO_2} = 234 ml/min, which checks with the allometric determination in (5.1.2) for the human adult. Carbon dioxide is generated in the body at about 230 ml/min, a slightly lower rate than oxygen absorption.

Oxygen dissolves poorly in blood plasma, but unites readily with hemoglobin in red blood cells, making the total effective blood solubility much higher, as shown in Fig. 5.1.3. This nonlinear relation is called a dissociation curve.

It is found, typically, that oxygen in arterial blood reaching the left ventricle has about 95 mm Hg partial pressure, a value slightly lower than the 103 mm Hg given in (5.1.7), because some blood is shunted past the alveoli. The mixed-venous blood arriving at the alveoli for the normal case we are considering has a partial pressure of oxygen that is typically about 37 mm Hg. These two oxygen tensions correspond to 97 and 78 percent saturations on the oxygen curve in Fig. 5.1.3a.

$$V_{O_2} = F_B*(0.86 - 0.68)*224 = 238 \text{ l/min} \tag{5.1.9}$$

where F_B = 5.60 l/min is the cardiac output, less about 10 percent because of the flow through the shunt (see Fig. 5.1.2), and 224 is the maximum number of milliliters of oxygen that can dissolve in 1 liter of blood. This result checks with that given by (5.1.8).

The shape of the curve for total blood solubility in Fig. 5.1.3(a) is so flat for the higher partial pressures (above about 50 mm Hg) that the input partial pressure of oxygen may vary markedly above this value with little effect on the concentration achieved. Note that the carbon dioxide saturation curve is affected by the oxygen level. In the same way, the oxygen saturation curve is affected by carbon dioxide level and also by blood temperature and pH (see Chapter 6 in West-74).

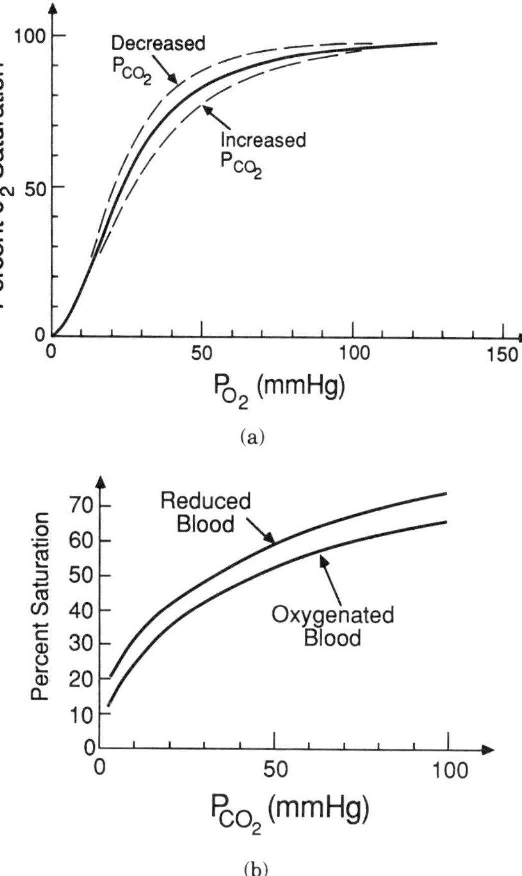

Figure 5.1.3 (a) Percent saturation of O_2 in blood as a function of its partial pressure, with effects of changes in CO_2.
(b) CO_2 saturation curves with effects of changes in O_2 content. (From West-74, with permission).

5.2 MODELING THE MECHANICS OF BREATHING

The mechanics of breathing is related to lung and pleural structures and to the muscles that force air to flow in and out. Also essential to a complete model are the gas exchanges between alveoli and blood capillaries in the lungs, transport of gases in the CV system, and absorption or release of gases by body tissue. We will begin by developing a rather simple linear pressure-flow model for the respiratory system and in the next section will add an associated oxygen transport module to enable the model to follow oxygen as it diffuses into the bloodstream. Oxygen transport throughout the CV system will be modeled later.

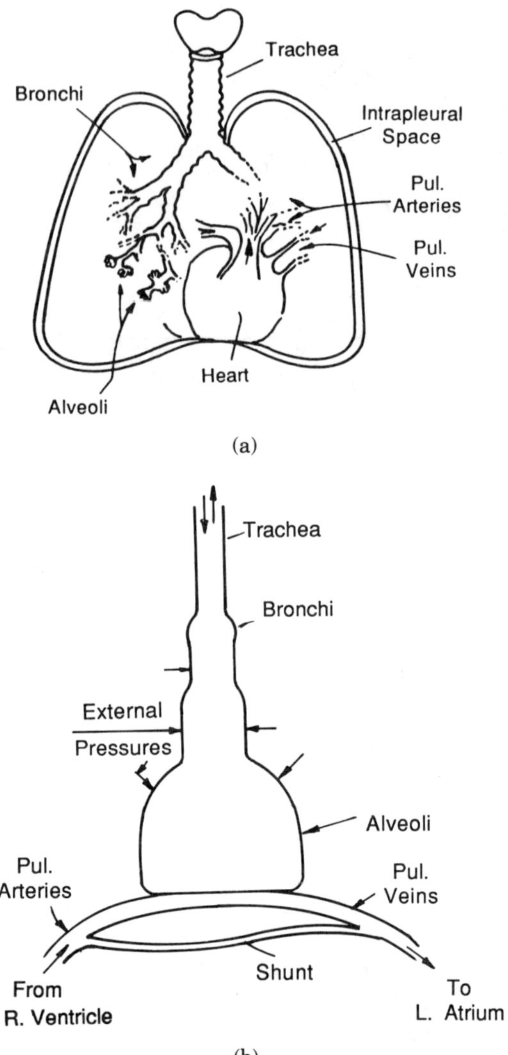

Figure 5.2.1. (a) The heart and lungs, together with the entire pulmonary circulation, are contained within the thoracic cavity.
(b) A respiratory model may be constructed by combining all parallel branches in both lungs and dividing this into four segments in series, (with the initial segment including the mouth as well as the larynx not shown).

In the respiratory system, the airways from the nose and mouth reach the intrapulmonary space in the thorax by way of the larynx and trachea (see Fig. 5.2.1a). The trachea divides repeatedly into more and more vessels of smaller and smaller size until the alveoli are reached

(Weibel-84). The pulmonary artery carries venous blood from the heart, which is also contained within the thoracic cavity. This artery also divides repeatedly, the smallest vessels being capillaries in intimate contact with alveoli. Carbon dioxide leaves the blood and enters the alveoli, ultimately leaving the body by way of the respiratory airways; oxygen goes in the opposite direction and, after entering the pulmonary capillaries from the alveoli by diffusion, is carried to the left heart and on to all parts of the body by the bloodstream.

Ventilation in the respiratory system requires the periodic contraction and relaxation of muscles associated with the rib cage and diaphragm. These alternations draw air in and expel it at about 11 to 14 times per minute (in the adult, at rest). In modeling the mechanics of this system, we combine the many vessels that are in parallel into a single conduit and choose only four series segments: the trachea, bronchi, and alveoli as shown in Fig. 5.2.1b, together with the mouth and nose (not shown). This system is represented in the fluid circuit model diagram of Fig. 5.2.2a, based on the work of Pedley and other more detailed models (Pedley-70, Horgan-68, Jodat-66, Fukui-72, Golden-73, and Jackson-73). It may be modified to have some of the features of these models. Here the inertances of the gas are neglected because they are rather unimportant compared with the resistances; linear approximations will be used

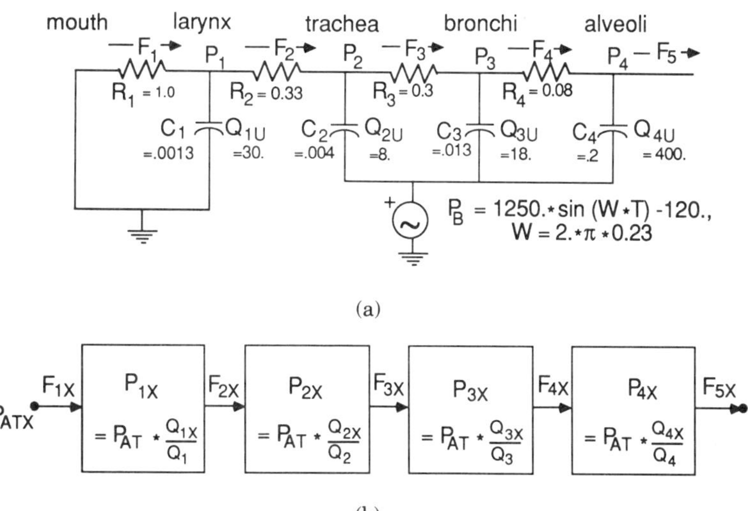

Figure 5.2.2. (a) A simple (4-segment) pressure-flow model for total gas in the respiratory system, shown in circuit form.
(b) An oxygen transport model for the same four segments. This model is, in effect, driven by the pressure-flow model, and the combination is a "multiple model."

for the resistances, which are somewhat nonlinear. The compliances, which consist of a combination of the effects of chest-wall elasticity and the compressibility of air, are also assumed to be linear and to include an unstressed volume, much as do arteries and veins. The pressure, P_B, produced by the chest and diaphragm muscles is assumed to vary sinusoidally, and no attempt has been made to model the muscles. This pressure is applied to the compliances, C_2, C_3, C_4, of the three segments that are within the chest cavity.

The final flow, F_5, in this model is the algebraic sum of the oxygen, carbon dioxide, and other gases that diffuse from the alveolar spaces into or out of the blood, and is normally quite small, because oxygen inflow is nearly equaled by carbon dioxide outflow.

The equations for air pressure and flow (in the model of Fig. 5.2.2a) are much like those for blood pressure and flow in the CV system. These equations are shown directly in ACSL program RESP-PF, together with parameter values. The element values used in this program were obtained from the references cited earlier and are in CGS units. Because the pressures used in respiratory studies are often given in cm H_2O, the last five equations are included to convert the pressures to these practical units; note that since they are needed only for output, they are included in the DYNAMIC rather than the DERIVATIVE section of the program, so that evaluation is required only once each communication interval (Cinterval).

```
PROGRAM   RESP-PF
   'CGS units are used'
 DYNAMIC
   Cinterval CINT= 0.05
   Constant TF=12.

  DERIVATIVE
   Algorithm IALG = 4          $ 'Runge Kutta 2'
   Maxterval MAXT =0.0005
   Nsteps NSTP = 1

     'Pressure-flow Equations
   Constant R1=1.0,Q1IC=40.,Q1U=430.,C1=.0013
   F1=(-P1)/R1
   Q1=INTEG(F1-F2,Q1IC)       $'Mouth and larynx'
   P1=(Q1-QU1)/C1

   Constant KB=1200.,KSB= -120.,FREQ=.23,PI=3.14159
   W=2.*PI*FREQ        $'T is in sec., W in rad/sec'
   PB=KB*SIN(W*T) + KSB
     'PB is pressure produced by resp. muscles'
```

```
        Constant R2=0.33,Q2IC=12.0,Q2U=8.,C2=.004
        F2=(P1-P2)/R2
        Q2=INTEG(F2-F3,Q2IC)      $'Trachea'
        P2=(Q2-QU2)/C2 + PB

        Constant R3=.3,Q3IC=29.,Q3U=22.,C3=.013
        F3=(P2-P3)/R3
        Q3=INTEG(F3-F4,Q3IC)      $'Bronchi'
        P3=(Q3-Q3U)/C3 + PB

        Constant R4=.08,Q4IC=508.,Q4U=400.,C4=.2,F5=0.
         'Assume total gas flow to blood, F5=0.0'
        F4=(P3-P4)/R4
        Q4=INTEG(F4-F5,Q4IC)      $'Alveoli'
        P4=(Q4-Q4U)/C4 +PB
        QT=Q1+Q2+Q3+Q4

       END $'Of Deriv.'
        TERMT(T .GE. TF)
      'Eqs. to convert PB etc. to PBM etc. in cmH20'
        PBM=PB*1.36/1332. $ P1M=P1*1.36/1332.
        P2M=P2*1.36/1332. $ P3M=P3*1.36/1332
        P4M=P4*1.36/1332.
      END $ 'Of Dynamic'

     END $ 'Of Program'
```

This P-F respiratory model is driven by a pressure generator: PB = KB*SIN(W*T) + KSB. Here the first term is a sinusoid of frequency 0.23/sec or 14/min and of amplitude 1200 CGS units (dynes/cm^2), with a small negative bias KSB = -120. When this model was operated (after a preliminary run to find initial conditions), the pressure PBM (equal to PB in cm H_2O where 1 cm H_2O = 981 CGS units) was plotted, together with the total lung volume:

$$QT = Q1 + Q2 + Q3 + Q4 \tag{5.2.1}$$

This oscillating volume QT (see Fig. 5.2.3a) has a peak-to-peak value slightly less than 500 ml; this is the tidal volume (sometimes indicated by V_T), and was referred to in the preceding section. It should be somewhat larger, about 600 ml, for an average adult male, which would require that PB be slightly increased.

The pressures P1M in the larynx and P4M in the alveoli (see Fig. 5.2.3b) are about half the value of the pressure PBM, and P2M and P3M will be found to be about the same. However, segment volumes (see Fig. 5.2.3c) show much variation, with the alveolar segment, which has by far

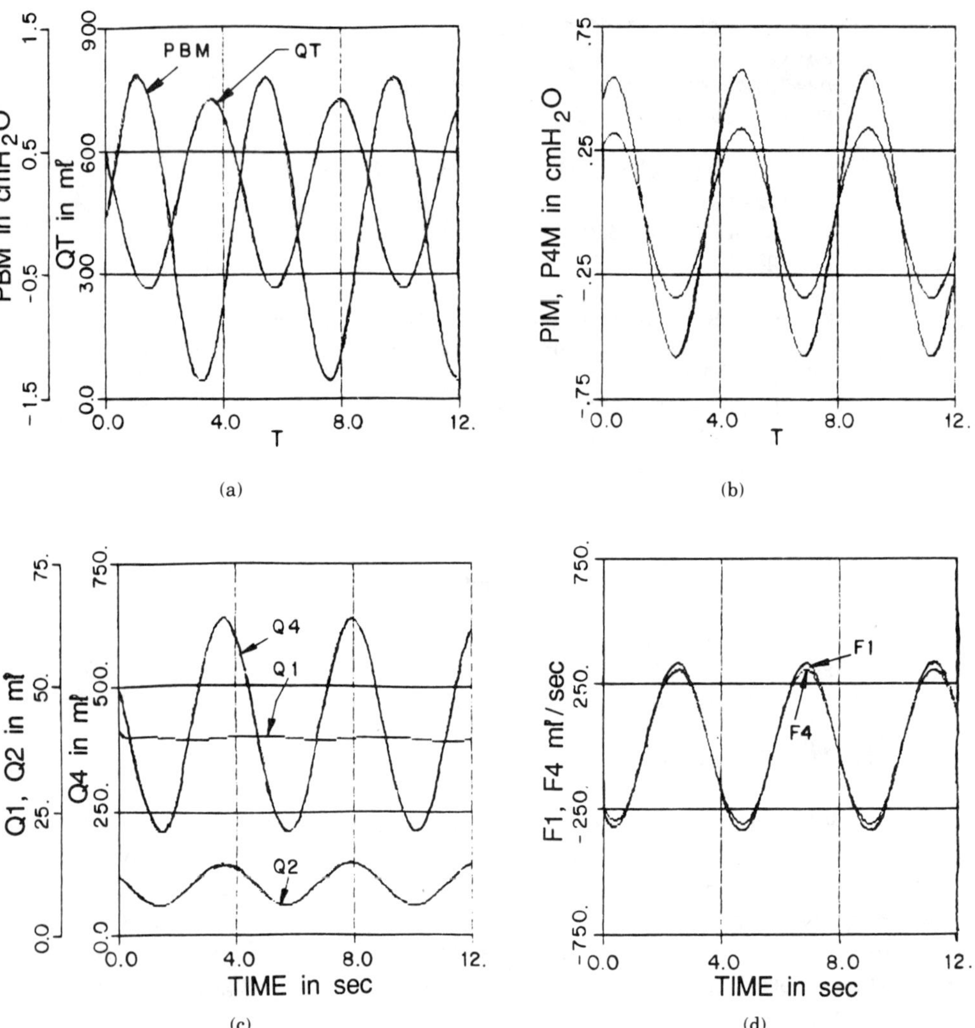

Figure 5.2.3. Some air pressures, volumes and flows obtained with the model RESP-PF.

the largest compliance, showing the largest volume oscillation. Two flows, F1 and F4, are shown in Fig. 5.2.3d and are nearly equal, as flow proceeds through the model to the large alveolar volume. The peak-to-peak value of the integral of F1 will also give the tidal volume, V_T.

Note that, although this pressure-flow model or an even simpler linear model may be satisfactory for many purposes, it may be desirable in some cases to include nonlinearities in R and C, and to use a more realistic pressure generation in place of CB. More parallel branch detail might be used, particularly if the ratio of ventilation to blood flow (the V_A/F ratio) varies in different parts of the lungs (West-70,74).

5.3 OXYGEN AND CARBON DIOXIDE TRANSPORT IN THE RESPIRATORY SYSTEM

Fluid-flow transport in the cardiovascular system was modeled in Section 3.3, with blood flow assumed to be constant and nonpulsatile. These assumptions may not be satisfactory if a defective heart valve causes blood to flow in retrograde fashion during part of the heart cycle, or if blood flow is affected by the substance being transported (e.g., halothane or morphine). In such cases the instantaneous blood flows and volumes of the pressure-flow model are needed in the transport model; this requires a combination of the two kinds of models, which we call a "multiple model" (Beneken-68). Multiple models are discussed in Section 1.1 and are developed in more detail in Chapter 6. Such a model for the respiratory system is shown in Fig. 5.2.2. It is essential here because air flow is not only pulsatile but also reverses direction with each cycle.

The first compartment of the oxygen transport model of Fig. 5.2.2b is shown in Fig. 5.3.1a; here the atmosphere appears on the left as an infinite compartment and source of oxygen with a partial pressure of 160 mm Hg. If air flow F1 proceeds to the right, then oxygen flow proceeds from the atmosphere to compartment 1; when F1 reverses its direction of flow, so does oxygen flow. In an ACSL program the partial pressure in gas flow between the atmosphere and the mouth may be determined by use of a function switch (FCNSW) driven by the sign of F1 (from the P-F model):

```
XX1 = FCNSW(F1, P1X, P1X, PATX)
```
(5.3.1)

The oxygen concentration in the atmosphere is normally 0.21, giving a partial pressure of $0.21 * 760 = 160$ mm Hg (at sea level), and in the first compartment it will be

$$\gamma_1 = Q_{1x}/Q_1 = P_{1x}/P_1 \tag{5.3.2}$$

from Henry's law. Usually, in dealing with gases, the concentration is not expressed, since partial pressure is a more useful variable. Thus the equations needed for compartment 1 in addition to Eq. (5.3.1) are, in ACSL form

```
F1X = (F1*XX1)/PAT
```
(5.3.3)

```
Q1X = INTEG( F1X - F2X, Q1XIC)
```
(5.3.4)

```
P1X = PAT * Q1X/Q1
```
(5.3.5)

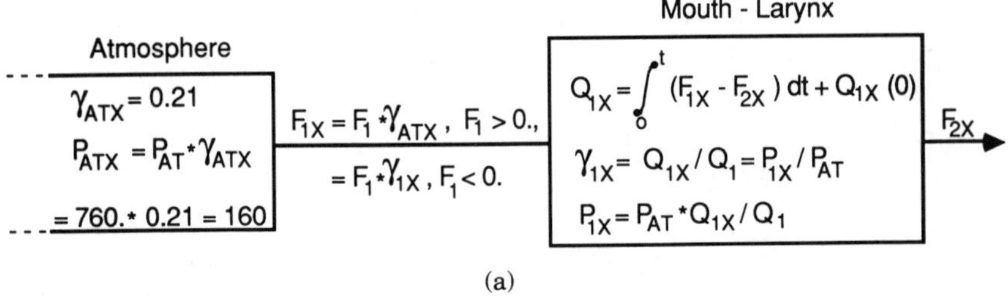

(a)

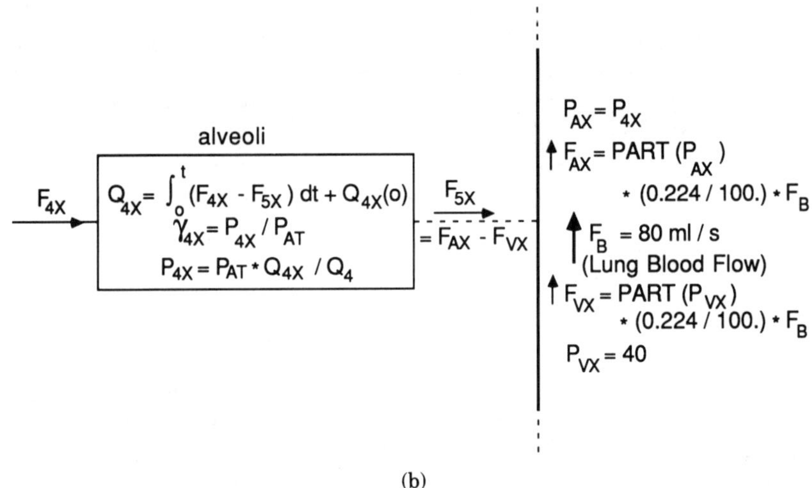

(b)

Figure 5.3.1. (a) Details of the first O_2 transport compartment (mouth-larynx) of the respiratory system of Fig. 5.2.2.
(b) Details of the fourth O_2 transport compartment (alveoli) showing O_2 diffusion flow into pulmonary blood flow, FB.

The ordinary sea-level numerical values for atmospheric pressure, PAT = 760 mm Hg, and for partial pressure of oxygen, PATX = 160, will be used, but the algebraic expressions may be needed if air pressures change (as in underwater diving). (Note that correction for uptake of water vapor is not used here.)

The airway input equation for the alveolar compartment is the same as that of the other compartments, but the oxygen output flow is by diffusion through alveolar-to-lung capillary membranes and requires different treatment. It has been shown (see Chap. 4 in Grodins-78), that oxygen outflow will be nearly that which makes the oxygen partial pressure in the pulmonary veins equal to that in the alveoli, PAX = P4X. This flow, FAX, must be related to the oxygen partition function PART(PAX), which gives the percent of maximum oxygen partial pressure in the capillaries leaving the alveoli, according to the equation

$$FAX = [PART(PAX)]*(0.224/100)*FB \tag{5.3.6}$$

The commands that must be added to the Derivative part of program RESP-PF to make it describe the multiple model of Fig. 5.2.2 are as follows:

```
'Transport equations start here; these equations'
'combined with those in RESP-PF give model RESP-OX'

Constant PATX=160.,Q1XIC=7.
'PATX is atmos. partial press of oxygen'
  XX1=FCNSW(F1,P1X,P1X,PATX)
  F1X=(F1*XX1)/760.
  Q1X=INTEG(F1X-F2X,Q1XIC)
  P1X=760.*Q1X/Q1

Constant Q2XIC=2.0
  XX2=FCNSW(F2,P2X,P2X,P1X)
  F2X=(F2*XX2)/760.
  Q2X=INTEG(F2X-F3X,Q2XIC)
  P2X=760.*Q2X/Q2

Constant Q3XIC=4.6
  XX3=FCNSW(F3,P3X,P3X,P2X)
  F3X=(F3*XX3)/760.
  Q3X=INTEG(F3X-F4X,Q3XIC)
  P3X=760.*Q3X/Q3

Constant Q4XIC=83.
  XX4=FCNSW(F4,P4X,P4X,P3X)
  F4X=(F4*XX4)/760.
  Q4X=INTEG(F4X-F5X,Q4XIC)
  P4X=760.*Q4X/Q4

Constant FB=80.,MAXX=.224,PVX=40.
'Bl. flow 80 ml/s, Max oxy.fraction in bl.=.224'
'PVX is partial press. of oxy. in mixed venous . . .
 blood in Pul. Artery,- assumed constant'
TABLE PART,1,13
/0.0,5.0,10.,20.,30.,40.,50.,60.,80.,90.,100.,150.,200., . . .
0.0,3.0,10.,33.,57.,74.,82.5,89.,95., 96.,98.,99.,99.5/
'This is a table for the oxy. partition fcn.,PART( )'

  PAX=P4X        $'Assume perfusion-limited oxy. uptake'
  FAX=PART(PAX)*.01*MAXX*FB
  FVX=PART(PVX)*.01*MAXX*FB
  F5X=FAX-FVX
  PPO=200.*T/TF $'Gen. partial press. oxy. for plotting'
  O2PC=PART(PPO)$'Oxy. sat. percent for plotting'
```

```
End $ 'Of Deriv.'
     TERMT(T .GE. TF)
   'PMs are pressures in cm of water'
     PBM=PB*1.36/1332.
     P1M=P1*1.36/1332.
     P2M=P2*1.36/1332.
     P3M=P3*1.36/1332.
     P4M=P4*1.36/1332.
END $ 'Of Dynamic'

END $ 'Of Program'
```

The combined program RESP-OX gives air *and* oxygen partial pressures, volumes, and flows corresponding to the human adult at rest. As a check, this program was operated for 12 sec, with results as shown in Fig. 5.3.2. In Fig. 5.3.2a, partial pressures of oxygen are shown for compartments 1, 3, and 4. Note that inspiration (as at T = 3) results in an oxygen peak pressure of 160 mm Hg in the first three compartments, but peaks are lower in the alveoli, where the pressure averages P4X $\approx$ 118 mm Hg. This would be lower, as would the peak in P3X if the outflows of water vapor and carbon dioxide were included in the model, and P4X would be closer to the alveolar value of 113 mm Hg given in (5.1.6).

Oxygen volumes in compartments 1, 2, and 4 are plotted in Fig. 5.3.2b and flows F1X and F4X in 5.3.2c. The flow into the blood, F5X, has a very small pulsation that can be seen only by plotting to an expanded scale. Its average value is 4.135 ml/s, or 0.248 l/min, which is close to the value given in (5.1.2). The oxygen diffusion is assumed to be *perfusion limited*—that is, the partial pressure of oxygen in the pulmonary veins approaches that in the alveoli, and more oxygen is taken up in proportion to any increase in blood flow. The constant nature of F5X is explained by the equation

$$\text{F5X} = \text{FAX} - \text{FVX} \tag{5.3.7}$$

in which FVX is the constant venous oxygen inflow to the lung capillaries, and FAX is rather constant as determined by the low slope of the upper part of the oxygen partition curve.

The oxygen partition curve, or oxyhemoglobin dissociation curve, as it is also called, is shown in Fig. 5.1.3a. A function generator, Y = PART(X), was set up in the ACSL program for this relationship; generation of a pressure ramp (called PPO in the program) was used to provide the abscissa and the PART( ) function to provide the ordinate, with the output O2PC expressed as percent of the maximum possible oxygen level in the blood, as shown in Fig. 5.3.2d. This curve varies somewhat as pH of the blood, or carbon dioxide level, or temperature of the blood changes;

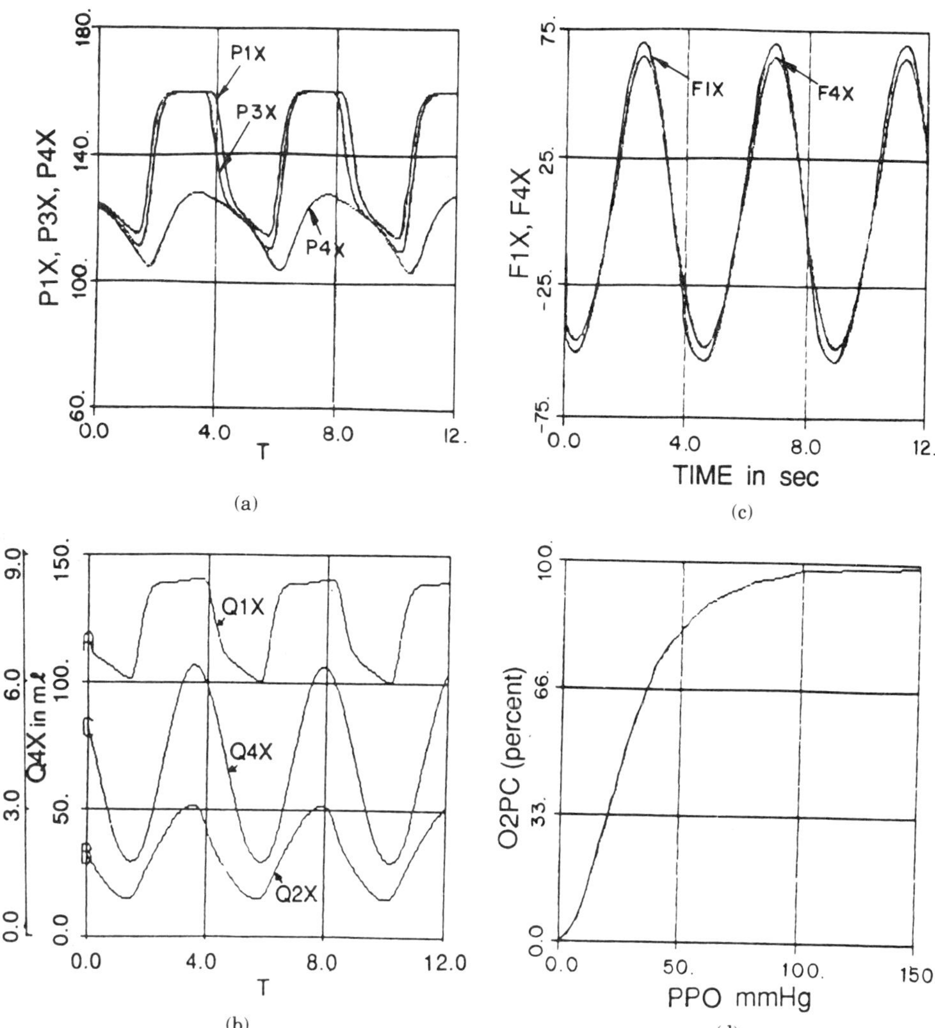

Figure 5.3.2. (a) Oxygen partial pressures in the respiratory tract.
(b) Oxygen volumes.
(c) Oxygen flows.
(d) Oxy-hemoglobin dissociation curve used in the model.

such changes may be included by using a function of more than one variable in the ACSL program, or computational expressions such those developed by (Spencer-79).

A model of carbon dioxide release may be set up in much the same form as the oxygen uptake model of Fig. 5.2.2, except that the carbon

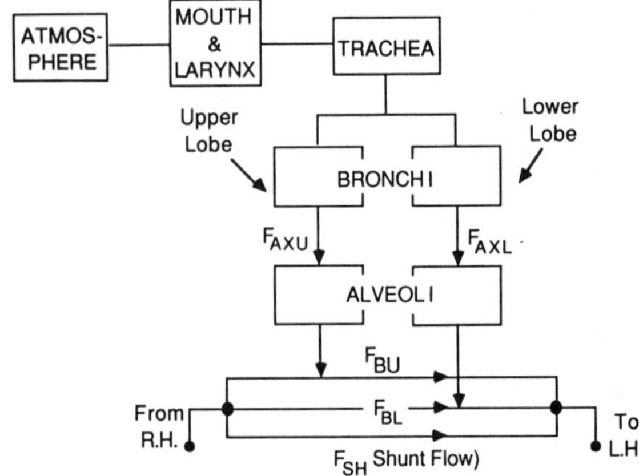

Figure 5.3.3. Oxygen (or CO_2) transport model with branching to upper and lower lobes of the lungs included. Similar branching would have to be introduced into the P-F model which drives the transport models. More compartments, including delays, might be used, and the two lungs modeled separately.

dioxide dissociation curve (shown in Fig. 5.1.3b) must be used inversely, since the flow is normally from blood into alveoli. Also, carbon dioxide transport in the blood is more complex, as shown by (Fukui-72). However, for normal humans, carbon dioxide partial pressures in the pulmonary capillaries and in the alveoli tend to reach equilibrium (Grodins-78) during the few milliseconds that blood takes to flow through these vessels (as in the case of oxygen). Thus, for the normal human adult at rest, a model with correct parameters will show that the carbon dioxide level of about 47 mm Hg in mixed-venous blood will be reduced to about 39 mm Hg in both alveoli and pulmonary veins (see Fig. 5.1.2).

The modeling of the transport of oxygen and carbon dioxide may be set up with more detail (see Fig. 5.3.3) in the respiratory system so that the upper lobes of the lung are distinguished from the lower to permit the introduction of at least an elementary spatial variation in the V/FB ratio, the ventilation rate to blood flow rate quotient, usually termed the V_A/Q ratio (West-70).

In the compartment models in Chapter 3 it was shown that in any given model some compartments might be perfect mixing chambers, but that plug-flow effects might require that other compartments be represented by DELAY functions (in ACSL). Thus, in the respiratory system model we have been using, at least one delay compartment might be added, if it could be shown that complete mixing in all four compartments is not justified. Unfortunately, the reversal of compartment flows of substances such as oxygen or carbon dioxide is much more difficult in DELAY compartments than in simple lags in ACSL.

5.4 KINETIC MODELS OF INERT GASES IN THE CARDIOVASCULAR SYSTEM

The preceding section deals with the rather difficult and nonlinear problem of oxygen uptake, using a respiratory model that is both multiple and pulsatile. In the multiple models to be discussed in Chapter 6, it will also be shown that the cardiovascular system may often be treated in nonpulsatile fashion (using the method shown in Section 4.6), and this simplification may be helpful in dealing with inert gas dynamics in the CV system. It is important at this point to examine elementary but important problems that arise in modeling the passage of inert gases through lung-blood and blood-tissue interfaces as well as through the heart and blood vessels. Such gases do not require nonlinear partition functions such as those of oxygen and carbon dioxide, but may be dealt with using solubility or partition constants (see Section 5.0).

Anesthetic gases are usually quite soluble in blood and tissue, and their flow across both lung-blood and blood-tissue diffusion barriers may, to a first assumption, be considered to be perfusion limited. This means that, as assumed for oxygen in Section 5.3, the partial pressure of any anesthetic gas in the pulmonary veins, excluding shunt flow, is nearly the same as in the alveoli; again, the term perfusion limited comes about because under this assumption the amount of gas taken up depends on the blood flow rate. Similarly, we will now assume that flow from or into tissue is rapid enough that concentration of gas in the venous side of the capillary bed equals that in the tissue it serves. However, a first improvement in the model described below might be to use the combined perfusion-diffusion scheme shown in Fig. 3.5.1c.

A simple transport model for dealing with the uptake of gases by the blood and then by tissues is shown in Fig. 5.4.1. A more detailed view of this model is shown in Fig. 5.4.2. Here only two compartments are shown in the blood circulation loop; it is easy to add more if needed, as in Chapter 3 examples, but the slower transients usually encountered in the transport of gases and pharmaceuticals do not require as much model detail as the more rapidly changing indicator transients. The total delay around the loop should still be about 39 sec for a normal adult. A shunt path for blood that does not closely pass active alveoli is included in the pulmonary part of the circulation.

In this model, since the gases transported are assumed to be inert (such as halothane or ethrane), it will be possible to use the equations given in Section 5.1, in which the partial pressures are linearly related to concentrations. Also, we will begin by considering the system from the alveoli on (Hynson-80). A respiratory multiple model, designed as in Section 5.3, can readily be added to this model.

If the dry gas concentration of an inert gas in the alveoli in this

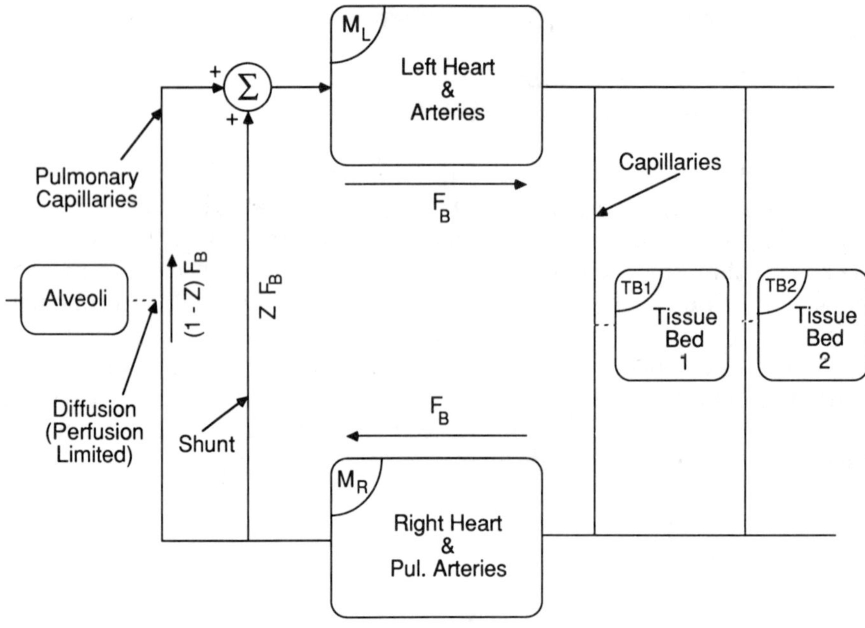

Figure 5.4.1. A simplified model for kinetics of gases in the body, with flow transport around the blood circulation loop, and diffusion (dashed lines) from alveoli to blood, and from blood to the tissue compartments.

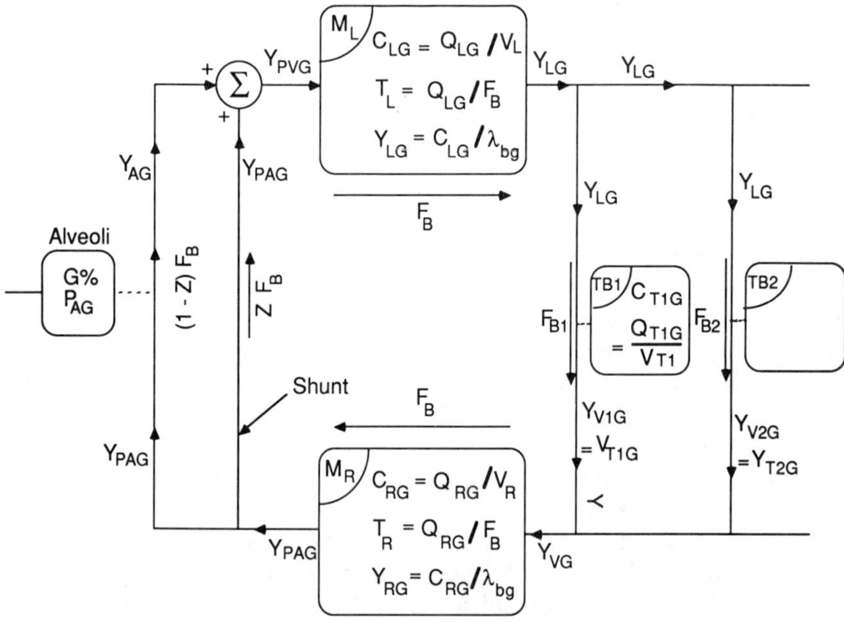

Figure 5.4.2. Details of gas partial pressures, flows and concentrations in the cardiovascular system, as modeled for gas transport in Fig. 5.4.1.

model is G percent, then the alveolar partial pressure (for sea-level atmospheric pressure) is

$$P_{AG} = 0.01 * G * (760 - 47) = 7.13 * G \text{ mm Hg} \qquad (5.4.1)$$

after correcting for water vapor saturation.

The partial pressure of gas in the blood leaving the lung capillaries that are close to the alveoli may be assumed to be the same as P_{AG}, because perfusion-limited flow occurs (Weibel-84, chap. 12). If some fraction Z of the total flow is a shunt flow, then the partial pressure in the pulmonary veins entering the left heart will be

$$P_{PVG} = Z * P_{PAG} + (1 - Z) * P_{AG} \qquad (5.4.2)$$

where P_{PAG} is the mixed-venous partial pressure of gas in the blood leaving the right heart via the pulmonary artery.

Many gases, particularly anesthetics, are quite soluble in blood; halothane has a solubility in blood, expressed as a gas-to-blood partition coefficient, of $\lambda_{bg} = 2.3$. Thus the concentration of gas in the pulmonary veins will be

$$C_{PVG} = P_{PVG} * \lambda_{bg}/P_{Atm} \qquad (5.4.3)$$

where P_{Atm} is atmospheric pressure.

In working with the transport of inert gases we can use either the concentration or the partial pressure; the latter is to be preferred, and this is even more the case when we deal with the transport of oxygen or carbon dioxide. It is convenient to work with a variable that we will call Y, the ratio of a partial pressure P to atmospheric pressure, $Y = P/P_{Atm}$; thus (5.4.3) may be written as

$$C_{PVG} = Y_{PVG} * \lambda_{bg} \qquad (5.4.4)$$

where

$$Y_{PVG} = P_{PVG}/P_{Atm} \qquad (5.4.5)$$

Here P_{Atm} can often be assumed to be 760 mm Hg, but may sometimes be quite different, especially for deep-sea divers or high altitude fliers.

As we follow the blood flow into compartment M_L in Fig. 5.4.2, the net input of gas will be $C_{PVG}*F_B - C_{LG}*F_B$, where F_B is cardiac output, or total blood flow through the compartment M_L, and C_{LG}, the concentration in M_L, may be determined by integrating net inflow over volume:

$$\begin{aligned} C_{LG} &= Q_{LG}/V_L \\ &= \int_0^t F_B*(C_{PVG} - C_{LG})/V_L \, dt + C_{LG}(0) \end{aligned} \qquad (5.4.6)$$

In Laplace transform notation, if F_B is constant

$$C_{LG} = C_{PVG}/(1 + sT_L) \qquad (5.4.7)$$

where $T_L = V_L/F_B$ (see Section 3.3).

Since the partial pressure, and thus the partial pressure ratio Y, are related to concentrations by $Y = C/\lambda_{bg}$, we also have, from (5.4.7)

$$Y_{LG} = Y_{PVG}/(1 + sT_L) \tag{5.4.8}$$

We will now consider the flow of gas into (and past) the i-th tissue bed compartment TB_i. Let the blood flow through its capillaries (their volume being neglected here) be F_{Bi}. The gas flow into the TB_i capillaries, with partial pressure ratio Y_{LG}, will be

$$F_{AiG} = C_{LG} * F_{Bi} \tag{5.4.9}$$

The net inflow of gas into tissue bed Ti with perfusion limiting will be such that pressures in the tissue bed and in the venous side of the capillaries will be equal:

$$Y_{TiG} = Y_{ViG} = C_{ViG}/\lambda_{TiG} \tag{5.4.10}$$

The flow of gas carried by blood on the venous side of the capillaries will be

$$\begin{aligned} F_{ViG} &= C_{ViG} * F_{Bi} \\ &= Y_{TiG} * \lambda_{TiG} * F_{Bi} \end{aligned} \tag{5.4.11}$$

This enables us to express the flow of gas into Ti from the capillaries as

$$\begin{aligned} F_{INiG} &= F_{AiG} - F_{ViG} \\ &= (Y_{LG}*\lambda_{BG} - Y_{TiG}*\lambda_{TiG})*F_{Bi} \end{aligned} \tag{5.4.12}$$

The volume of gas in the tissue bed is

$$Q_{iG} = \int_0^t \mathrm{F}_{INiG}\, dt + Q_{iG}(0) \tag{5.4.13}$$

The gas flow from all veins into the right heart compartment M_R will be

$$\begin{aligned} F_{VG} &= \sum_i F_{ViG} \\ &= \sum_i Y_{TiG} * \lambda_{TiG} * F_{Bi} \end{aligned} \tag{5.4.14}$$

Using $C_{VG} = Y_{VG} * \lambda_{BG}$ and $F_{VG} = F_B*C_{VG}$, it may be shown that

$$Y_{VG} = \sum_i Y_{TiG} * \lambda_{TiG} * (F_{Bi}/F_B) * \lambda_{BG} \tag{5.4.15}$$

The net inflow to the right heart will result in a concentration

$$C_{\mathrm{RG}} = \int_0^t \mathrm{F_B} * (C_{\mathrm{VG}} - C_{\mathrm{PAG}})/V_{\mathrm{R}}\, dt + C_{\mathrm{RG}} \qquad (5.4.16)$$

And, for F constant, as in M_L:

$$Y_{\mathrm{PAG}} = Y_{\mathrm{VG}} \;/\; (1 + sT_{\mathrm{R}}) \qquad (5.4.17)$$

where $T_{\mathrm{R}} = V_{\mathrm{R}} \;/\; F_{\mathrm{B}}$.

This may be extended to many tissue compartments and may also be duplicated (and interconnected) into a multiple model if more than one inert gas is to be transported (see Chapter 6). Note also that M_L and M_R may be partially replaced by delay compartments, as required to give more correct appearance times.

5.5 CONTROL OF THE RESPIRATORY SYSTEM

The respiratory control system is much more complex than cardiovascular control (see Section 4.5). This can be seen in the simplified model diagram of Fig. 5.5.1, which shows that control of the heart must be combined with control of the respiratory apparatus. Note also that the output of the central nervous system depends on four main inputs:

1. P_aO_2, the partial pressure of O_2 in arterial blood.
2. P_aCO_2, the partial pressure of CO_2 in arterial blood.
3. pH_a, the acidity or alkalinity of the arterial blood. This term depends partly on the weak acid that results when CO_2 dissolves in plasma to form H_2CO_3.
4. pH_{CSF}, the pH of the cerebrospinal fluid. This term responds more slowly to changes in CO_2 level in the blood than does pH_a.

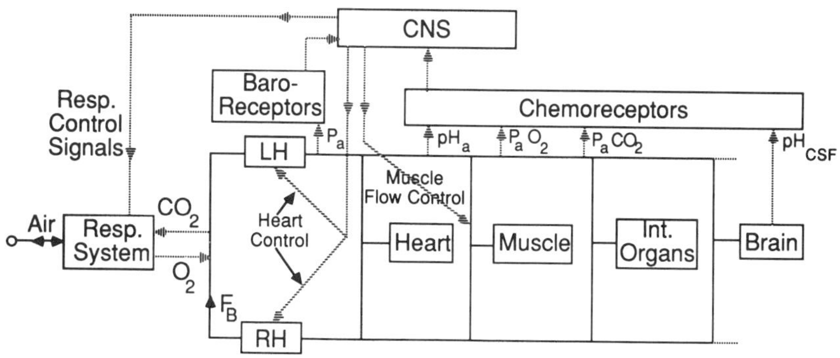

Figure 5.5.1. Block diagram of the respiratory and cardiovascular systems, with feedback control of ventilation and cardiac output.

Models of this system have been set forth by many leading respiratory system physiologists and bioengineers (Grodins-67,78, Duffin-72, Horgan-68, Jackson-73, Fukui-72, Dickinson-77, Saunders-80, and Murray-Smith-88), and more complex new models appear in Swanson (Swanson-90). Here a simple model will be outlined in which only carbon dioxide transport and chemoreceptor output from carbon dioxide in the blood will be considered. However, this simplification can give some meaningful results, especially for the changes that result when the fraction of carbon dioxide in the inspired air is changed.

A first model of respiratory control might be based on the four-segment lung model of Fig. 5.2.2, with carbon dioxide replacing oxygen as the transported gas, together with the cardiovascular transport model of Fig. 5.4.2, with carbon dioxide as the transported gas. To this combination of submodels a CNS signal path from chemoreceptors in the muscle compartment to the breathing muscles should be added, to control the rate of strength (or depth) of breathing. The carbon dioxide partition curve as given in Fig. 5.1.3b will also be needed, with percent saturation (in blood) as input and partial pressure as output. The resultant model would resemble that of Milhorn but with more physical modeling of the respiratory submodel (Milhorn-65,66). It would also resemble the model of Fukui, (Fukui-72) except that a non-pulsatile CV model is used.

PROBLEMS

5.1. A diver working near the surface of the sea (assume a pressure of 760 mmHg) is supplied with a gas mixture containing equal pressures of oxygen and helium, with water vapor at 4 mmHg pressure.

(a) With the aid of Table 5.0.2, estimate the diver's alveolar partial pressures, explaining any approximations.

(b) Estimate the partial pressures in the diver's expired air.

5.2. Oxygen solubility in blood plasma is 0.3 ml of O_2 per 100 ml of blood. From Fig. 5.1.3(a) showing total percent of oxygen saturation in blood, find the fraction due to solution in plasma only, if $P_{O_2} = 50$ mm Hg.

5.3. Make a gradual sweep in the frequency of breathing in the model RESP-PF by setting FREQ = (0.5 + T/60.0) * .23, and using TF = 60.0, to go from half to twice the breathing rate used in RESP-PF as given in the text, in 8 steps. Observe the effect of this changing rate upon F4 and QT, and explain.

5.4. The tidal volume QT, as obtained with the model RESP-PF has a peak-to-peak value of 500, which is somewhat low for a normal adult, awake and at rest. Use a parameter sweep program to try increases in the depth of breathing from KB = 1200 to 1600 in steps of 50, and determine by interpolation the value that should be used to give QT = 600. Check that your value is correct by using a single run of RESP.PF.

5.5. Explain, using sketches of flow versus time, the necessity of using function switches in program RESP-OX.

5.6. (a) Use the multiple model program RESP-OX to check the oxygen partial pressures P4X, flow FLX and volume Q4X shown in Fig. 5.3.2.

(b) Use the gradual sweep of breathing rate of Problem 5.3 in RESP-OX, and observe and explain its effects on Q4X, and F1X.

(c) Use the stepwise parameter sweep of KB to change the breathing pressure in RESP-OX, and observe and explain its effects as in (b).

5.7 Set up a model of a respiratory control system as suggested in the last paragraph of Section 5.5.

REFERENCES

BENEKEN, J. E. W. AND V. C. RIDEOUT, "The use of multiple models in cardiovascular system studies: transport and perturbation methods," *IEEE-TBME* Vol. BME-15, pp. 281–89; Oct. 1968.

BROWN, J. H. U. AND D. S. GANN, *Engg. Principles in Physiology,* Vol. I, Part V; New York: Academic Press; 1973.

COMROE, J. H., *Physiology of Respiration,* Chicago: Year Book Medical Publishers Inc.: 1965.

COONEY, DAVID O., *Biomedical Engg. Principles,* Chap. 10; New York: Marcel Dekker, Inc.; 1976.

DICKINSON, C. J., *A Computer Model of Human Respiration,* Baltimore: University Park Press; 1977.

DUFFIN, J., "A mathematical model of the chemoreflex control of ventilation," *Resp. Physiol.,* Vol. 15, pp. 277–301; 1972.

———, *Physics for Anaesthetists,* Springfield, IL: Chas. C. Thomas; 1976.

FUKUI, YASUHIRO, "A Study of the Human Cardiovascular-Respiratory System using Hybrid Computer Modeling," Ph.D. thesis, University of Wisconsin; 1972.

GOLDEN, J. F., J. W. CLARK, JR., AND P. M. STEVENS, "Mathematical modeling of pulmonary airway dynamics," *IEEE-TBME,* Vol. 20, No. 6, pp. 397–404; Nov. 1973.

GRODINS, F. S., J. BUELL AND A. J. BART, "Mathematical analysis and digital simulation of the respiratory control system," *J. Appl. Physiol,* Vol. 22, p. 260; 1967.

GRODINS, F. S., AND S. M. YAMASHIRO, *Respiratory Function of the Lung and its Control,* New York: Macmillan; 1978.

GUYTON, A. C., *Textbook of Medical Physiology,* Philadelphia: Saunders; 1976.

HORGAN, J. D. AND R. L. LANGE, "Chemical control in the respiratory system," *IEEE-TBME,* Vol. 15, No. 2, pp. 119–27; April 1968.

HYNSON, J. M., "Model Studies for the Design of a Servoanesthesia System," M.S. thesis, University of Wisconsin; 1980.

JACKSON, A. C. AND H. T. MILHORN, "Digital computer simulation of respiratory mechanics," *Computers Biomed. Res.*, Vol. 6, pp. 27–56; 1973.

JACQUEZ, J. A. *Respiratory Physiology,* New York: McGraw-Hill; 1979.

JODAT, R. W., J. D. HORGAN AND R. L. LANGE, "Simulation of respiratory mechanics," *Biophys. J.*, Vol. 6, pp. 773–85; 1966.

LARSON, C. P., "Solubility and Partition Coefficients," Chap. 1 in *Uptake and Distribution of Anesthetic Agents,* E. M. Papper and R. J. Kitz, (Eds.), New York: McGraw-Hill; 1963.

MILHORN, H. T., JR., *The Application of Control Theory to Physiological Systems,* Philadelphia PA: W. B. Saunders Co.; 1966.

______, R. BENTON, R. ROSS AND A. C. GUYTON, "A mathematical model of the human respiratory control system," *Biophys. J.*, Vol. 5, p. 27; 1965.

MURRAY-SMITH, D. J. AND E. R. CARSON, "The modelling process in respiratory medicine," *The Respiratory System,* pp. 296–333, D. G. Cramp & E. R. Carson (Eds.), London: Croom Helm; 1988.

NUNN, J. F., *Applied Respiratory Physiology with Special Reference to Anaesthesia,* London: Butterworths; 1977.

PAPPER, E. M. AND R. J. KITZ, *Uptake and Distribution of Anesthetic Agents.* New York: McGraw-Hill; 1963.

PEDLEY, T. J., R. C. SCHROTER AND M. F. SUDLOW, "The prediction of pressure drop and variation of resistance within human bronchiole airways," *Resp. Physiol.*, Vol. 9, pp. 371–86; 1970.

SAUNDERS, K. B., H. N. BALI AND E. R. CARSON, "A breathing model of the respiratory system: the controlled system," *J. Theor. Biol.*, Vol. 84, pp. 135–61; 1980.

SPENCER, J. L., ET AL., "Computational expressions for blood oxygen and carbon dioxide concentrations," *Ann. Biomed. Eng.*, Vol. 7, No. 1, pp. 59–66; 1979.

STEWARD, A., ET AL., "Solubility coefficients for inhaled anaesthetics for water, oil and biological media," *Brit. J. Anaeth.*, Vol. 45, pp. 282–293; 1973.

SWANSON, G. D., ET AL., *Respiratory Control: Modelling Perspective.* New York: Plenum; 1990.

THEWS, GERHARD, AND HELMUT HUTTEN, "Biophysics of respiratory gas transport," Sec. 12.6 in *Biophysics,* Walter Hoppe et al, (Eds.); Berlin: Springer-Verlag, 1983.

WEST, J. B. *Ventilation/Blood Flow and Gas Exchange,* Oxford: Blackwell; 1970.

______, *Respiratory Physiology—The Essentials,* Baltimore: Williams & Williams; 1974.

WEIBEL, E. R., *The Pathway for Oxygen: Structure and Function in the Mammalian Respiratory System,* Cambridge, Mass.: Harvard University Press; 1984.

YAMAMOTO, W. S., "Computer simulation of ventilatory control by both neural and humoral CO_2 signals," *Am. J. Physiol.* 238 (*regulatory integrative comp. physiol.* 7): R28–R35; 1980.

6 Multiple Modeling

6.0 BASIC PRINCIPLES OF MULTIPLE MODELING

The flow of blood in the cardiovascular system normally serves to carry blood cells, hormones, nutrients, and ions (such as Na^+), as well as gases in solution, throughout the body. If a pharmaceutical substance is introduced into a vein or artery, blood flow also transports the substance. Such mass transport is discussed in the compartment transport models of Chapter 3 for the case where the blood flow could be assumed to be constant or of known variability. If the substances introduced into the bloodstream affect the strength and/or pulse rate of the heart, or in some other way change blood flow, then a pressure-flow model is needed to simulate such changes. The combination of the pressure-flow and transport models, each modeling the CV system in a different way, is an example of what is called a multiple model (Beneken-68). Such modeling may be useful in the study of gas transport in the respiratory system or in combinations of the respiratory and cardiovascular and other systems. An elementary example of this kind of multiple model, used to study oxygen transport in the respiratory system, was introduced in Chapter 5 (see Fig. 5.2.2).

The pulsations in the cardiovascular system are ordinarily more rapid than those in the respiratory system, and the transport of an indicator (and indicator dilution) in the cardiovascular system may require a rather detailed multiple model. Such modeling is examined in Section 6.1. There it is noted that in cases where there is no interest in such rapid changes, the multiple model may be simplified considerably by using the nonpulsatile CV model introduced in Section 4.6.

A much more complex multiple model (of the dynamics of anesthesia) appear in block form in Fig. 1.0.1. Here it is shown that P-F submodels of the anesthesia machine, the respiratory system, and the cardiovascular system might be used to drive transport models for oxygen and anesthetic, giving nine submodels without counting tissue compartments, the central nervous system, and external computer-control modeling. Models of this type are discussed in more detail in later sections of this chapter.

Multiple models are also useful in the study of the uptake and effects of various pharmaceutical substances (Masusawa-88, Smith-72) and anesthesiology trainers, as mentioned in Section 1.2 and discussed in Section 6.3.

6.1 MULTIPLE MODELING OF TRANSPORT IN THE ARTERIAL SYSTEM

A rather simple pressure-flow model of the left heart and systemic arteries was introduced in Chapter 4 (see Fig. 4.2.5 and program LH-PF-3). This same model will be used for simulation study of an inert substance introduced into the left atrium as it is transported through the systemic capillary beds. We will begin the modeling by assuming that a perfect mixing chamber may be used to correspond to each compliance in the P-F model, as shown in Fig. 6.1.1. The upper part of the figure is the pressure-

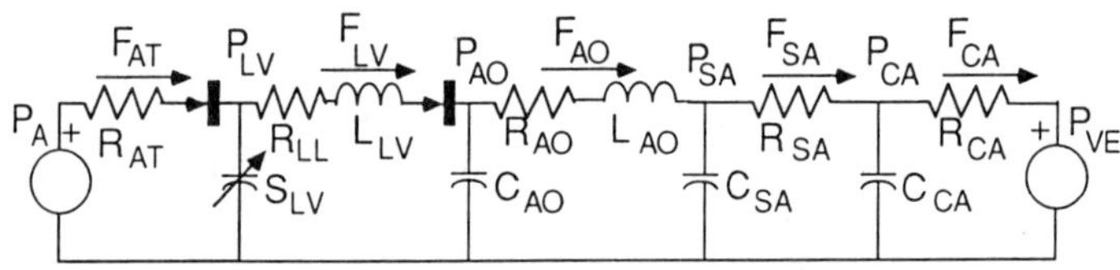

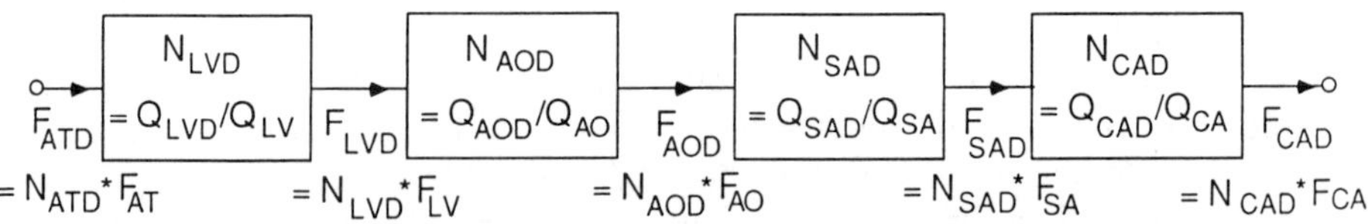

Figure 6.1.1. A multiple model of the left heart and systemic arteries.

flow part of the model, with the same detail and parameters as in Fig. 4.2.5; the compartmented transport model is shown in the lower part of the figure.

The equations for the P-F model, appearing in ACSL program LH-PF-3 in Section 4.2, will be rewritten for the case where the unstressed volume is included in the initial and other total volumes. This change is necessary because the total volume in each compartment is needed to determine the concentration correctly. The new ACSL program, with the volumes QV and so on now representing total volumes, has initial condition volumes increased by the amount of the unstressed volumes, QLVU = 0.0, QAOU = 85.0, QSAU = 250.0, QCAU = 1150.0; this program, which we call MULMOD3 because it is based on LH-PF-3, is as follows:

```
PROGRAM  MULMOD3
   Constant PATM=6.0, PVEM=3.0
 INITIAL
   PAT= PATM*1332.          $ PVE= PVEM*1332.
END $ 'of Initial'
DYNAMIC
  Cinterval CINT= 0.02
  Constant TF=20.0
  DERIVATIVE
    Algorithm IALG = 5     $ 'Runge Kutta 4'
    Maxterval MAXT =0.001 $ Nsteps NSTP = 1

    LOGICAL XX
   Constant TH=0.8, TS=0.3, SLD=55., SLS=1950.0
   Constant PI=3.14159, K1=.9, K2=0.3, B=1.05
    X = T - ZOH(T,0.,0.,TH)
    XX=(X .LE. TS)
    STW= RSW(XX,X,0.0)
    SSW=K1*SIN(PI*STW/TS)-k2*SIN(2.*PI*STW/TS)
    ACT= BOUND(0.,1.0,B*SSW)
    SLV= SLD*(1.-ACT) + SLS*ACT

 'Pressure-flow equations'
  Constant RAT=5., QLVIC= 145., QLVU=0.0
   FAT= BOUND(0.0,5000.,(PAT- PLV)/RAT)
   QLV= INTEG((FAT-FLV),QLVIC)
   PLV= (QLV-QLVU)*SLV

  Constant RLV=5.0,LLV=0.5,RAO=5.,LAO=.5, . . .
   CAO=.00015, QAOIC-100., QAOU-85.
   FLV= LIMINT((PLV-PAO)/LLV - RLV *FLV/LLV,0.,0.,5000.)
   QAO= INTEG((FLV-FAO),QAOIC)
   PAO= (QAO-QAOU)/CAO
   FAO= INTEG((PAO-PSA)/LAO - RAO*FAO/LAO,0.0)
```

```
    Constant CSA= .0003, RSA= 50.,QSAIC-281.,QSAU-250.
     QSA= INTEG(FAO-FSA,QSAIC)
     PSA= (QSA-QSAU)/CSA
     FSA= (PSA-PCA)/RSA

    Constant CCA=0.0022, QCAIC=1038.,QCAU=810.,RCA=1150.
     QCA= INTEG(FSA-FCA,QCAIC)
     PCA= (QCA-QCAU)/CCA
     FCA= PCA/RCA

   'Transport Equations'
    Constant AMP = .01, T1=.08, T2=1.6
     NATD = AMP*PULSE(T1,200.,T2)
     FATD = NATD * FAT

     QLVD = INTEG(FATD-FLVD, 0.0)
     NLVD = QLVD/QLV
     FLVD = FLV*NLVD

     QAOD = INTEG(FLVD - FAOD, 0.0)
     NAOD = QAOD/QAO
     FAOD = FAO*NAOD

     QSAD = INTEG(FAOD - FSAD, 0.0)
     NSAD = QSAD/QSA
     FSAD = FSA*NSAD

     QCAD = INTEG(FSAD - FCAD, 0.0)
     NCAD = QCAD/QCA
     FCAD = FCA*NCAD
   END $ 'of Deriv.'
     PLVM= PLV/1332.
     PAOM= PAO/1332.
     PSAM= PSA/1332.
     PCAM= PCA/1332.
     TERMT (T .GE. TF)
     Q= QLV + QAO + QSA + QCA
  END $ 'of Dynamic'
 END  $ 'of Program'
```

Note that the transport equations are included at the end of the DERIVATIVE section of the program, and that total blood volume, Q (of left heart, arterial system, and systemic capillaries), is calculated. This total volume will be a constant and equal to the sum of the initial volumes in this model unless some change is made in the model that affects total blood volume.

The program MULMOD3 gives results as shown in Fig. 6.1.2. (Re-

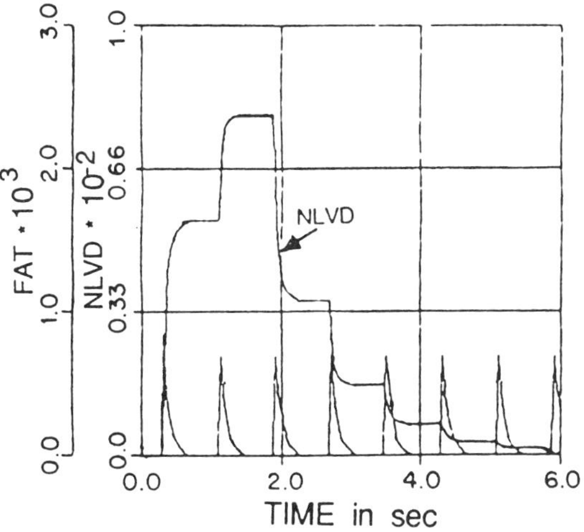

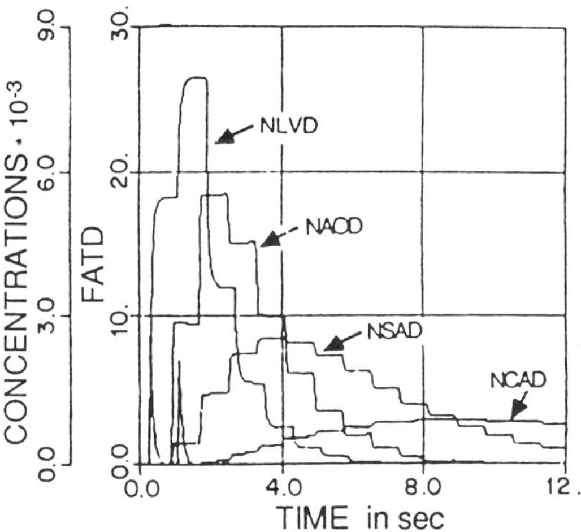

Figure 6.1.2. Responses of the multiple model MULMOD3 to a single input pulse of drug D of length 1.6 sec.
(a) Concentration in the ventricle, NLVD, and blood flow FAT into the ventricle.
(b) Plots of all concentrations, and of the 2-pulse drug flow FATD.

sults obtained in Section 4.2 for LH-PF-3 could also be obtained from this multiple model, since the LH-PF-3 model was used for the P-F part of MULMOD3.) In this model the inflow of some drug, *D*, into the left atrium is assumed to be a square pulse of amplitude AMP = 0.01, beginning at T1 = 0.8 sec and ending at 2.4 sec giving a two-pulse input for FATD, the flow of the drug into the ventricle through the mitral valve. A plot of the left ventricular concentration (NLVD) and the blood flow (FAT) in Fig. 6.1.2a clearly shows the steps in concentration with each heartbeat, and the coincidence of the ventricular concentration changes with the pulses in blood flow. Figure 6.1.2b shows the concentrations in all the compartments of the model in Fig. 6.1.1. It can be seen that the peak is later in downstream segments, and also lower, because of dispersion in the mixing chambers.

All of the compartments in the drug transport part of Fig. 6.1.1 are mixing chambers in this model. We know, from other studies in Chapter 3, that at least one transport delay compartment might be used here to give a correct appearance time. It is not easy to include the effects of blood volume changes in an ACSL DELAY, but ignoring such changes would not cause serious error. If blood flow direction should alternate because of a leaky (incompetent) aortic valve, the operation of the DELAY compartment would be quite unsatisfactory. A multicell delay compartment model has been designed for this kind of application, however (Rideout-70), and could, with some effort, be set up in ACSL.

Note that this model can be extended to a complete cardiovascular loop, which might be based on model PF-1 in Chapter 4. If the changes in the rate of infusion of the substance to be transported were slow, a nonpulsatile heart model (see Section 4.6) might be used (Rideout-88, Tham-88, 90).

6.2 MULTIPLE MODELING IN THE STUDY OF CONGENITAL HEART DEFECTS

Infant heart defects such as the transposition of the great arteries (TGA) are difficult to study in animals because they occur so seldom. TGA defects occur in human newborns at the rate of about 1 in 8000 births, but are usually noticed at once because the infants are distressed and may be 'blue' from lack of oxygen. Blackstone *et al* made analog computer model studies of the pressure-flow dynamics of such infants before and after the Mustard operation for correction of this defect (Mustard-64, Blackstone-82a), in infants of one to two years of age. The Mustard operation essentially consists of an exchange of the low-pressure atrial inputs; another operation in which the great arteries are switched to correct transposition (Jatene-76) may also be used.

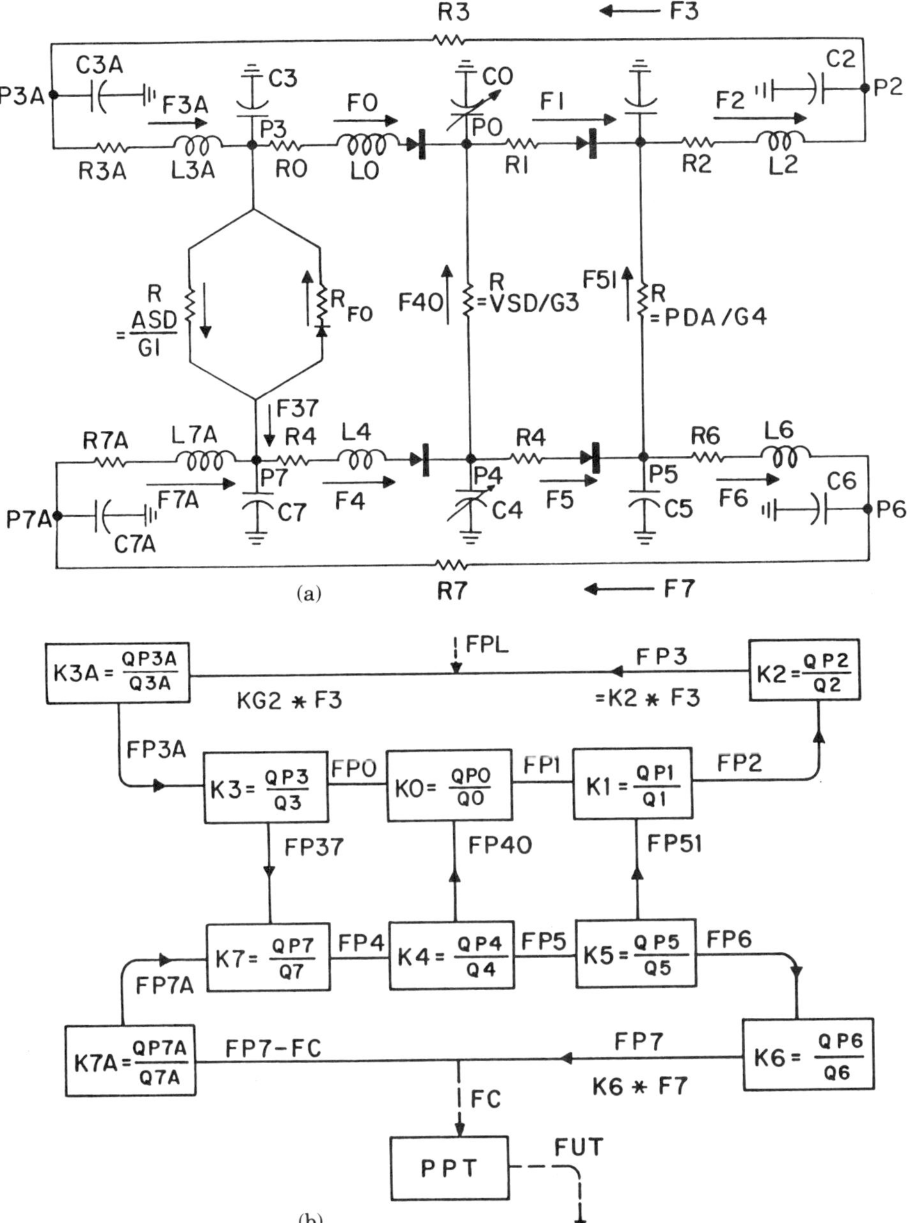

Figure 6.2.1. (a) Pressure-flow model of a TGA infant. Here the basic defect is a transposition of the aorta and the pulmonary artery, with the result that there are two somewhat independent loops, one through the lung capillaries (resistance R3), and the other through the body capillaries (resistance R7). Note the interconnections between the two loops, the PDA (patent ductus arteriosus) and FO (Foramen Ovale), which tend to close at birth, in normals, and possibly a VSD; the ASD (atrial septal defect) may be present at birth, but usually is created by balloon septostomy. from (Blackstone-84), with permission.
(b) Oxygen transport model, driven by the P-F model in (a).

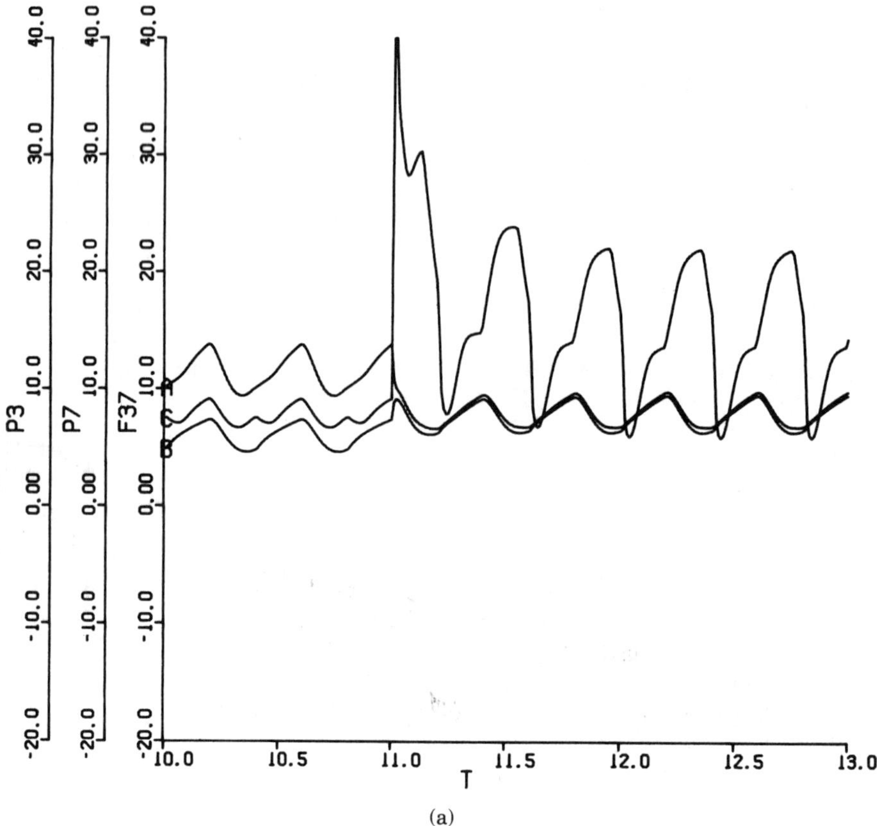

(a)

Figure 6.2.2. Effects of balloon septostomy in a TGA infant on blood pressures and flows. A small ASD was suddenly created at T = 11 sec., causing an increase in F37 (curve C).

The TGA defect often requires a simpler palliative operation shortly after birth. This is *atrial septostomy,* and is best explained with the aid of the pressure-flow model diagram of Fig. 6.2.1a. This operation, made with a balloon at the end of a catheter, requires first that a catheter containing the deflated balloon be inserted through the large veins into the right atrium and on through the foramen ovale, a small opening between the atria that normally closes shortly after birth. The balloon is then filled with air and pulled back sharply to make a large opening in the atrial septum.

It may be seen in the P-F model in Figure 6.2.1a, that although the balloon septostomy would allow some mixing of blood between the two circuits, maintenance of the patent ductus might be beneficial as well; this maintenance is possible with the aid of drugs (prostaglandins) to

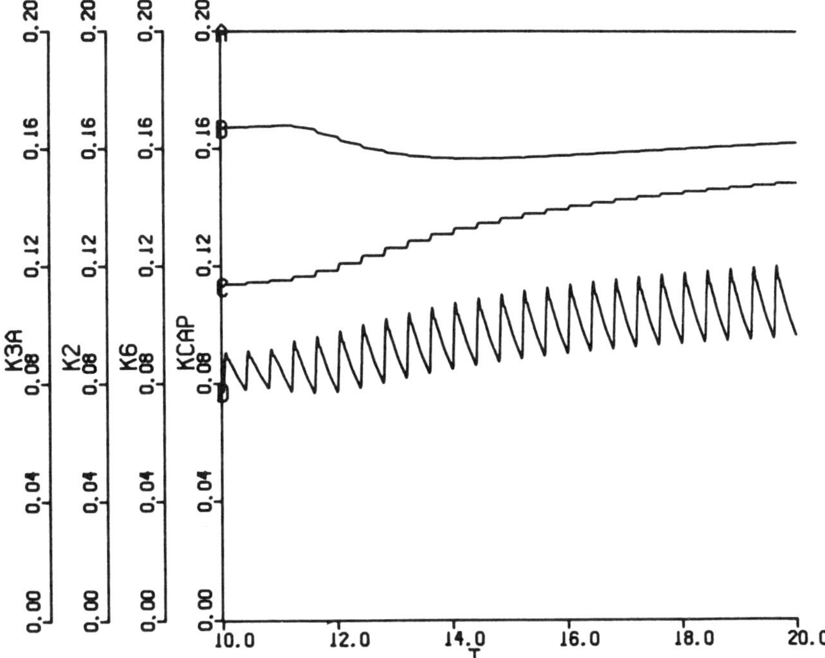

Figure 6.2.3. Oxygen concentration ratios in the model of Fig. 6.2.1 corresponding to flow changes at T = 11.0 in Fig. 6.2.2. Note the rising O_2 concentration in K6 (curve C).

prevent the normal closing of the PDA. (We will ignore the VSD, which might also help oxygenation of blood going to the body capillaries, because it is a dangerous defect, and when found to be present, it is usually closed as soon as possible.) It might also be expected that a pulsatile model is essential for modeling studies of this system, and indeed that it might be advantageous to also add atrial pumping to the model.

It is important to note in connection with setting up this model and determining system parameters that, despite the TGA defect, the circulation is normal during fetal life, when the lung capillaries have a high resistance, the ductus arteriosus is open and (with fetal right atrial pressure larger than that on the left), the foramen ovale is also open (Ganong-89, Chapter 32).

An ACSL program was used to study the model of Fig. 6.2.1 (Blackstone-82b,84). Typical results were those obtained with an open PDA and a small VSD as the equivalent of a balloon atrial septostomy was performed at T = 11.0 to greatly reduce the resistance to flow between the atria. In Fig. 6.2.2 it may be seen that the transatrial flow of blood (F37) is much increased by the septostomy both in its average and oscillatory content, and thus should carry more oxygen from the pulmonary circuit to the systemic circuit.

In Fig. 6.2.3 transients of the ratio of partial pressure to blood volume (corresponding to concentration) are shown. They tend to change more slowly than blood flows, after the septostomy at T = 11.0, as is typical of cardiovascular transport. But, as would be expected, the concentration in the aorta (K6) increases, and that in the pulmonary artery (K2) decreases because of the circulation of oxygenated blood through a loop involving the PDA and the new ASD.

Thus it was shown that the atrial septostomy improved oxygen levels in body tissues particularly with maintenance of a patent ductus. It appears that simplification of the model by use of a nonpulsatile pressure-flow model (Blackstone-84, Rideout-88) is not desirable because the oscillatory flows across the open atrial septum and elsewhere may be quite important in oxygen transport.

6.3 MULTIPLE MODELING IN ANESTHESIA STUDIES

Early modelers of anesthesia (Mapleson-64) were aware of the need to link blood flow and drug transport, but the computers then available did not make it possible to set up complex multiple models. After the appearance of the hybrid computer, large multiple models such as that of Fukui began to appear; later on, such modeling was specifically applied to anesthesia (Zwart-72, Smith-72, Fukui-72, 82a, 82b). Schils used a simpler model in the development of his scheme for computer control of anesthesia, and Hynson used a hybrid computer to determine the parameters of this simpler model from a more complex multiple model developed by Beduhn (Beduhn-79, Hynson-80, Schils-83, 87). These and other modeling efforts were important in the efforts made to develop computer control methods for administration of anesthetics and relaxants (Lampard-73, Westenskow-85).

Tham set up a model to study not only the dynamics of the effects of halothane on the heart and blood vessels but also its effects on the parameters of the barocontrol system (Tham-90). In Tham's model, shown without full detail in Fig. 6.3.1, the pressure-flow model is nonpulsatile (see Section 4.6). The interconnections show that the heart is weakened by coronary halothane concentration, but the halothane concentration in the brain affects the barocontrol loop and some of the parallel pathway resistances. Tham's model is unusual for its many CNS system interconnections, which made possible its application to studies of the dynamic responses of this complex nonlinear system (Tham-88). Models much like this one have increasingly been used for classroom and laboratory dem-

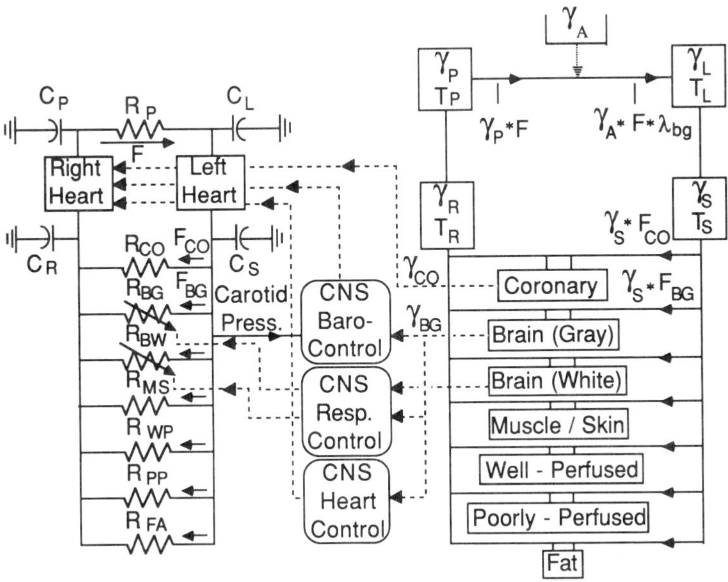

Figure 6.3.1. Tham's multiple model for the study of the effects of halothane on the heart and circulatory system, including its effects on the baro-control loop (from Tham-88, with permission).

onstrations of complex biological systems; a pioneer in such modeling is Dickinson, (Dickinson-77).

The field of anesthesiology, with its wide range of application (to the greatest variety of patients and most surgical procedures), is one that has led to the most efforts in the development of computer model-based trainers. These models have taken many forms (Denson-69, Gaba-88, Philip-86, Schwid-86, 87). The training programs of Ty Smith and H. Schwid contain multiple models that permit the important inclusion of the P-F system, driving a number of transport models for the many drugs (some of which interact with one another) used in the typical induction.

PROBLEMS

6.1. **(a)** Run the multiple model of the left heart and arterial system, MULMOD3, and check concentration responses against those given in Fig. 6.1.2(b). Rerun with heart rate doubled and explain results.

(b) This partial model is open-loop with no recirculation, and thus the integration of drug flows anywhere along its path should equal the amount of drug infused (see Section 3.4). Verify this by integrations of NLVD and NSAD.

6.2. If the aortic valve is insufficient with back flow resistance four times forward resistance, make a qualitative prediction (before running the model) as to the effects of this defect on FLV, PLVM and NSAD. Then modify the multiple model MULMOD3 to represent this insufficiency, and run the model. Compare results with the original system and with your predictions.

6.3. **(a)** Set up a multiple model using the non-pulsatile pressure-flow model PF-NP of Section 4.6, together with a transport loop with compartments M_L, M_S, M_R, and M_P corresponding to the four compliances in Fig. 4.6.2. Using a 2.4-second input of some inert substance at the input to the left heart compartment, M_L, find the concentration responses and compare results with those given for MULMOD3; explain differences.

(b) Introduce a DELAY function in place of half of the systemic compartment M_S, so that an "appearance time" is introduced into the concentration responses. Compare the concentration curves obtained with those using the compartment transport model discussed in Section 3.4, and explain differences.

6.4. Multiple models are useful in systems involving the circulation for cases where the drug infused changes the blood flow by its influence upon the heart, or upon blood vessel flow resistance. Thus, halothane anesthetic tends to weaken the heart (see Section 6.3). This may be approximated in the model of Problem 6.3 by causing the drug concentration level in compartment M_S to decrease left ventricle max systolic stiffness (or to increase G_2). Try this and note the effects.

REFERENCES

BEDUHN, D. L., "A New Model of Anesthetic Uptake and Distribution" (M.S. Thesis, University of Wisconsin-Madison), 1979.

BENEKEN, J.E.W. AND V. C. RIDEOUT, "The use of multiple models in cardiovascular system studies: transport and perturbation methods," *IEEE Trans. Biomed. Eng.*, Vol. 15, pp. 281–89; 1968.

BLACKSTONE, E. H., AND V. C. RIDEOUT, "Model studies of blood pressure and flow and of oxygen transport in infants with TGA," *Proc. Tenth IMACS World Congress on System Simulation and Computation;* 1982.

———, "Mathematical modeling and computer simulation of oxygen transport in infants with TGA," *Proc. Third Southern Biomed. Eng. Conf;* New York: Pergamon Press, 1984.

———, AND D. L. BEDUHN, "Simulation analysis of interatrial transposition of venous return (Mustard's operation," *Ann. Biomed. Eng.*, Vol. 10, pp. 193–218; 1982.

DENSON, J. S., AND S. ABRAHAMSON, "A computer-controlled patient simulator," *JAMA;* Vol. 208, No. 3. pp. 504–08; 1969.

DICKINSON, C. J., *A Computer Model of Human Respiration,* Baltimore, MD: University Park Press; 1977.

FUKUI, YASUHIRO, "A Study of the Cardiovascular-Respiratory System using

Hybrid Computer Modeling," (Ph.D. thesis, University of Wisconsin) Madison; 1972.

———, AND N. TY SMITH, "Interaction among ventilation, circulation and the uptake and distribution of halothane—use of a hybrid compute: I. The basic model," *Anesthesiology,* Vol. 54: pp. 107–18; 1981a.

———, "Interaction among ventilation, circulation and the uptake and distribution of halothane: II. The effects of carbon dioxide," *Anesthesiology,* Vol. 54, pp. 119–24; 1981b.

GABA, D. M., AND A. DEANDA, "A comprehensive anesthesia simulation environment: Re-creating the operating room for research and training," *Anesthesiology,* Vol. 69, pp. 387–94; 1988.

GANONG, W. F., *Review of Medical Physiology,* (14th ed.) Los Altos, CA: Appleton & Lange; 1989.

HYNSON, J. M. "Model Studies for the Design of a Servoanesthesia System," (M.S. thesis, University of Wisconsin) Madison; 1980.

JATENE, A. D., ET AL., "Anatomic correction of transposition of the great vessels," *J. Thoracic and Cardiovasc. Surg.;* Vol. 73, pp. 363–70; 1976.

LAMPARD, D. G., J. R. COLES, AND W. A. BROWN, "Electronic digital computer control of ventilation and anesthesia," *Anaesth. and Intensive Care;* Vol. 1, p. 382; 1973.

MAPLESON, W. W., "An electric analogue for uptake and exchange of inert agents and other agents," *J. Appl. Physiol,* Vol. 19; pp. 1193–1195; 1964.

MASUSAWA, T., Y. FUKUI, T. DOHI, AND N. T. SMITH, "Simulation model of cardiovascular response for drug administration," *J. Clin. Monit.,* Vol. 4, p. 150; 1988.

MUSTARD, W. T. ET AL., "The surgical management of transposition of the great vessels," *J. Thoracic Cardiovasc. Surg.,* Vol. 48, pp. 953–58; 1964.

PHILIP, J. H., "Gas Man—An example of goal-oriented computer-assisted teaching which results in learning," *J. Clin. Monit. Comput.,* Vol. 3, pp. 165–173; 1986.

RIDEOUT, V. C., "Cardiovascular system simulation in biomedical engineering education," *IEEE Trans. Biomed. Eng.;* BME-21, March, 101–107: March 1972.

RIDEOUT, V. C. AND R. L. SCHAEFER, "Hybrid computer simulation of the transport of chemicals in the circulation," *Proc. AICA Conf. on Hybrid Computing,* pp. 348–354, Sept., 1970.

RIDEOUT, V. C. AND R. Q. Y. THAM, "A nonpulsatile multiple model for pharmacokinetic simulation," *Proc. 1988 Rocky Mountain Bioeng. Symp.;* ISA Paper 88-028; 1988.

SCHILS, G. F., "A Study of Anesthesia" (Ph.D. Thesis, University of Wisconsin-Madison), 1983.

SCHILS, G. F., F. J. SASSE AND V. C. RIDEOUT. "Automatic control of anesthesia using two feedback variables,: *Annals BME,* 15, 19–34; 1987.

SCHWID, H. A., "A flight simulator for general anesthesia training," *Computers Biomed. Res.,* Vol. 20, pp. 64–75; 1987.

———, C. WAKELAND, AND N. TY SMITH, "A simulator for general anesthesia," *Anesthesiology,* Vol. 65, No. 3A, p. A475; Sept. 1986.

SHAHER, R. M. AND B. S. L. KIDD, "VSD and PDA in Transposition of the Great Arteries," *Circulation Res.,* Vol. 37, p. 232; 1968.

SMITH, N. TY, A. ZWART, AND J.E.W. BENEKEN, "Interaction between circulatory effects and the uptake and distribution of halothane: use of a multiple model," *Anesthesiology,* Vol. 37, pp. 47–58; 1972.

THAM, ROBERT Q. Y. THAM, "A Study of the Effects of Halothane on the Canine Cardiovascular System and Baroreceptor Control," (Ph.D. thesis, University of Wisconsin) 1988.

———, F. J. SASSE, AND V. C. RIDEOUT, "Large-scale Multiple Model for the Simulation of Anesthesia," in *Advanced Simulation in Biomedicine,* D. P. F. Möller, (Ed.); New York: Springer Verlag; 1990.

WESTENSKOW, D. R. ET AL., "Volatile anesthetic delivery using an uptake model and feedback control," pp. 168–74 in H. Stoeckel (Ed), *Quantitation Modelling and Control in Anesthesia;* New York: Thieme, Inc.; 1985.

ZWART, A., N. TY SMITH, AND J.E.W. BENEKEN, "Multiple model approach to the uptake and distribution of halothane: the use of an analog computer," *Computers Biomed. Res.,* Vol. 5, pp. 228–38; 1972.

7

Heat Flow and Thermoregulation

7.0 INTRODUCTION

In higher forms of life, the internal body temperature is maintained at a rather constant level, despite changes in the external environment, to help provide conditions favorable to metabolism and other necessary processes within blood and tissue. Thus, for the human, an internal temperature close to 37°C is normally maintained by a thermoregulatory feedback system, despite large changes in ambient temperature and other environmental factors (Benzinger-61, Seagrave-71, Bligh-73). In order to understand thermoregulation and be able to design equipment to aid in the maintenance of temperature in hospital patients and aerospace pilots, it may be desirable to model the generation and flow of heat in the body together with the thermoregulatory system.

In recent years the use of *hypothermia* as an aid in anesthesia and muscle relaxation (Cooper-60, Curtis-85) has led to multiple modeling in simulation studies involving thermoregulation (Slate-77). More recently, *hyperthermia* has been employed as a means of attacking cancer, using rather simple means for heating when the extremities of limbs are involved and rather sophisticated diathermy with shortwaves and microwaves as well as ultrasonic heating for cancer in other parts of the body. Here, again, modeling and computer simulation have been used in the study of this kind of therapy, which is sometimes employed in conjunction with chemotherapy (Iberall-72, Chan-73, Jain-80, Strohbehn-84).

Heat flow within the body occurs by diffusion in tissues and by blood flow transport in veins and arteries. Heat energy is generated within the body in a number of ways, some of which are included, together with other thermal effects, in the following classification:

1. *Obligatory*
   Gains: Basal metabolism
   Muscle action of heart and respiratory system
   Losses: Respiratory (evaporation and heating of air)
   Evaporation of "insensible" perspiration
2. *Involuntary Control*
   Gains: Thermogenesis in muscle due to shivering
   Increased metabolism in response to cold
   Losses: Evaporation of perspiration released by sudamotor control
   Gains and losses: Due to conduction, convection, and radiation from the skin; also effects of circulatory changes.
3. *Voluntary Action*
   Gains: Due to muscle action
   Gains or losses: Due to ingestion of hot or cold liquids
   System parameter changes: By adding or removing clothing
   Changing of heat or air movement in environment

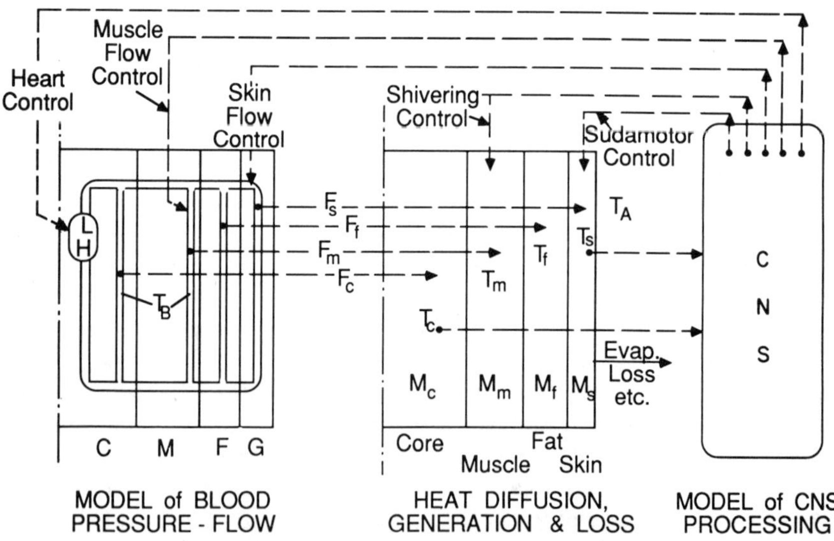

Figure 7.0.1. Multiple model of the generation and loss of heat in the body, and its diffusion and transport by blood flow; also included is the CNS processor that acts as the plant controller in the thermoregulatory control loop.

Figure 7.0.1 is a multiple model illustrating the flow, generation, and loss of heat in various ways, together with the associated nerves that transmit temperature signals from skin and body core to the central nervous system for processing. This processing, in response to cold temperatures, may cause an increase in metabolism in muscles as a result of shivering; in response to warm temperatures, sweating may result in cooling due to increased evaporation. Other efferents may affect heart output and change regional flows by vasodilation or by vasoconstriction. Thus the nerves carrying temperature signals are part of a multivariable negative feedback system that provides temperature regulation in the body.

7.1 THERMAL UNITS AND THEIR USE IN SIMPLE MODELING

The basic unit of heat energy in the SI system (see Section 2.6) is the kilocalorie (kcal), which is the heat required to raise a liter of water at 4°C by 1°C. A more accurate definition is

$$1 \text{ kcal} = 4184 \text{ J (joules)} \tag{7.1.1}$$

The derived unit for rate of heat flux is

$$\begin{aligned} 1 \text{ kcal/hr} &= 4184/3600 \\ &= 1.162 \text{ W (watt, or joule/s)} \end{aligned} \tag{7.1.2}$$

The basal metabolism or energy consumption of the body of a normal adult at rest is about 40 kcal/hr$*$m^2. Thus, for a normal 68-kg adult of, say, 1.8 m^2 skin area, basal metabolism is approximately

$$H_b = 40 * 1.8 = 72 \text{ kcal/hr} \tag{7.1.3}$$

A common source of heat in the body is the oxidation of glucose ($C_6H_{12}O_6$). One mole of glucose (180 g) can combine with oxygen to produce 6 moles of water and 6 moles of carbon dioxide, together with 673 kcal of heat energy, according to the equation

$$C_6H_{12}O_6 + 6\ O_2 \rightarrow 6\ H_2O + 6\ CO_2 + 673 \text{ kcal} \tag{7.1.4}$$

This energy, the free energy value for glucose, corresponds to 673/180 = 3.74 kcal/g, and the "respiratory quotient" or ratio of CO_2 moles produced per mole of O_2 is unity.

Fats may also be oxidized in the body and will produce a somewhat higher free energy per gram of about 9 kcal/g, at a respiratory quotient of about 0.7 (Cooney-76, Cameron-78). These values may be slightly less where oxidation is not complete. Digestion of food is quite complex, with simple molecules being used to synthesize important high-energy compounds such as ATP (adenosine diphosphate), which can be utilized by muscle to do work (Baldwin-67).

7.2 DIFFUSION OF HEAT IN THE BODY

The Fourier heat conduction equation or diffusion equation expresses the dynamics of heat balance in solids (Bird-60, Seagrave-71, Stolwijk-66, Wissler-64, Atkins-69, Huckaba-80). This equation may be compactly expressed as

$$\rho * c * (\partial T/\partial t) = \nabla k \nabla T + H \tag{7.2.1}$$

where

ρ = density (g/cm^3)
c = specific heat [kcal/(°K*kg)]
k = heat conductance [kcal/(hr*cm*°K)]
T = temperature (°K)
t = time (hr)
H = net inflow rate of heat other than by diffusion [kcal/(hr*cm)]

Often k may be treated as a constant, and if Cartesian coordinates are used, Eq. (7.2.1) becomes

$$\rho * c * (\partial T/\partial t) = k * (\partial^2/\partial x^2 + \partial^2/\partial y^2 + \partial^2/\partial z^2)T + H \tag{7.2.2}$$

If we are concerned with diffusion in one space dimension, as in a semi-infinite slab, then for k constant

$$\rho * c * (\partial T/\partial t) = k * (\partial^2 T/\partial x^2) + H \tag{7.2.3}$$

For radial (one-dimensional) heat flow in concentric cylinders, the diffusion equation is

$$\rho * c * (\partial T/\partial t) = k * (\partial^2 T/\partial r^2 + (1/r) * \partial t/\partial r) + H \tag{7.2.4}$$

For radial heat flow in concentric spherical shells

$$\rho * c * (\partial T/\partial t) = k * (\partial^2 T/\partial r^2 + (2/r) * \partial T/\partial r) + H \tag{7.2.5}$$

The human body does not conveniently fit any coordinate system, but cylindrical coordinates provide an approximate fit, and spherical coordinates have sometimes been used for the head (Gordon-76). Nevertheless, the form of the trunk, which is the most important thermal part of the body, is so irregular that one-dimensional slabs (Eq. (7.2.3)) have often been used since their introduction by Stolwijk and Hardy (Stolwijk-66). The layers used are typically core, muscle, fat, and skin, plus a central blood "pool" from which blood flow carries heat to all segments.

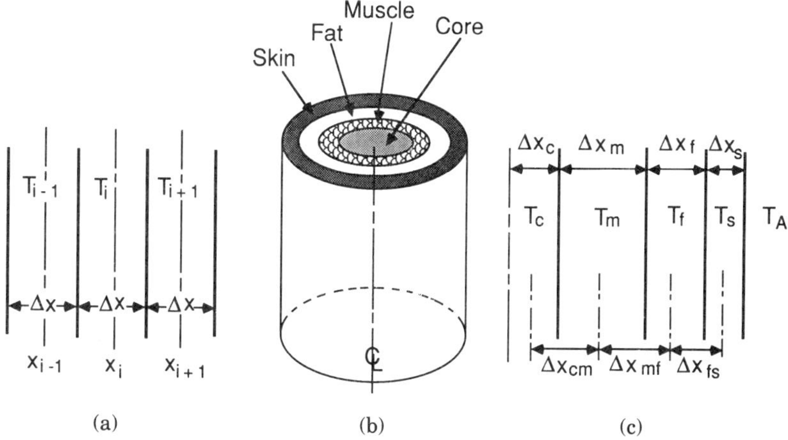

Figure 7.2.1. (a) Finite layers in a semi-infinite slab of uniform material. (b) Finite concentric layers in a cylinder used to simulate the human trunk. (c) Slab representation corresponding to the radial distance in (b).

The use of Cartesian coordinates in place of cylindrical coordinates is justified for the outer layers because the radius is large enough that the term (in (7.2.4)) involving $1/r$ is negligible, and in the core the internal organs and central blood pool make it too irregular to permit this term to be given much meaning. Note that we are somewhat restricted here by the choice of the finite difference methods used; *finite element* methods (Martin-73) are more difficult but permit models to be set up to follow more closely the forms of the body. These methods have been used in modeling related to hyperthermia treatments (Hahn-84, Strohbehn-84, Charny-87, 88).

Figure 7.2.1a shows a slab of uniform material broken into finite layers of equal thickness Δx to permit a finite difference approximation to be developed for the space dimension. In this case, if k is constant and $H = 0$ in (7.2.3), then at x_i

$$\left.\frac{\partial T}{\partial t}\right|_i = \alpha * \left.\frac{\partial^2 T}{\partial x^2}\right|_i \quad \text{where } k/(\rho * c) = \alpha$$

$$\doteq \frac{\alpha}{\Delta x} * \left(\left.\frac{\partial T}{\partial x}\right|_{i+0.5} - \left.\frac{\partial T}{\partial x}\right|_{i-0.5} \right)$$

$$\doteq \frac{\alpha}{\Delta x} * \left(\frac{T_{i+1} - T_i}{\Delta x} - \frac{T_i - T_{i-1}}{\Delta x} \right)$$

or

$$dT_i/dt = \alpha * \{T_{i-1} + T_{i+1} - 2 * T_i\}/(\Delta x)^2 \tag{7.2.6}$$

This formulation becomes somewhat more complex if each layer is a different material, as shown in Figs. 7.2.1b and 7.2.1c. If the layers are assumed to be core, muscle, fat, and skin, as shown, with layer temperatures T_c, T_m, T_f, and T_s, and an outside ambient temperature T_a, then (7.2.1) may be used to find the difference-differential equation corresponding to (7.2.6).

Let us begin by considering the muscle layer, as follows:

$$\begin{aligned}\rho_m{*}c_m{*}\partial T_m/\partial t &= \partial/\partial x(k{*}\partial T/\partial x)|_m + H_m \\ &\doteq \{(k{*}\partial T/\partial x)|_{mf} - (k{*}\partial T/\partial x|_{cm}\}/\Delta x_m + H_m \\ &\doteq k_{mf}{*}(T_f - T_m)/(\Delta x_{mf}{*}\Delta x_m) \\ &\qquad - k_{cm}{*}(T_m - T_c)/(\Delta x_{cm}{*}\Delta x_m) + \mathrm{H_m}\end{aligned} \tag{7.2.7}$$

where the Δx's are as shown in the figure, and units are as shown for (7.2.1). The algebraic sum of heat input and output rate H_m should include the basic metabolism m_m, extra metabolism due to shivering m_{sh} and to exercise m_{ex}, (all per unit volume) together with heat brought in by blood flow to the muscle, $f_m{*}(T_b - T_m)$.

The entire Eq. (7.2.7) may be multiplied through by the volume of muscle V_m in the part of the body being considered. If we then define and use the following quantities, a simpler and more convenient formulation of the muscle layer equations will result:

$C_m = V_m{*}c_m{*}\rho_m$ (total heat capacitance of the muscle layer)

$M_m + M_{sh} + M_{ex} = V_m{*}(m_m + m_{sh} + m_{ex})$ (total muscle metabolism)

$F_m{*}(T_b - T_m) = f_m{*}V_m{*}\ T_b - T_m)$ (total heat from blood)

$K_{mf} = k_{mf}{*}V_m/(\Delta x_{mf}{*}\Delta x_m)$ (total thermal conductance, $m - f$)

$K_{cm} = k_{cm}{*}V_m/(\Delta x_{cm}{*}\Delta x_m)$ (total thermal conductance, $c - m$)

Equation (7.2.7) may now be written as

$$\begin{aligned}C_m{*}dT_m/dt = K_{mf}{*}(T_f - T_m - K_{cm}{*}(T_m - T_c) \\ + M_m + M_{sh} + M_{ex} + F_m * (T_b - T_m)\end{aligned} \tag{7.2.8}$$

The equation for core temperature may be written in similar fashion; note that it has only a single (basal) metabolism term, and that a term for evaporation loss from the lungs, E_l, is included:

$$C_c{*}dT_c/dt = -K_{cm}{*}(T_c - T_m) + M_c + F_c{*}(T_b - T_c) - E_l \tag{7.2.9}$$

For the fat layer

$$\begin{aligned}C_f{*}dT_f/dt = K_{mf}{*}(T_m - T_f) - K_{fs}{*}(T_f - T_s) + M_f \\ + F_f{*}(T_b - T_f)\end{aligned} \tag{7.2.10}$$

The skin layer includes a constant "insensible" evaporative heat loss, E_{si}, plus the additional loss, E_{sn}, resulting from the sweating controlled by CNS feedback; there may also be radiation loss, RAD, and convection loss, CON:

$$C_s*dT_s/dt = K_{fs}*(T_f - T_s) - K_{sa}*(T_s - T_a) + M_s - E_{si} - E_{sf} - \text{RAD} - \text{CON} + F_s*(T_b - T_s) \qquad (7.2.11)$$

These equations may be used for each part of the body considered; thus a somewhat reduced model might have head, trunk, arms (combined), and legs (combined), for a total of 16 equations. An additional equation is needed for the central blood pool:

$$C_b * dT_b/dt = \sum_j \text{F}_j * (T_j - T_b) \qquad (7.2.12)$$

Note that differences have been taken in the space dimension, but not in the time dimension, so that difference-differential equations have been written. If the model is to be written in Fortran for solution, differences must be taken in time as well as space (Smith-65); however, if ACSL or some similar program is used, the differencing in time will occur in the ACSL program and will be translated into Fortran. In ACSL the Δt step size will be given by the choice of MAXT in the fixed step-size algorithms.

Various formulas have been used for the skin heat losses in (7.2.11); these include the loss due to CNS-controlled sweating (Hwang-77, Colin-70):

$$E_{sn} = 1.84*A*V^{0.37}*(P_s - P_A) \qquad (7.2.13)$$

where A is skin area exposed (m^2), V is wind velocity (m/s), and P_A is partial pressure of water vapor in air and P_s is saturated water vapor pressure at skin temperatures (both in mm Hg).

The radiation loss is:

$$\text{RAD} = 5.58*(T_s - T_e)*A \qquad (7.2.14)$$

where T_e is the temperature of the environment.

The convection loss is:

$$\text{CON} = 6.23*(P_A/760)^{0.6}*\text{V}^{0.6}*(T_s - T_a) \qquad (7.2.15)$$

Note that throughout the equations in this section, the temperatures appear as differences, and may be Kelvin or Celsius or referred to some convenient reference temperature.

7.3 COMPUTER SIMULATION OF A SIMPLE MODEL

A simple model consisting of a single cylinder, or a slab, may be set up using the five equations, (7.2.9) to (7.2.12). Numerical values for the trunk, head, arms (combined with hands), and legs (with feet) are shown

TABLE 7.3.1

Segment	A Area, m^2	W_i Mass, kg	C_i Heat Capacity, kcal/°C	K_{ij} Conductance, kcal/°C hr	M_i Basal Metabolism, kcal/hr	E_{si} Basal Evaporating, kcal/hr	F_i Basal Blood Flow, l/hr
Trunk							
Core	0.0	12.18	9.82	1.37	45.38	9.00	210.00
Muscle	0.0	17.90	16.15	4.75	5.00	0.0	6.00
Fat	0.0	7.07	4.25	19.80	2.13	0.0	2.56
Skin	0.6804	1.35	1.21	4.53	0.40	3.25	2.10
Head							
Core	0.0	3.01	2.22	1.38	12.84	0.0	45.00
Muscle	0.0	0.37	0.33	11.40	0.10	0.0	0.12
Fat	0.0	0.37	0.22	13.80	0.11	0.0	0.13
Skin	0.1326	0.27	0.24	0.88	0.08	0.63	1.44
Arms							
Core	0.0	2.51	1.55	6.70	0.78	0.0	0.94
Muscle	0.0	3.44	3.10	18.55	1.15	0.0	1.38
Fat	0.0	1.12	0.67	36.10	0.20	0.0	0.24
Skin	0.3482	0.67	0.60	2.30	0.18	0.63	2.50
Legs							
Core	0.0	7.37	4.47	23.00	2.36	0.0	2.85
Muscle	0.0	10.26	9.23	30.10	2.88	0.0	3.45
Fat	0.0	2.60	1.56	78.10	0.47	0.0	0.57
Skin	0.6998	1.44	1.30	4.66	0.39	3.47	5.85
Central Blood		2.50					

in Table 7.3.1. Note that the quantities for the two arms are combined, as are those for the two legs. These values are for an adult male, based on data from Stolwijk and Hardy (Stolwijk-66, 77, Slate-77).

Numerical values for a single cylinder or slab model may be approximated by adding corresponding quantities for needed parameters from Table 7.3.1; these appear in the ACSL program THERMO, which follows. Note that this model has been simplified to a single set of layers using the sum of the numerical values from the table for different parts of the body.

```
PROGRAM THERMO
 DYNAMIC
   Constant TSTOP-8.          $ 'Time in hours'
   TERMT(T .GE. TSTOP)
   Cinterval CINT = 0.1
  DERIVATIVE
   Algorithm IALG = 4         $ '2nd order RK'
   Maxterval MAXT = .005      $ Nsteps NSTP = 1
'Calculate core temp.'
   Constant KCM= 32.45,CC=18.06,FBC= 258.8
   Constant  MC= 71.36,EL= 9.0, ESC= 7.98,TCI= 36.0
   TC = INTEG((KCM*(TM-TC)+ MC + . . .
             FBC*(TB-TC)-EL-ESC)/CC, TCI)
'Calculate muscle temp.'
   Constant KMF= 64.8, CM=28.81,FBM= 10.95
   Constant MM= 9.13, TMI=35.0
   TM = INTEG((KMF*(TF-TM)-KCM*(TM-TC)+ MM + . . .
             MSH+FBM*(TB-TM)/CM, TMI)
'Calculate fat temp.'
   Constant KFS=147.8, CF=3.35, FBF=3.50
   Constant MF= 2.91, TFI= 33.7
   TF = INTEG((KFS*(TS-TF)-KMF*(TF-TM+ MF + . . .
             FBF*(TB-TF))/CF, TFI)
'Calculate skin temp.'
   Constant CS= 3.35, KSA= 7.71, FBS= 11.89
   Constant MS= 1.05, ESS= 7.98, TSI= 34.0
   TS = INTEG((KFS*(TF-TS)-KSA*(TS-TA)+ MS + . . .
             FBS*(TB-TS)- ESS - ESW)/CS, TSI)
'Calculate blood temp.'
   Constant CB= 2.25, TBI= 36., MB=10.
   TB = INTEG((FBC*(TC-TB) +FBM*(TM-TB) +FBF*(TF-TB) . . .
             =FBS*(TS-TB)+MB)/CB, TBI,
'Set up ambient temp. variation T,A; times & amounts'
   Constant TAI =25., T1=2.,T2=4.,T3=6.
   Constant DTA1=10., DTA2=-20., DTA3=10.
   P= T-T1 $ Q= T-T2 $ R= T-T3
   TA2 =TA1 + FCNSW(P, 0.0, 0.0, DTA1)
```

```
      TA3 =TA2 + FCNSW(Q, 0.0, 0.0, DTA2)
      TA = TA3 + FCNSW(R, 0.0, 0.0, DTA3)
   'Set up shiver and sweat feedback terms'
      Constant K1=26.,K2=0.4, TCRM=37.8,TSRM=34.
      X =(K1*(TCRM-TC) +K2*(TSRM-TS))*(TSRM-TS)
      MSH = BOUND(0.0, 500., X)
      Constant K3=200.,K4=25.,TCRW-36.5,TSRW=33.5
      Y =K3*(TC-TCRW) +K4*(TS-TSRW)
      ESW = BOUND(0.0, 500., Y)
     END $ 'of Derivative'
    END $ 'of Dynamic'
   END $ 'of Program'
```

In program THERMO, in addition to the five equations for the diffusion and blood flow transport of heat, two equations (also based on work by Stolwijk) are included for control feedback. The first provides a means for activation of a shivering reaction in muscle based on a function of skin and core temperatures. This equation, which is quite nonlinear, is

$$X = (K_1*(37.8 - T_C) + K_2*(34.-T_S))*(34.-T_S) \qquad (7.3.1)$$

X is limited to positive values using an ACSL Bound command to give the shivering thermogenesis, M_{sh}, which is added to the normal muscle metabolism, M_m, in the T_M equation.

Another equation in this program yields the evaporative skin cooling, that tends to occur due to increased sweating when skin and core temperatures are high; here we use the limited output of Y, where

$$Y = K_3*(T_C - 36.5) + K_4*(T_S - 33.5) \qquad (7.3.2)$$

The quantity Y, when bounded to positive values, gives E_{sw}, the evaporative heat loss from the skin layer. E_{sw} appears as a negative term in the T_S equation, as does the insensible perspiration loss E_{ss}.

The model is exposed to a normal outside or ambient temperature T_A, initially at 25°C, and initial temperatures of the various layers in the body were determined by preliminary runs, with T_A fixed at this value. In the experimental run, shown in Fig. 7.3.1, a function was set up using function switches to raise T_A from 25° to 35° after two hours and then to lower it to 15° after two more hours. At time T = 6 hr, T_A was returned to 25°C.

Figure 7.3.1a shows that the simulated system has a core temperature that is held within a range of about 35.8° to 36.8° by the feedback control, despite variations in ambient temperature T_A ranging from 15° to 35°. Resultant temperatures shown for all layers in Fig. 7.3.1b indicate that the layers nearer the outside show more variation in temperature and have a lower average temperature.

Figure 7.3.1c shows the cooling effect of the sweating less E_{sw},

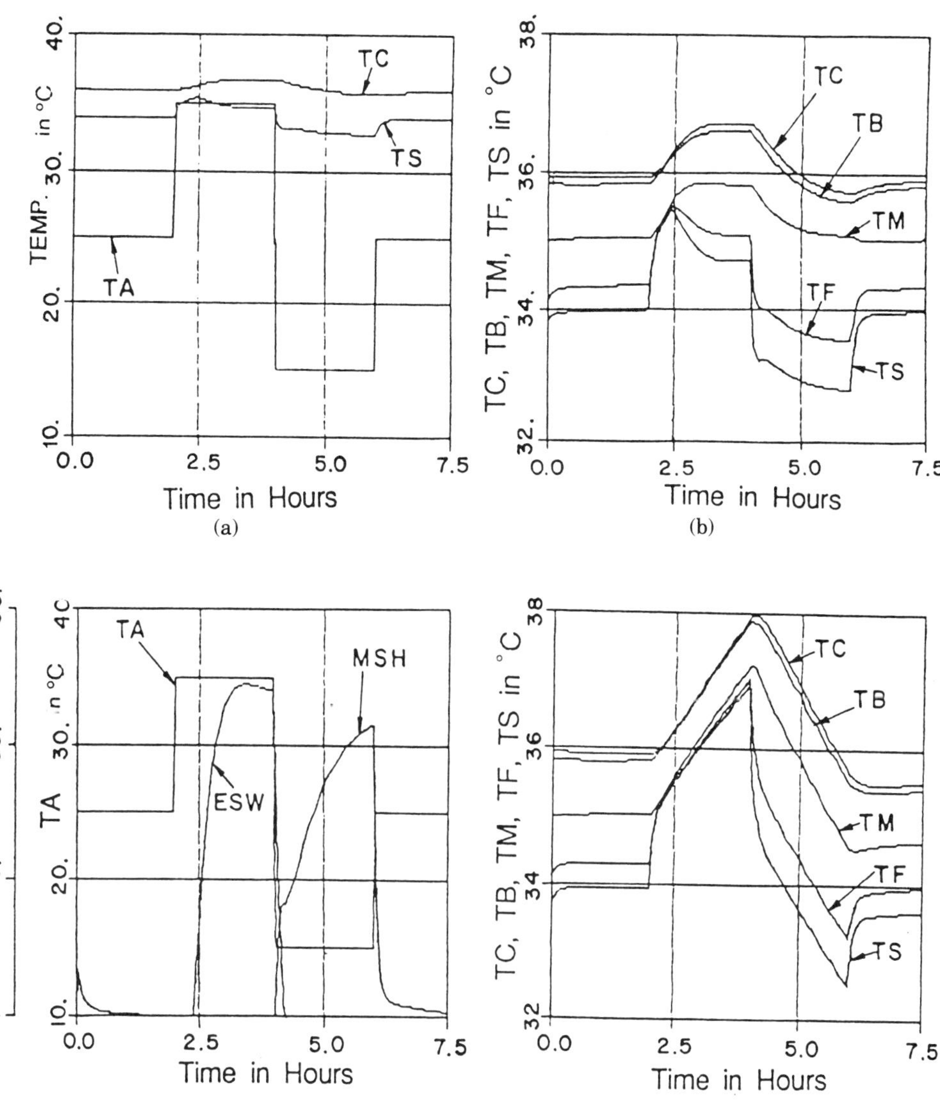

Figure 7.3.1. (a) Skin Temperature T_S, and core temperature T_C, in response to an ambient temperature pattern, T_A.
(b) Temperatures T_S, T_M, T_F, T_B and T_S responding to the same T_A, but plotted to a more limited abscissa scale.
(c) Feedback heat flows E_{sw} (loss due to sweating) and M_{sh} (gain due to shivering).
(d) Temperatures as in (b) when feedbacks E_{sw} and M_{sh} are zero.

which appears principally when temperature is high. It tends to cause reduced skin temperature, resulting in a reduction in T_S after $T = 2.5$; this, in turn, tends to hold down the temperature of inner layers, as determined partly by diffusion but mostly by blood transport of heat. This figure also shows the shivering thermogenesis term M_{sh}, which appears when T_A is low, for $4 < T < 6$, and tends to raise muscle temperatures during this period.

In Fig. 7.3.1d, the temperatures of the four layers when feedback is removed may be seen to have large and rapid responses to T_A, as compared to those in part b.

7.4 HEAT FLOW AND THERMOREGULATION IN INFANTS

Heat flow and thermoregulation in infants may be important to model for a number of reasons, including the design and use of incubators for infants at risk and the study of the use of hypothermia during open-heart operations. Numerical values of parameters needed for modeling are somewhat more difficult to obtain for infants, and their regulatory systems may not be well developed. Furthermore, infants have something of thermal regulatory importance that adults do not, namely *brown fat*. This is a fat layer mostly on the back and shoulders that can generate heat, being used up as it does so, unlike ordinary white fat, which mainly acts as a passive insulator (Heim-71, Harding-71).

Finding thermal data relating to infants is not easy; a number of sources were discovered by Plummer, and a table of values for neonates (see Table 7.4.1) that he used in his work is reproduced here (Plummer-74). The regulatory system scheme used in the adult model may be scaled for use in the infant. Note that the data for hands are combined with arms, and those for feet with legs, as in the adult (see Table 7.3.1). Some use may be made of allometric relationships (see Section 2.7), but this can only be relied on for changing infant data to correspond to a child of different size.

7.5 MULTIPLE MODELING AND OTHER PROBLEMS IN THERMAL SIMULATION

More detailed representation of the body is possible (Gordon-76), and the use of finite element methods may assist in this (Charny-87). The effects of clothing may also be included (Ho-75). Reviews and lists of references

TABLE 7.4.1

Segment	A Area, cm²	W_i Mass, g	C_i Heat Capacity, kcal/°C	K_{ij} Conductance, kcal/°C hr	M_i Basal Metabolism, kcal/hr	E_{si} Basal Evaporating, kcal/hr	F_i Basal Blood Flow, l/hr
Trunk							
Core	0.0	552	0.360	1.19	1.83	0.487	17.56
Muscle	0.0	451	0.406	3.00	0.14		0.16
Fat	0.0	134	0.080	5.69	0.04		0.10
Skin	629	120	0.108		0.04	0.139	0.62
Head							
Core	0.0	275	0.203	1.56	1.56		13.2
Muscle	0.0	27	0.024	2.93	0.008		0.01
Fat	0.0	54	0.032	2.51	0.016		0.02
Skin	267	54	0.049		0.016	0.059	0.261
Arms							
Core	0.0	127	0.077	0.806	0.036		0.045
Muscle	0.0	321	0.289	2.00	0.097		0.116
Fat	0.0	119	0.071	3.69	0.035		0.043
Skin	504	119	0.107		0.035	0.139	0.494
Legs							
Core	0.0	193	0.114	1.12	0.058		0.073
Muscle	0.0	408	0.367	2.44	0.122		0.147
Fat	0.0	118	0.077	4.61	0.039		0.054
Skin	562	118	0.115		0.039	0.149	0.551
Central Blood		107	0.094		3.90		

regarding thermal modeling are available (Iberall-72 and Hwang-77), as well as interesting and valuable studies on model validation (Damato-68, Konz-77, Stolwijk-77). Others have dealt with specific problems that are not often recognized, such as countercurrent effects (Mitchell-68) and problems of heat exchange during cardiopulmonary bypass (Curtis-85).

True multiple models for thermal studies should include a pressure-flow model of blood circulation in addition to the thermal diffusion and regulatory systems discussed in preceding sections. However, such multiple models might use nonpulsatile cardiovascular modeling, because heat transients (like those of anesthesia) are slow compared to heart and blood pulsation. Transport models for pharmacokinetics modeling might also be included.

In an ambitious model, Slate set up a multiple model for study of infants during hypothermia and anesthesia during open-heart surgery (Slate-77a,b). A diagram depicting the form and important interconnections in his model is shown in Fig. 7.5.1.

PROBLEMS

7.1. **(a)** In problems related to the heating of auditoriums, a "rule of thumb" is to assume that each human (seated, and at rest) produces heat energy at a 100-watt rate. Check this against the basal metabolism for the adult human given in Section 7.1.

(b) Determine how long the oxidation of a one-ounce candy bar (assumed to be the same as glucose) would suffice to supply the basal metabolism of an adult human at rest.

7.2. **(a)** The human adult thermoregulatory model THERMO lumps all sections of the body together (see Table 7.3.1). Run this model and check temperature outputs for the given variations in ambient temperature, T_A, against those given in Fig. 7.3.1.

(b) Change the fat layer in THERMO to have double its thickness, and again run it and compare temperatures with those given in Fig. 7.3.1.

7.3. Change the skin layer in this model into two layers of equal thickness, but with blood flow only in the inner layer. Assume that vaso-dilatation and constriction of the skin blood vessels is proportional to the temperature of the outer skin layer (within limits) and again run the model and compare results with those in Fig. 7.3.1.

7.4. **(a)** Make the model more accurate and detailed by dividing it into two anatomical parts, a head and the rest of the body. Modify THERMO to make this change, and again run it and check against Fig. 7.3.1, with discussion and explanation of changes noted in response.

(b) Put a layer of clothes on the body of the model in (a), and assume that this layer is equivalent to the skin layer without metabolism, sweat

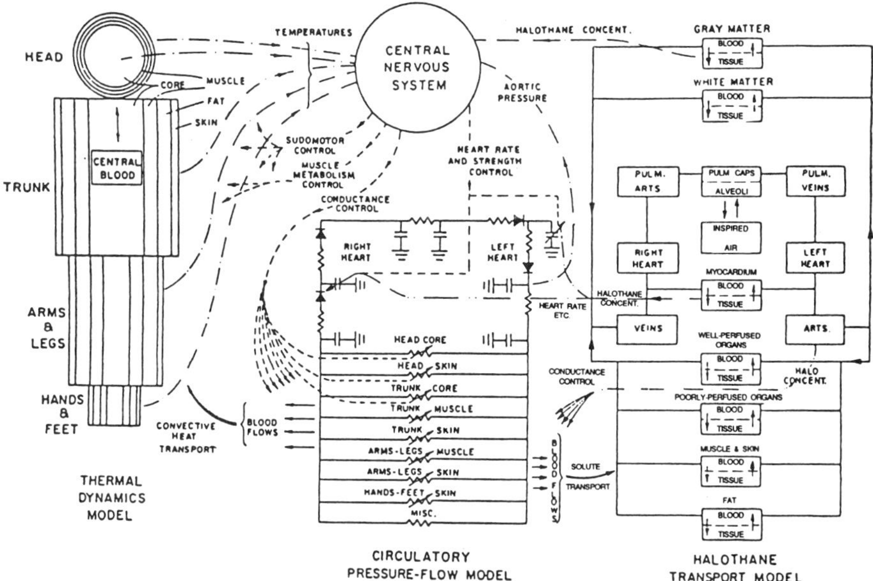

Figure 7.5.1. Model of an infant including effects of hypothermia and anesthesia. (Slate-77b, with permission).

glands or blood flow. Also assume that it is porous enough to allow skin evaporation to continue unchanged. Again run this program and check against the results in (a).

7.5. Use the data for an infant in Table 7.4.1 to set up a program corresponding to THERMO, with sweating and shivering controls (scaled for an infant) included. Compare temperature responses with those of the normal adult.

REFERENCES

ATKINS, A. R. AND C. H. WYNDHAM, "A study of temperature regulation in the human body with the aid of an analogue computer," *Pflugers Arch.*, Vol. 307, pp. 104–119; 1969.

BALDWIN, ERNEST, *Dynamic Aspects of Biochemistry,* Fifth Edition, Cambridge: Cambridge University Press; 1967.

BENZINGER, T. H., "The Human Thermostat," *Scientific American,* pp. 2–10, Jan. 1961.

BIRD, R. B., W. E. STEWART AND E. N. LIGHTFOOT, *Transport Phenomena,* New York: Wiley & Sons; 1960.

BLIGH, JOHN, *Temperature Regulation in Mammals and other Vertebrates,* Amsterdam: North-Holland; 1973.

CAMERON, J. R. AND J. G. SKOFRONICK, *Medical Physics,* New York: John Wiley & Sons; 1978.

CHAN, ANDREW K., ET AL., "Calculation by the method of finite differences of temperature distribution in layered tissues," *IEEE Trans. Biomed Eng.,* Vol. BME-20, No. 2, pp. 86–90; March, 1973.

CHARNY, C. K., M. J. HAGMANN, AND R. L. LEVIN, "A whole body thermal model of man during hyperthermia," *IEEE Trans. Biomed. Eng.,* BME-34, No. 5, pp. 375–87, May 1987.

CHARNY, C. K. AND R. L. LEVIN, "A whole body thermal model of man with a realistic circulatory system," *IEEE Trans. Biomed. Eng.,* Vol. 35, No. 5, pp. 362–71, May 1988.

COLIN, JEAN, ET AL., "Combined effect of radiation and convection," Chap. 7 in *Physiological and Behavioral Temperature Regulation,* J. D. Hardy et al. (Eds); Springfield, IL: Charles C. Thomas; 1970.

COONEY, DAVID O., *Biomedical Engineering Principles,* New York: Marcel Dekker, Inc.; 1976.

COOPER, K. E. AND D. N. ROSS, *Hyperthermia in Surgical Practice,* Philadelphia: F. A. Davis Co.; 1960.

CURTIS, R. M. AND G. J. TREZEK, "Analysis of heat exchange during cooling and rewarming in cardiopulmonary bypass procedures," in *Heat Transfer in Medicine and Biology,* Vol. 2, A. Schitzer and R. C. Eberhart, (Eds.), New York: Plenum Press, 1985.

DAMATO, A. N., ET AL., "Cardiovascular response to acute thermal stress (hot dry environment) in unacclimated normal subjects," *Am. Heart J.,* Vol. 76, pp. 769–74; Dec. 1968.

GORDON, R. G., R. B. ROEMER, AND S. M. HORVARTH, "A mathematical model of the human thermoregulatory system—transient cold response," *IEEE Trans. Biomed. Eng.,* Vol. BME-23, pp. 434–44; Nov. 1976.

HAHN, G. M., "Hyperthermia for the engineer: a short biological primer," *IEEE* - TMBE; Vol. BME-31, No. 1, pp. 3–8; 1984.

HARDING, P. G. R., "The metabolism of brown and white adipose tissue in the fetus and newborn," *Clin. Obstet. Gynecol.,* Vol. 14, pp. 685–709; 1971.

HEIM, T., "Thermogenesis in the newborn infant," *Clin. Obstet. Gynecol.*; Vol. 14, pp. 780–821; 1971.

HO, S. P., AND S. S. T. FAN, "Effect of clothing on the temperature distribution of human thermal system," *Comput. Biol. Med.,* Vol. 5, pp. 203–19; 1975.

HUCKABA, C. E. AND H.-S. TAM, "Modeling the Human Thermal System," Chap 1 in *Advances in Biomedical Engineering,* Part 1, New York: Marcel Dekker Inc., David O. Cooney, (Ed.); 1980.

HWANG, C-L. AND S. A. KONZ, "Engineering models of the human thermoregulatory system—a review," *IEEE Trans. Biomed. Eng.,* Vol. BME-24, No. 4, pp. 309–25; July 1977.

IBERALL, A. S., "Comments on 'A Review on Mathematical Models of the Human Thermal System,'" *IEEE Trans. Biomed. Eng.*, Vol. 18, p. 67; Jan. 1972.

JAIN, RAKESH K., "Heat transfer in tumors: Characterization and applications to thermography and hyperthermia," Chap. 2 in *Advances in Biomedical Engineering,* Part 1; New York: Marcel Dekker; David O. Cooney, (Ed.); 1980.

KONZ, S., ET AL., "An experimental validation of mathematical simulation of human thermoregulation," *Comput. Biol. Med.*, Vol. 7, pp. 71–82; 1977.

MARTIN, H. C. AND G. F. CAREY, *Introduction to Finite Element Analysis,* New York: McGraw-Hill; 1973.

MITCHELL, J. W. AND J. E. MYERS, "An analytical model of the countercurrent heat exchange phenomena," *Biophys. J.*, Vol. 8, pp. 897–911; 1968.

PLUMMER, S. J., "A Hybrid Computer Model of the Full-Term Human Neonate's Thermoregulatory System," (M.S. thesis, University of Wisconsin) 1974.

SEAGRAVE, R. C., *Biomedical Applications of Heat and Mass Transfer,* Ames, Iowa: Iowa State University Press; 1971.

SLATE, JOHN B., "A Model of the Human Thermoregulatory and Cardiovascular Systems During Anesthesia and Hypothermia," (M.S. thesis, University of Wisconsin) 1977.

———, V. C. RIDEOUT AND E. H. BLACKSTONE, "Simulation of thermoregulation and anesthesia in the human," *Proc. 1977 Summer Computer Sim. Conf.*, pp. 471–76; 1977.

SMITH, G. D., *Numerical Solution of Partial Differential Equations,* New York: Oxford Univ. Press; 1965.

STOLWIJK, J. A. J. AND J. D. HARDY, "Temperature regulation in man—a theoretical study," *Pflugers Arch.*, Vol. 291, pp. 129–62, 1966.

———. "Control of body temperature," pp. 45–67, in *Handbook of Physiology—Reactions to Environmental Agents,* D. H. K. Lee, (Ed.): Bethesda: Am. Physiol. Soc.; 1977.

STROHBEHN, J. W. AND R. B. ROEMER, "A survey of computer simulations of hyperthermia treatments," *IEEE Trans. Biomed. Eng.*, Vol. BME-31, No. 1, pp. 136–49; 1984.

WISSLER, E. H., "A mathematical model of the human thermal system," *Bull. Math. Biophys.*, Vol. 26, pp. 147–66; 1964.

8

Some Physiological and Prosthetic System Models

8.0 INTRODUCTION

Many different physiological systems or groups of systems have been modeled, and descriptions of these models have appeared in the medical and bioengineering literature. Only a few models are discussed here, with a view toward illustrating their wide variety and the different modeling styles that have been found useful. The usefulness of such programs as ACSL in dealing with nonlinear systems is emphasized.

Prosthetic systems now include, in addition to the rather familiar limb prostheses, a growing number of systems designed for automated drug infusion, as well as aids for vision and hearing. It was mentioned (in Section 2.3) that systems for automating drug infusion may require rather sophisticated design methods. Such systems, together with the highly developed noninvasive measuring schemes of today, require that knowledge and skill in physics and chemistry and many branches of engineering be combined with medical science. Only a few systems can be described here, and emphasis will be given to the most difficult part, the modeling of the relevant physiological systems.

8.1 MODELS OF BODY FLUID VOLUME REGULATION

The system for regulation of body fluid volume (also called the water balance system) is important to an understanding of diseases such as hypertension and their causes. At first, this system may seem to be a simple one, but on closer examination it may be seen to involve many other systems. As discussed in Section 2.5, the modeling of such complex systems may begin with the use of formal methods such as interpretive structural modeling, described by Sage (Sage-77), or more *ad hoc* methods may be used. Often models are built up from a simple initial form by adding those components and interconnections found to be important, with a final reduction of the model to the minimum size (*parsimonious* modeling) essential to the objectives of the modeler.

Some models have appeared that illustrate the complexity of fluid volume regulation, with its interrelationships to the renal, respiratory, and cardiovascular systems, including effects of mechanical, endocrine, and neural interaction. Such models include those by (Abbrecht-80) and (Ikeda-79), as well as the very large and involved Guyton-Coleman model (Guyton-67,72), which has been studied (Meij-73) and reviewed (Sagawa-75) in some detail. It is best to begin with the simplest possible model of this system, used by Guyton to illustrate the interrelationship between water balance and hypertension.

Figure 8.1.1 shows the Guyton-Coleman model as a single-loop feed-

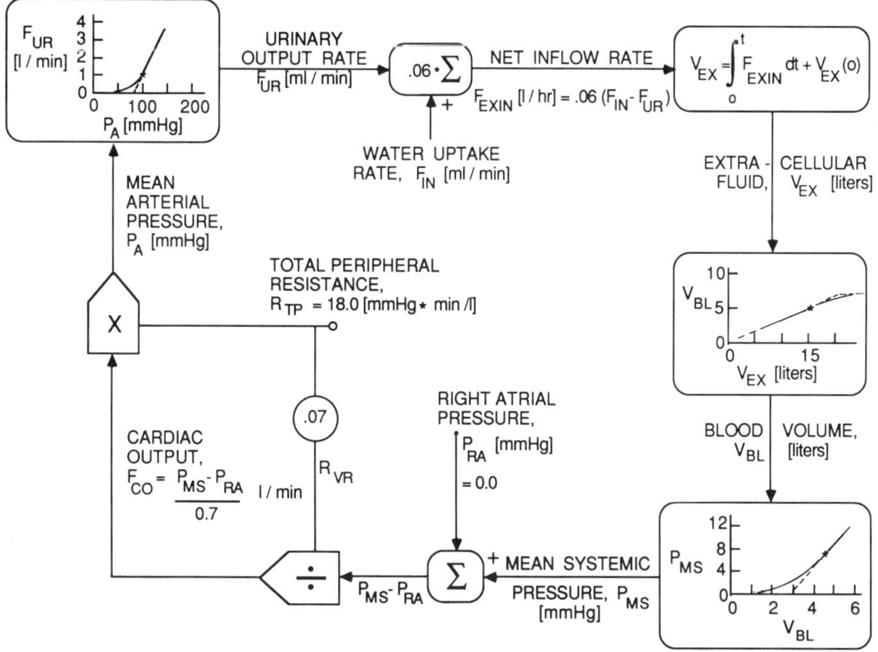

Figure 8.1.1. The Guyton-Coleman body fluid balance system in simple single-loop form. Points of operation in steady state are marked on the nonlinear transfer function curves.

back system, with simple (and necessarily incomplete) single-variable nonlinear relationships for the renal, blood volume, and mean systemic pressure systems. A multiplication and a division convert the mean systemic pressure P_{MS} to mean arterial pressure P_A in a simplified example of what is fondly referred to as "Guytonian mechanics" (Guyton-75, Chau-84, Coleman-90).

The only time-dependent block in this model is an integrator that sums the difference between rates of water uptake F_{IN} and urinary output F_{UR}, to give the extracellular volume V_{EX}. This integration is very important, making the system a type 1 control system (see Appendix C) and providing infinite gain in the loop in steady state, tending to hold $F_{UR} = F_{IN}$.

This model may be linearized about some narrow range of operation and studied as a linear control system. Dotted straight lines have been drawn through the normal operating points (each marked by an X), tangential at these points to the nonlinear curves in the block diagram of Fig. 8.1.1. Equations corresponding to these lines, with upper and lower limits (UL and LL) indicated and units shown are as follows:

Blood volume V_{BL} (in liters):

$$V_{BL} = 0.33 * V_{EX} \; \{\text{UL at } V_{BL} = 6.0\} \tag{8.1.1}$$

Mean systemic pressure (in mm Hg):

$$P_{MS} = 3.5 * (V_{BL} - 3) \; \{\text{LL at } P_{MS} = 0.0\} \tag{8.1.2}$$

Cardiac output (in liters/min):

$$F_{CO} = (P_{MS} - P_{RA})/R_{VR} = (P_{MS} - P_{RA})/(.07 * R_{TP})$$

Mean arterial pressure (in mm Hg):

$$P_A = F_{CO} * R_{TP}$$

The last two equations may be combined, and, assuming right atrial pressure $P_{RA} = 0$, this yields the mean arterial pressure P_A:

$$P_A = P_{MS} / .07 \tag{8.1.3}$$

Urinary output rate F_{UR} (in ml/min):

$$F_{UR} = 0.05 * (P_A - 80) \; \{\text{LL at } F_{UR} = 0.0\} \tag{8.1.4}$$

The water uptake rate F_{IN} is also in ml/min, and the net flow into extracellular space, in liters/hr, is

$$F_{EXIN} = 0.06 * (F_{IN} - F_{UR}) \tag{8.1.5}$$

where $60/1000 = 0.06$ is the conversion factor from ml/min to liters/hr.

The final (and most important) equation is the integration that yields extracellular volume V_{EX}, in liters:

$$V_{EX} = \int_0^t F_{EXIN}\, dt + V_{EX}(0) \tag{8.1.6}$$

where t is in hours, and the initial volume $V_{EX}(0)$ is yet to be determined.

The effect of feedback in the steady state will be to make F_{UR} equal to F_{IN}. Equations (8.1.1) to (8.1.6) may then be expressed as follows:

$$\begin{aligned} V_{EX} &= V_{EX}(0) \\ V_{BL} &= V_{EX}/3.0 \\ P_{MS} &= 3.5 * (V_{BL} - 3.0) \\ P_A &= P_{MS}/0.07 \\ F_{UR} &= (P_A - P_{AZ}) * 0.05 = 1.0 \end{aligned} \tag{8.1.7}$$

where $F_{IN} = 1.0$, $P_{RA} = 0.0$, and $P_{AZ} = 80$.

The solution of (8.1.7) yields the following steady-state values:

$$P_A = 100.0,\ P_{MS} = 7.0,\ V_{BL} = 5.0, \text{ and } V_{EX} = 15.0 \tag{8.1.8}$$

These results, as well as transient responses, may be obtained with the ACSL program B-FLUID for body fluid dynamics, based on (8.1.1) to (8.1.6). (Note that BOUND commands have been included for the limits shown in (8.1.1), (8.1.2), and (8.1.4), together with other limits that are realistic but probably will not be needed.)

```
PROGRAM B-FLUID
   Constant TF = 48.
 DYNAMIC
   Cinterval CINT = 0.1
  DERIVATIVE
   Algorithm IALG = 4    $'Runge-Kutta 2'
   Maxterval MAXT = .05  $ Nsteps NSTP=1
  'Equations'
   VBL = BOUND( 0.0, 6.0, VEX/3.0)
   PMS = BOUND( 0.0, 25.0, 3.5*(VBL - 3.0))
   PA  = PMS/0.07
   'FCNSW changes PAZ to PAX at T=0.0, and to PAY at TP'
   Constant PAX=80.0, PAY=80.0, TP=180.0
   PAZ= FCNSW(T-TP, PAX, PAX, PAY)
   FUR = BOUND( 0.0, 25.0, .05*(PA-PAZ))
   FEXIN = 0.06 * (FIN - FUR)
   VEX = INTEG( FEXIN, VEXIC)
   Constant VEXIC =15.0, A=0.0, FINIC=1.0, TI=4.0, FINAD=0.5
   FIN = FINIC + A*FCNSW( T-TI, 0.0, 0.0, FINAD)
  'Use A=1. to increase water uptake by FINAD at TI'
  END $'Of Deriv.'
```

```
    TERMT (T .GE. TF)
    PMSE  = .1332*PMS          $'European or SI'
    PAE   = .1332*PA           $'units in kilopascals'
  END   $'Of Dynamic'
END     $'Of Program'
```

The system described by this program is linear if none of the limits are entered. Its linear operation may be checked by introducing a small step increase in water uptake and checking the results against a simple linear analysis. If we set $A = 1$ at run time, all variables should hold constant only until $T = T_I = 4$ hr, and then changes should occur as water uptake F_{IN} is suddenly stepped up from its normal value of 1 to 1.5 ml/min. Results of such a run are shown in Fig. 8.1.2a. Here the variables

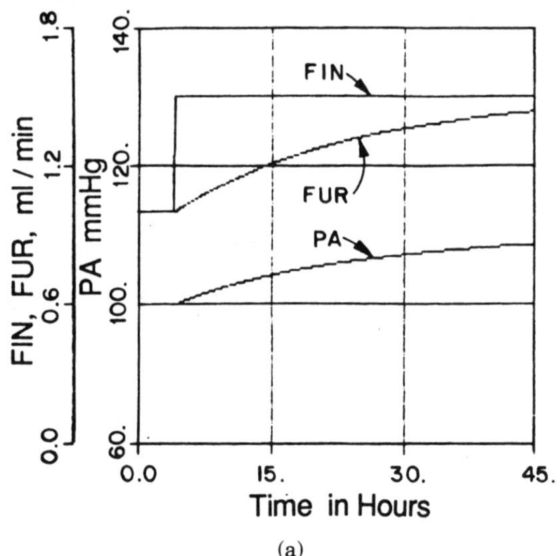

(a)

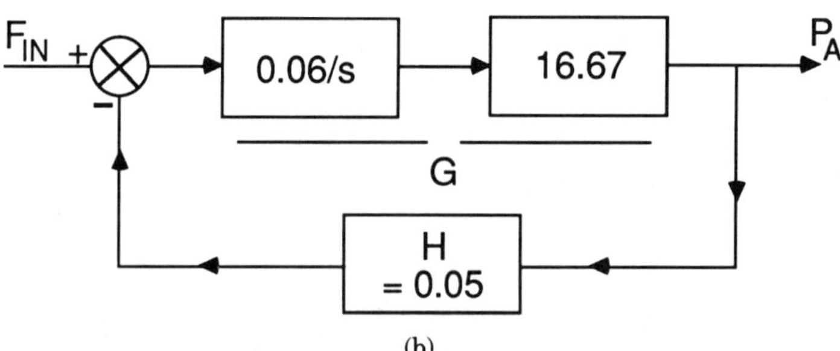

(b)

Figure 8.1.2. (a) Program B-FLUID responding to a step increase in water uptake FIN at T = 4.0 hrs.
(b) Simple equivalent linear control system for the system of Fig. 8.1.1.

are initially at the values given by (8.1.8), as shown for F_{UR} and P_A. After the step increase in F_{IN} at $T = 4$, P_A tends to increase to a value that raises F_{UR} to 1.5 ml/min to equal F_{IN} in a $(1 - \epsilon^{-t/\tau})$ manner, where τ is a time constant. Such an increase, at $t = \tau$, will reach $100*(1 - 1/\epsilon) = 63.2$ percent of its final increase. An examination of either the curve for F_{UR} or P_A indicates that τ is about 20 hrs.

The value of τ will now be calculated for the linearized system using the control loop shown in Fig. 8.1.2b. This figure was obtained from the linear equations derived from (8.1.1) to (8.1.6) by a further linearization technique in which we consider only small excursions (ΔV_{BL} for change in blood volume and so on) about the operating points shown in Fig. 8.1.1:

$$\begin{aligned}
\Delta V_{BL} &= \Delta V_{EX}/3 \\
\Delta P_{MS} &= 3.5*\Delta V_{BL} \\
\Delta P_A &= \Delta P_{MS}/0.07 \\
\Delta F_{UR} &= 0.05*\Delta P_A \\
\Delta F_{EXIN} &= 0.06*(\Delta F_{IN} - \Delta F_{UR}) \\
\Delta V_{EX} &= \Delta F_{EXIN}/s \qquad \text{(in Laplace notation)}
\end{aligned} \tag{8.1.9}$$

Combining these to find a control loop with ΔF_{IN} as input and ΔP_A as output gives the system shown in Fig. 8.1.2b in which the forward gain and feedback gain are

$$G = 1.0/s \text{ and } H = 0.05 \tag{8.1.10}$$

Thus the response to an input step of ΔF_{IN} of $F_{INAD} = 0.5$ will be (see Appendix C)

$$\begin{aligned}
\Delta P_A &= \frac{G}{1 + G*H} * \Delta F_{IN}/s \\
&= \frac{0.5}{s(s + 0.05)}
\end{aligned} \tag{8.1.11}$$

This response, in the time domain, may be obtained from this equation by use of Laplace transform pair 7 (in Appendix B):

$$\begin{aligned}
\Delta P_A &= (0.5/0.05)*(1 - \epsilon^{-0.05t}) \\
&= 10*(1 - \epsilon^{-t/20})
\end{aligned} \tag{8.1.12}$$

Thus the time constant is 20.0 hrs, and the final value of ΔP_A is 10.0 mm Hg. These values check with the computed results in Fig. 8.1.2a.

An interesting nonlinear result may be obtained with the computer model in which it is used to find the effect of changes in the response of the kidney to changes in P_A (which might be caused by changes in flow

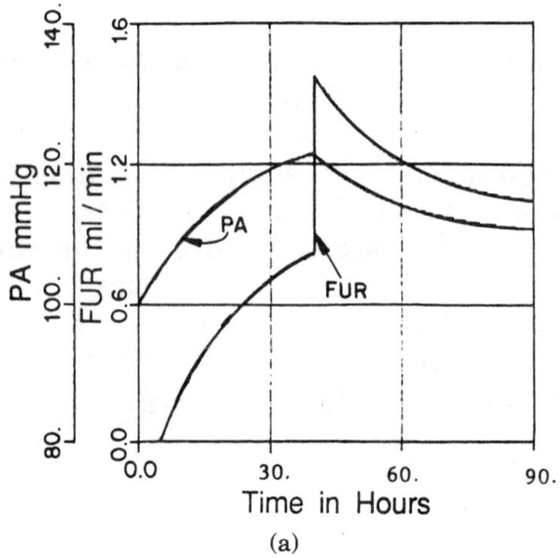

(a)

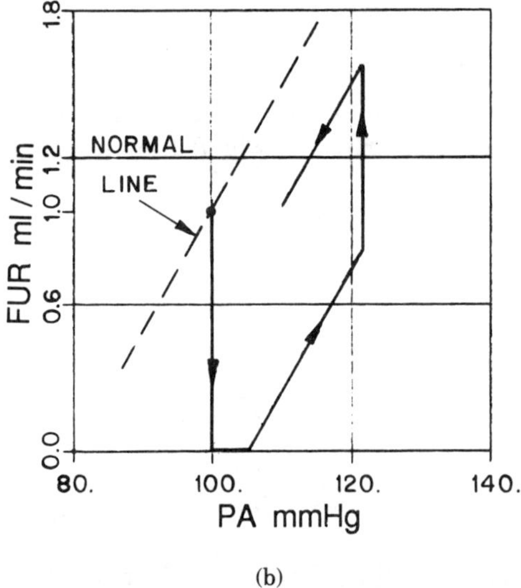

(b)

Figure 8.1.3. (a) Time response if the response curve for FUR vs. PA (see Fig. 8.1.1) is suddenly shifted to the right (without a change in slope) by setting PAZ = 105. at T = 0. This runs the arterial pressure up from 100. to about 125. at T = 40.0; the value of the pressure offset, PAZ is then reduced to 90.0 and pressure falls, but some hypertension remains.
(b) Phase plane plot corresponding to responses in (a). Here the old transfer function curve is shown aas a dashed line, and arrows indicate the direction of changes with time on the solid line.

resistance in the renal arteries). This may be done by the following run-time command:

```
SET TP=40.0, PAX=105.0, PAY=90.0, TF=90.0
```

This command will change the pressure offset PAZ from 80 to 105 mm Hg at $T = 0.0$, then back to 90 at $T = 40$. The resultant transients start at $T = 0$ and are plotted versus time in Fig. 8.1.3a. In Fig. 8.1.3b, a "phase plane" plot of F_{UR} vs. P_A shows a locus of the entire response.

It must be emphasized that this single-loop model is much too simple to represent body fluid regulation, except in the most elementary manner. Other control loops must be added before the model can be seriously used (Guyton-67,72,75, Sagawa-75). However, it serves to illustrate the concepts and use of linearization, with its advantages in finding a closed-form solution for small signals, and indicates how the computer simulation with nonlinearities included may be checked.

A next step in development of the model discussed here might be to include better representation of curvatures in the nonlinear functions, using table-defined functions such as the one introduced in Chapter 5.

8.2 INTRA-AORTIC BALLOON PUMPING

Temporary support for a weakened left ventricle can be provided by *intra-aortic balloon pumping* or *counterpulsation* (Philippe-80, Plummer-89). This procedure may be used after a myocardial infarction has occurred causing cardiogenic shock. Shock may lead to a vicious cycle in which release of catecholamines results in increased afterload, reduced cardiac output and thus reduced coronary flow that in turn causes further weakening of the heart. Preload (atrial pressure) increases as the cycle progresses, and complete failure and death may occur.

The balloon counterpulsation scheme is one in which a balloon (of 30 to 40 cc expanded volume) is inserted via the femoral artery into the descending aorta. This balloon is attached to a pump through a catheter, and actuating signals cause balloon inflation (with carbon dioxide or helium) from just after systole until nearly the end of diastole. With a balloon-pumping system in place and operating, the downstream flow is increased and reverse flow to the heart during diastole is impeded, thus reducing the pressure at the aortic root during diastole. As a result the cardiac output increases, but the heart does less work, and thus may be able to recover somewhat from shock.

Modeling studies are useful to determine the advantages of balloon pumping and to study some of the problems that can occur (Jelinak-72, Clark-73, 80).

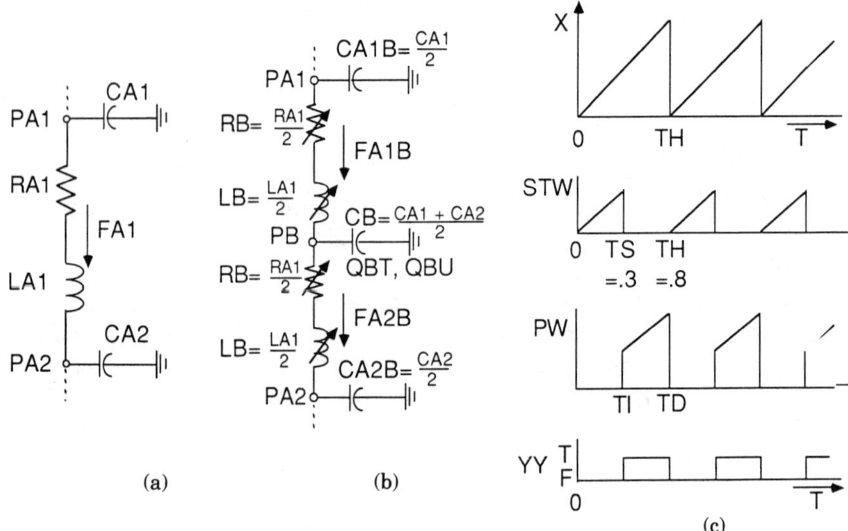

Figure 8.2.1. (a) Original first aortic branch in PF-1.
(b) Balloon pumping T-section to replace first aortic branch.
(c) Sequence for determining balloon inflation logic signal YY (usually initiated in the model at some later time TBP).

A model from Section 4.3, PF-1, can be used for a preliminary modeling study of balloon pumping; with modifications, it will be named PF-1-BP. The only change is to insert a balloon model at a point (see Fig. 4.3.5) corresponding to the upper part of the aorta, between compliances CA1 and CA2 (with pressures PA1 and PA2). The series R-L branch (see Fig. 8.2.1a) was replaced by a T-section (shown in Fig. 8.2.1b) with half of the compliance of CA1 and CA2 placed in a new compliance CB and the remaining halves now called CA1B and CA2B. The parameters RA1 and LA1 are split as shown. The parameters (for the balloon deflated) are as follows:

```
CA1B = .00009, CA2B = .00012
QA1BU = 18.1,  QA2BU = 21.0
CB = (CA1 + CA2)/2 = .0002
RB = RA1/2 = 2.5
LB = LA1/2 = 0.25
QBU = (QA1U + QA2U)/2 = 59.1
TI = 0.305, TD = .79, TBP = 16.0, RR = 0.5
```

The last line refers to balloon inflation time, TI, just past the end of systole in each cycle, balloon deflation time, TD, near the end of diastole, and the time of pump turn-on, TBP. The constant RR is the maximum ratio of balloon radius to aortic radius.

Within DERIVATIVE the logic signal YY is set up to be TRUE when cycle time is between TI and TD and less than TBP, using:

```
YY =(X .GE. TI) .AND. (X .LE. TD) .AND. (T .GE. TBP),
```

where X is the sawtooth timing signal used in both PF-1 and in PF-1-BP, as shown in Fig. 8.2.1c. Some computations are also needed (see Section 4.1) to find the values of the varying parameters (indicated by an added subscript, V) when the balloon is inflated to half its possible radius (RR = 0.5). Also note that wall damping (RPW1) is included in series with CA1B.

```
RY = RSW( YY, RR, 1.0) $ '(RY will follow the radius change)'
RX = REALPL ( TX, RY, 1.0) $ '(gives some smoothing of RY)'
Constant TX = 0.1
RBV = RB / (RX)**4
LBV = LB / (RX)**2
CBV = CB * (RX)**3
QBUV= QBU/ (RX)**2
```

The flow equations for FA1 and FA2 in DERIVATIVE in PF-1 should be omitted, and the following new or modified equations introduced:

```
PA1 = (QA1 - QA1BU)/CA1B + KP1*RPW1*(FLV-FA1B)
FA1B = (1./LBV)*INTEG( PA1 - PB - RBV*FA1B, 0.0)
QA1 = INTEG( FLV - FA1B, QA1BIC)
PB  = (QB - QBUV)/CBV
FA2B = (1./LBV)*INTEG( PB - PA2 - RBV*FA2B, 0.0)
QBP = INTEG( FA1B - FA2B, QBIC)
PA2 = (QA2 - QA2BU)/CA2B
QA2 = INTEG( FA2B - FA2, QA2BIC)
```

In test experiments with PF-1-BP an infarction of the left ventricle was set up to occur at T = 4.8, with LS being reduced from 2500.0 to 750.0; results of this and of balloon pumping being started at T = 16.0 are shown in Fig. 8.2.2. In this figure it can be seen that downstream aortic pressure and stroke volume showed a good recovery after a few beats of balloon pumping.

Stroke volume and cardiac work were measured during systole, using a *moded* integrator (MODINT) with XX as a control signal to reset the MODINT each beat so that integration was over the systolic period only. The required command is

```
SV = MODINT( FLV, 0.0, .T., XX)
```

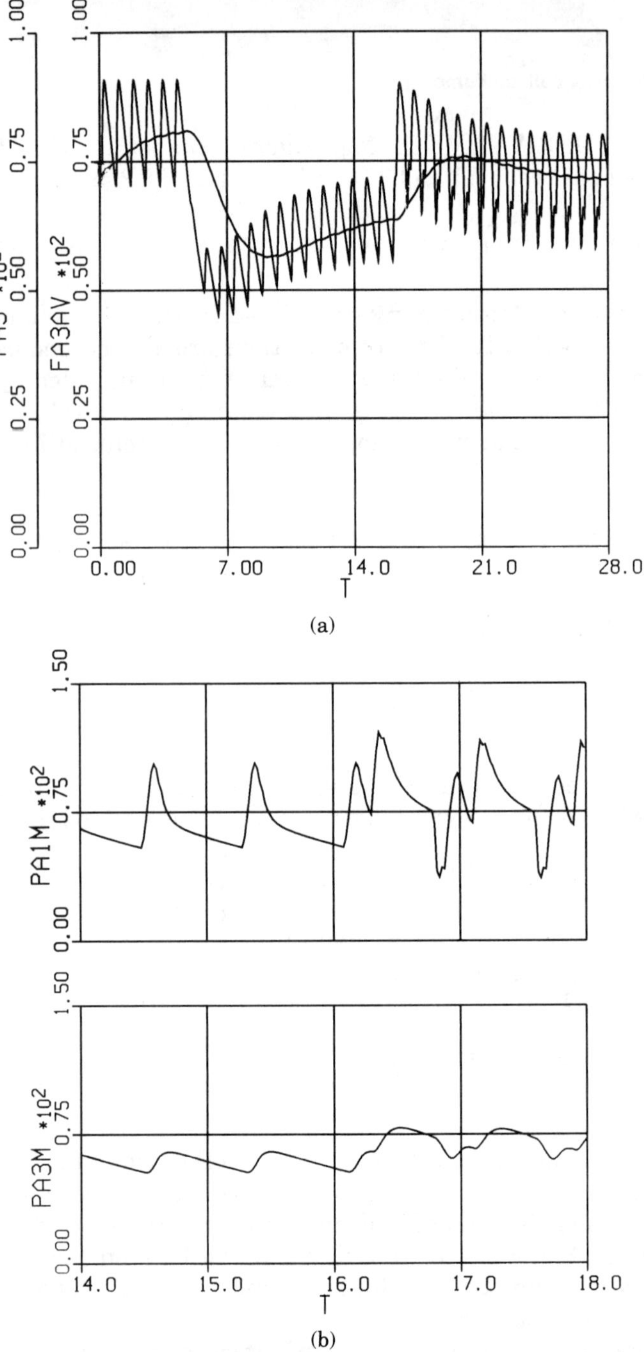

Figure 8.2.2. Some model outputs obtained with model PF-1-BP showing the effects of balloon pumping (after T = 16.0) upon cardiovascular variables after a myocardial infarction (at T = 4.8).
(a) Aortic flow FA3 downstream from the balloon with a plot of filtered FA3 (FA3AV) superimposed.
(b) Details of PA1M and PA3M around the time (16.0 sec) that pumping begins. Note the strong counterpulse appearing within diastole.

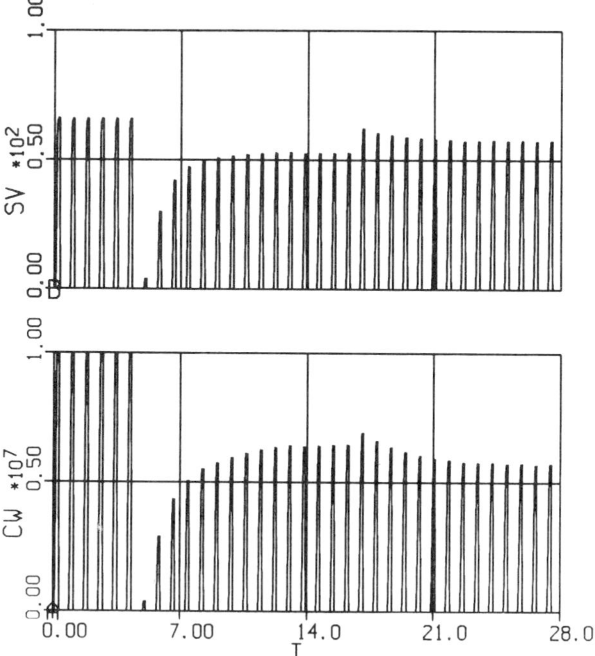

Figure 8.2.3. Plots of LV stroke volume SV (in ml), and cardiac work CW (in dyne cm.), when an infarction at 4.8 sec is followed by balloon pumping at 16 sec.

Similarly, cardiac work during each beat was measured using

```
CW = MODINT( PLV*FLV, 0.0, .T., XX)
```

Results from model PF-1-BP shown in Fig. 8.2.3 indicate that reduced cardiac work and increased stroke volume resulted from the use of counterpulsation. Modeling studies of this kind may be important in the design of control systems for balloon pumping and for optimization (Barnea-90, Zelano-90).

8.3 GLUCOSE-INSULIN MODELS

A presentation of a computer model of the glucose-insulin system was made by Stolwijk and Hardy in 1974 (Stolwijk-74). Randall, who later included a Basic-language model of this system in his biomodeling text (Randall-80), points out that the Stolwijk-Hardy model, expressed in both Fortran and analog computer form, was one of the first models to appear with computer coding included in a major medical text. The system was also presented (see Fig. 8.3.1) in hydraulic analog form.

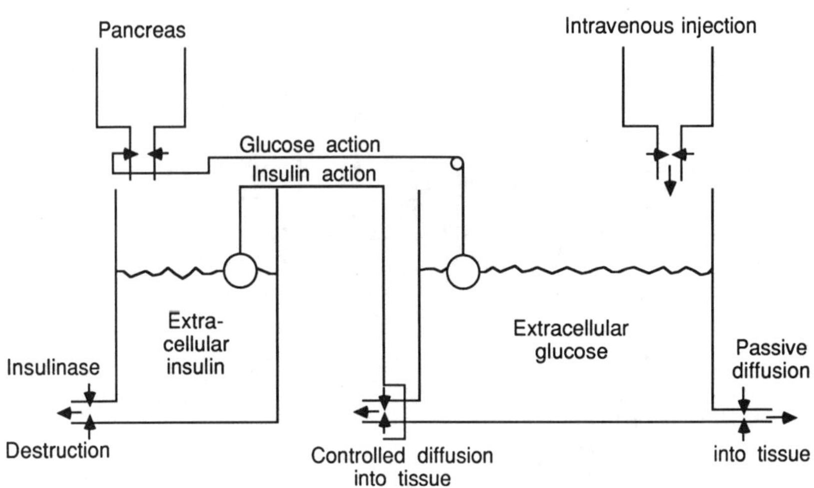

Figure 8.3.1. Hydraulic analog of insulin-glucose regulation (from Stolwijk-74 with permission). In this model it may be seen that feedback from glucose level to insulin supply results from glucose activation of the pancreas, while insulin level completes the feedback path by controlling the major flow of glucose into tissue.

The Stolwijk-Hardy model is presented here as an ACSL program and its analysis is included as an example of a negative feedback system containing a strong nonlinearity. Nomenclature has been changed to correspond to the general scheme discussed in Chapter 2, with the first letter in each variable name corresponding to the kind of variable (F for flow, C for concentration, and so on) and the second letter, or first subscript, for the substance (G for glucose, I for insulin) and so forth. The model is a simple one, but serves to illustrate basic features of the system, including its response to a sudden increase in glucose input for a short period. It also serves as an example of the use of a combination of analytical and computer approaches in a nonlinear system. More detailed and useful computer models of this system have been described (Albisser-80, Carson-76).

The system, shown in block form in Fig. 8.3.2, is a multiple model in which the pool of extracellular fluid is shown twice, once for glucose (with concentration C_G) and once for insulin (concentration C_I). These concentrations are obtained by integration of net flows in and out (mass balance), divided by the effective volumes of the extracellular fluid for these two substances, $V_G = 150$ and $V_I = 150$. (These volumes have been divided by 100, so that their units are mg% and mU%.)

The concentrations (in units of mg/mg% for C_G and mU/mU% for C_I) are given by

$$C_G = \int_o^t ((F_{GL} + F_{GI} - F_{GF} - F_{GR} - F_{GC})/V_G)\ dt \qquad (8.3.1)$$

$$C_I = \int_o^t ((F_{IP} - F_{IF})/V_I)dt \qquad (8.3.2)$$

where t is in hours, and the flows are all in mg/hr in the first equation and mU/hr in the second. The flows are given by

$F_{GL} = 8400$, the normal flow rate from the liver (assumed constant) into the glucose compartment.

$F_{GI} = 80{,}000$, for a pulse lasting from $T_1 = 1.0$ to $T_2 = 1.5$ hr

$F_{GF} = K_1 * C_G = 24.7 * C_{GF}$ is the first-order decay of glucose, effectively an outflow.

$F_{GR} = K_2 * (C_G - C_{G2}) = 72 * (C_G - 250)$, limited or bounded by 0 and 10^5, the "renal spill," occurring only when $C_G > 250$.

$F_{GC} = K_3 * C_G * C_I = 13.9 * C_G * C_I$

$F_{IP} = K_4 * (C_G - C_{G4}) = 14.3 * (C_G - 51)$, bounded by 0 and 10^5, the insulin inflow from the pancreas, occurring only when $C_G > 51$ mg/hr.

$F_{IF} = K_5 * C_I = 76.0 * C_I$ is the first-order insulin loss.

The steady-state values and a linearized model of the variations from steady state may now be determined by a more formal method than

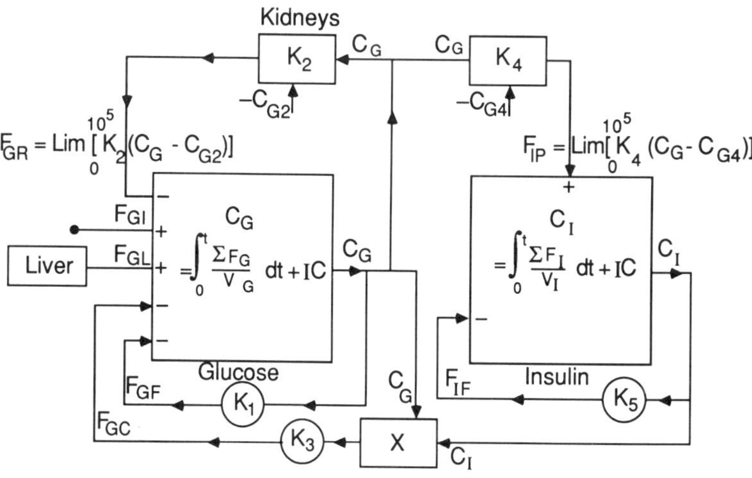

Figure 8.3.2. Block diagram of the glucose-insulin system.

that used in the preceding section. First of all, each dependent variable may be expressed as a steady-state quantity (indicated by adding a zero subscript) plus a varying delta quantity, $C_{GO} + \Delta C_G$, and so on. Equations (8.3.1) and (8.3.2) then become

$$\frac{d}{dt}(C_{GO} + \Delta C_G) = (F_{GLO} + \Delta F_{GL} + F_{GIO} + \Delta F_{GI} - F_{GFO} - \Delta F_{GF} - F_{GRO} - \Delta F_{GR} - F_{GCO} - \Delta F_{GC})/V_G \quad (8.3.3)$$

$$\frac{d}{dt}(C_{IO} + \Delta C_I) = (F_{IPO} + \Delta F_{IP} - F_{IFO} - \Delta F_{IF})/V_I \quad (8.3.4)$$

In steady state all delta quantities are zero, and since the derivatives of constants are also zero, we have

$$0.0 = F_{GLO} + F_{GIO} - F_{GFO} - F_{GRO} - F_{GCO} \quad (8.3.5)$$

$$0.0 = F_{IPO} - F_{IFO} \quad (8.3.6)$$

These can be solved using the parameter values given above, and assuming that infusion is zero (so that $F_{GIO} = 0.0$) and that flow F_{GRO} is zero (below the lower limit for F_{GR}) and that flow F_{IP} is within its limits, (all assumptions that should be checked later when steady-state values have been obtained.)

Substitution of numerical values into (8.3.5) and (8.3.6) gives

$$0.0 = 8400 + 24.7{*}C_{GO} + 13.9{*}C_{GO}{*}C_{IO} \quad (8.3.7)$$

$$0.0 = 14.3{*}(C_{GO} - 51) - 76{*}C_{IO} \quad (8.3.8)$$

Solving these simultaneously gives

$$C_{GO} = 81.0 \text{ and } C_{IO} = 5.645 \quad (8.3.9)$$

If the steady-state equations are subtracted from (8.3.3) and (8.3.4), only the delta or variable quantities remain, and thus the equations for a small input disturbance ΔF_{GI} are

$$d\Delta C_G/dt = (\Delta F_{GI} - K_1{*}\Delta C_G - K_3{*}C_{GO}{*}\Delta C_I - K_3{*}C_{IO}{*}\Delta C_G - K_3{*}\Delta C_G{*}\Delta C_I)/V_G \quad (8.3.10)$$

$$d\Delta C_I/dt = (K_4{*}\Delta C_G - K_5{*}\Delta C_I)/V_I \quad (8.3.11)$$

These equations are linear, except for the one product term involving $\Delta C_G{*}\Delta C_I$; since this is expected to be a product of two small quantities it may be neglected (although this may have to be checked as ΔF_{GI} is made larger). With this term omitted, the equations are linear, with constant coefficients and zero initial conditions, and Laplace transform methods may be used to find closed-form solutions. In the Laplace *s*-domain, (8.3.10) and (8.3.11) become

$$s\Delta C_G = \Delta F_{GI}(s) - (K_1 + K_3{*}C_{I0}){*}\Delta C_G - (K_3{*}C_{G0}){*}\Delta C_I \tag{8.3.12}$$

$$s\Delta C_I = K_4{*}\Delta C_G - K_5{*}\Delta C_I \tag{8.3.13}$$

These equations may be written as

$$\Delta C_G = \frac{\Delta F_{GI}(s) - (K_3{*}C_{G0}){*}\Delta C_I}{(s + a)} \tag{8.3.14}$$

$$\Delta C_I = \frac{K_4{*}\Delta C_G}{(s + b)} \tag{8.3.15}$$

where $a = K_1 + K_3{*}C_{I0}$, $b = K_5$, and the feedback loop has the form shown in Fig. 8.3.3.

The open-loop forward gain (see Appendix C) may be expressed as

$$G = K/((1 + sT_a){*}(1 + sT_b) \tag{8.3.16}$$

with feedback gain $H = K_3{*}C_{G0}$ and $K = K_3/(a{*}b)$

$$T_a = 1/a = 1/(K_1 + K_3{*}C_{I0}),\ T_b = 1/b = 1/K_5$$

The closed-loop gain is

$$\Delta C_I/\Delta F_{GI} = G/(1 + GH)$$

$$= K/(1 + K{*}H + s(T_a + T_b) + s^2T_a{*}T_b) \tag{8.3.17}$$

If ΔF_{GI} is some known simple function such as a step at $t = 0$, $\Delta F_{GI} = 100/s$, the response ΔC_I may easily be determined from (8.3.17). Also, the open-loop gain may be used to study stability of this system. (Because it only reaches 180 degrees of phase shift at infinite frequency, it will always be stable; however, its response may be quite oscillatory if the zero frequency gain is high.)

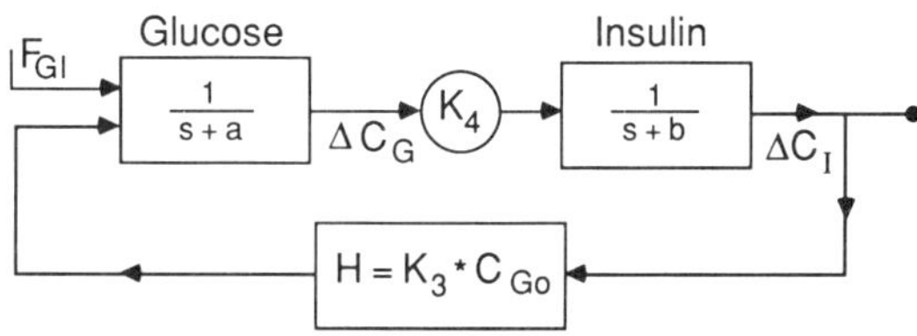

Figure 8.3.3. Linear approximate form of the glucose-insulin feedback loop for small inputs.

Solutions of the linearized equations for this system may also be used to check the ACSL or other language program used for the study of the complete nonlinear system. An ACSL program called GLUC-TOL (for glucose tolerance test) is shown below for the system of Eqs. (8.3.1) and (8.3.2)

```
PROGRAM GLUC-TOL
 DYNAMIC
   Cinterval CINT = .05
   Constant TF = 8.
   TERMT(T .GE. TF)

  DERIVATIVE
   Algorithm IALG = 4
   Maxterval MAXT = .01
   Nsteps NSTP = 1
   Constant FGL = 8400.          $'Gluose rate, from liver'
   FGI = A*PULSE (T1, 500., TP) $'Glucose injection rate'
   Constant T1 = 1.0, TP = 0.5, A = 80000.
   FGF = K1*CG                   $'First-order loss rate'
   Constant K1 = 24.7
   FGR = BOUND(0.0, 10000.,K2*(CG-CG2)) $'Renal spill'
   Constant K2 = 72.0, CG2 = 250.
   FGC = K3 * CG * CI            $'Controlled loss rate'
   Constant K3 = 13.9
   FIP = BOUND(0., 10000.,K4*(CG-CG4)) $'Insulin - pancreas'
   Constant K4 = 14.3, CG4 = 51.0
   FIF = K5 * CI                 $'First-order ins. loss rate'
   Constant K5 = 76.0
   CG = INTEG((FGL + FGI - FGF - FGR - FGC)/VG, CGIC)
                                  'Glucose concentration'
   CI = INTEG((FIP - FIF)/VI, CIIC)
                                  'Insulin concentration'
   Constant CGIC = 81.0, CIIC = 5.645, VG=150.0, VI= 150.0
  END
 END
END
```

In this program the initial conditions for the two integrations are set to the values determined by algebraic solution of the steady-state equations, as given in (8.3.9); they could also have been determined by initial guesses followed by a long run of the program with FGI held at zero (set A = 0.0 at run-time).

This program was allowed to run as given above for a final time of TF = 8.0 for normal pancreas (results in Fig. 8.3.4) and for a pancreas with reduced pancreas output (Fig. 8.3.5). The concentrations hold steady during the half-hour preliminary run before the input pulse of glucose showing that the initial conditions are correct. In all cases the concentration CG rises rapidly during the glucose input flow, then drops rapidly as a result of the increased CI. Both concentrations display some undershoot of the initial (and final) values, with a mild oscillation.

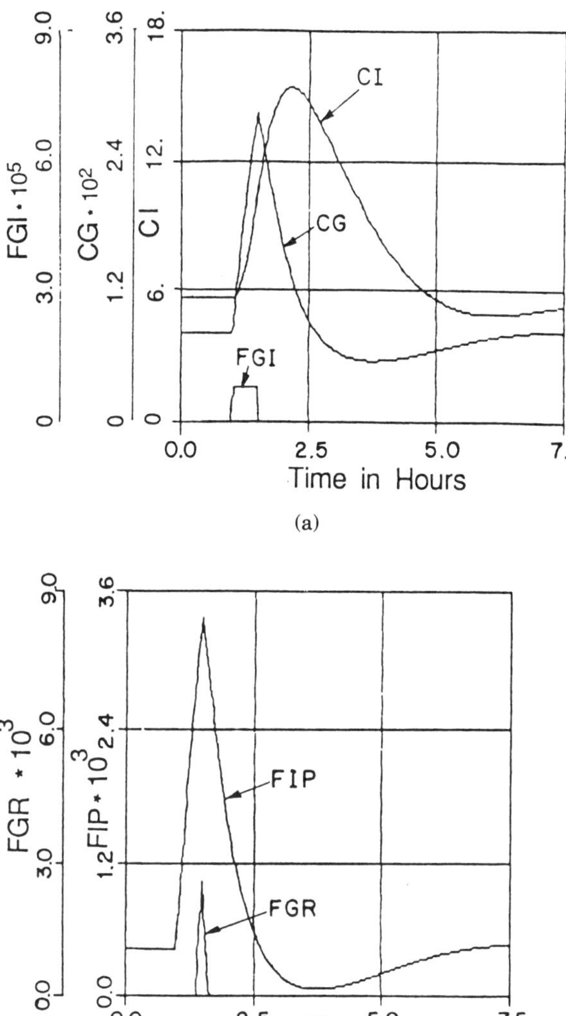

Figure 8.3.4. (a) Input pulse FGI and concentrations CG and CI, for a normal pancreas, obtained with program GLUC-TOL (Glucose Tolerance Test). (b) Normal flows from bounded limiters, FGR and FIP.

8.4 SOME OTHER PHYSIOLOGICAL AND PROSTHETIC MODELS

Endocrine system models, as discussed by McIntosh and McIntosh, may be developed and applied as in the case of the glucose-insulin model of Section 8.3 (McIntosh-80, Carson-82).

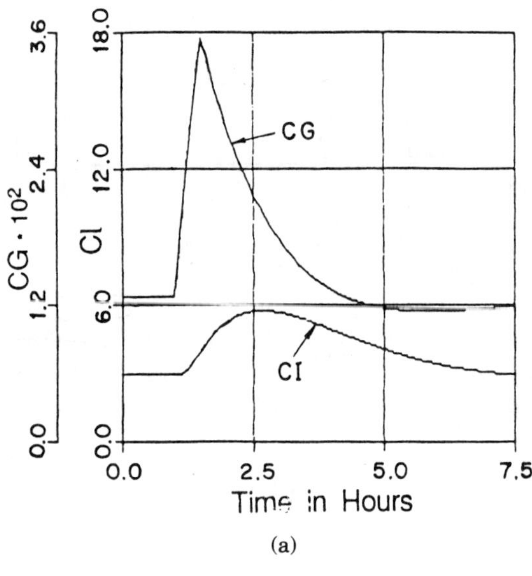

(a)

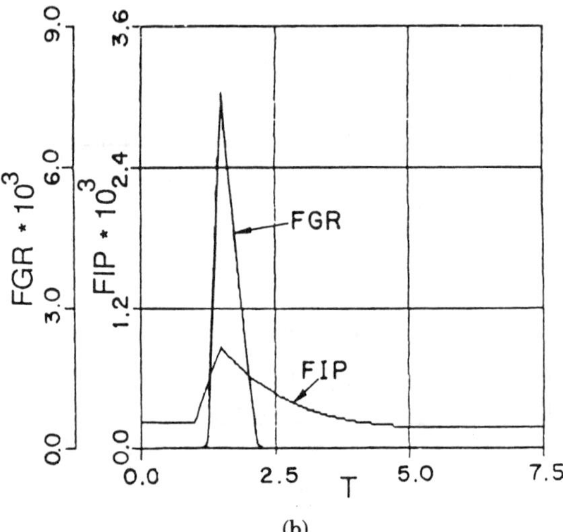

(b)

Figure 8.3.5. *(continued)*
(a) Concentrations if pancreas outflow is reduced five times (K4 = 2.86).
(b) Flows from bounded limiters corresponding to (a).

Models of pharmacokinetics may be devised, using simple compartmental schemes or the more physically based models of Bischoff and Dedrick (see references in Chapter 3). These models, describing the movement of the drug through the body, may be combined with pharmacodynamic models, which describe the reaction of the body to the drug

(Scheiner-79). Also, modeling studies of computer-controlled drug delivery schemes have appeared (Sheppard-80, Slate-79, Koivo-78, and Voss-86).

The administration of anesthetics and of associated drugs, such as those needed for muscle relaxation, lead to special problems in modeling, particularly when computer control is used (Lampard-73, Fukui-82, Ohlson-82, Jaklitsch-87, Tucker-85, and Schils-87). The use of multiple modeling in such systems may be important, and has been discussed in Chapter 6.

The modeling of kidney function offers problems because of its complexity (Chandhoke-81). An important prosthesis, the artificial kidney, has also been modeled (Abbrecht-78). Multiple modeling (using three interconnected models) has been used to follow the fluid flow within the kidney as well as the transport of NaCl and hippuran (Gianunzio-71).

The use of programs such as ACSL is advantageous in modeling any system with external computer control, partly because of the ease with which the computer and its program may be simulated.

PROBLEMS

8.1. The Guyton-Coleman model of fluid balance (Fig. 8.1.1) is described by Equations (8.1.7). These equations are set up in ACSL form in program B-FLUID. Response to a small (0.5 ml/min) step increase in water intake is shown in Fig. 8.1.2. Find the responses of the system to larger input changes of −1.0 and +2.0 ml/min, and discuss your results, giving some thought to the effects of system nonlinearities.

8.2. Model B-FLUID was used to show the effects of sudden increases in PAZ from 80.0 to 105.0, followed by a change back to 90.

(a) Repeat this experimental run and check your results against those shown in Fig. 8.1.3.

(b) Change PAZ from 80.0 to 60.0 at T=0 and then back to 70.0 at T=40, and show plots as in Fig. 8.1.3(b) for this case, and discuss.

(c) Use tables to introduce more smoothly varying nonlinear functions (to obtain FUR, VBL, and PMS), and compare output plots with those in Fig. 8.1.3.

8.3 Program PF-1-BP in Section 8.2 is a balloon-pumping version of PF-1. Make changes of plus or minus 0.15 sec in the on and off times TI and TD of the balloon pump and show the effects of these changes on pressures and flows. Discuss these results, keeping mind that the model has a fixed heart rate, and that normal variations in heart rate and systolic period may give rise to practical problems.

8.4. Modify PF-1-BP to include flow work, similar to cardiac work, but measured downstream from the balloon; again use a MODINT to reset the integrator with each beat.

8.5. The Stolwijk-Hardy glucose-insulin model shown in Figs. 8.3.1 and 8.3.2 is modeled in program GLUC-TOL;

(a) Run the model in its normal healthy condition, and check your results against Figs. 8.3.4(a) and (b).

(b) Use a parameter sweep modification of GLUC-TOL to reduce K4 in the equation for insulin outflow, FIP, from its normal value of 14.3 in six steps of 0.75 times. Plot the sequence of responses for CG, CI, FGR, and FIP and discuss the changes, and the effects of nonlinearities upon these output curves.

(c) For the case shown in Figs. 8.3.5(a) and (b) (where K4 is reduced by five times), show the effect of an injection of insulin at 2.5 hours.

REFERENCES

ABBRECHT, P. H. AND N. W. PRODANY, "A model of the patient-artificial kidney system," *IEEE-TBME,* Vol. BME-18, No. 4, pp. 257–64; 1978.

ABBRECHT, P. H., "Regulation of extracellular fluid volume and osmolality," *Ann. BME,* Vol. 8, pp. 461–72; 1980.

ALBISSER, A. M. ET AL, "Hypercomplex models of insulin and glucose dynamics—do they predict experimental results?," *Ann. BME,* Vol. 8, pp. 539–57; 1980.

BARNEA, O., ET AL, "Cardiac energy considerations during intra-aortic balloon pumping," *IEEE-TBME;* Vol. 37, No. 2, pp. 170–81; 1990.

CARSON, E. R. AND D. G. CRAMP, "A systems model of blood glucose control," *Intl. J. Bio-Med. Comp.,* Vol. 7, p. 21; 1976.

CARSON, E. R., C. COBELLI AND L. FINKELSTEIN, *"The Mathematical Modeling of Metabolic and Endocrine Systems,"* New York: Wiley & Sons; 1982.

CHANDHOKE, P. S. AND G. M. SAIDEL, "Mathematical model of mass transport throughout the kidney," *Ann. BME,* Vol. 9, No. 4, pp. 263–302; 1981.

CHAU, N. P., AND M. E. SAFAR, "Computer modeling in cardiovascular research: Guyton models and essential hypertension," in *"Computer Modeling of Complex Biological Systems,"* I. Iyengar and S. Sitharama (Eds.); Boca Raton, FL: CRC Press Inc.; 1984.

CLARK, JOHN W., JR. ET AL. "On the feasibility of closed loop control of intra-aortic balloon pumping," *IEEE-TBME,* Vol. BME-20, No. 6; pp. 404–12; 1973.

CLARK, J. W. ET AL, "Automatic control of a series-parallel circulatory assist system in severe uni- or biventricular failure," *Ann. BME,* Vol. 8, pp. 57–74; 1980.

COLEMAN, T. G. AND W. J. GAY, "Simulation of typical physiological systems," pp. 41–69 in *Advanced Simulation in Biomedicine,* D. Moller (Ed.), New York: Springer-Verlag; 1990.

FUKUI, Y., N. TY SMITH AND R. A. FLEMING, "Digital and sampled-data control of arterial blood pressure during halothane anesthesia," *Anesth. and Analgesia,* Vol. 61, No. 12; Dec. 1982.

GIANUNZIO, J. W., "A Multiple Model Study of Flow and Transport in the Cardiovascular-Renal System," (Ph.D. Thesis, University of Wisconsin-Madison) 1971.

GUYTON, A. C. AND T. G. COLEMAN, "Long-term regulation of the circulation: interrelationships with body fluid volumes," Chap. 11 in *Physical Bases of Circulatory Transport: Regulation and Exchange,* E. B. Reeve and A. C. Guyton (Eds.); Philadelphia: W. B. Saunders; 1967.

GUYTON, A. C., T. G. COLEMAN AND H. J. GRANGER, "Circulation: overall regulation," *Annual Rev. Physiol.,* Vol. 34, pp. 13–46; 1972.

GUYTON, A. C., A. E. TAYLOR AND H. J. GRANGER, "Quantitative analyses of body fluid regulation," Chap. 22 in *Circulatory Physiology II: Dynamics and control of the Body Fluids,* Philadelphia: W. B. Saunders; 1975.

IKEDA, NORIAKI ET AL, "A model of overall regulation of body fluids," *Ann. BME,* Vol. 8, pp. 431–44; 1979.

JAKLITSCH, R. R., AND D. R. WESTENSKOW, "A model-based self-adjusting two-phase controller for vecuronium-induced muscle relaxation during anesthesia," *IEEE-TBME,* Vol. BME-34, No. 8, pp. 583–94; 1987.

JELINEK, J., "Hemodynamics of counterpulsation: the study of a lumped-parameter computer model," *Jl. Biomechanics,* Vol. 5, pp. 511–19; 1972.

KOVIO, A. J., V. F. SMOLLEN AND R. V. BARILE, "An automated drug administration system to control blood pressure in rabbits," *Math. Biosci.,* Vol. 38, pp. 45–56; 1978.

LAMPARD, D. G., J. R. COLES AND W. A. BROWN, "Electronic digital computer control of ventilation and anesthesia," *Anaesth. & Intensive Care,* Vol. 1, p. 382; 1973.

MCINTOSH, J. E. A. AND R. P. MCINTOSH, *Mathematical Modeling and Computers in Endocrinology,* New York: Springer-Verlag; 1980.

MEIJ, S. H., "Hybrid simulation of the circulation and its overall regulation in the human body," *Laboratorium voor technische Naturkunde,* Delft; 1973.

OHLSON, K. B., D. R. WESTENSKOW AND W. S. JORDAN, "A microprocessor based feedback controller for mechanical ventilation," *Ann. BME,* Vol. 10, pp. 35–48; 1982.

PHILIPPE, E. ET AL, "Microprocessor control of intra-aortic balloon pumping," *Ann. BME,* Vol. 8, pp. 209–24; 1980.

PLUMMER, P. M., "Biomedical engineering fundamentals of the intra-aortic balloon Pump," *Biomedical Instrumentation & Technology,* pp. 452–59; 1989.

RANDALL, J. E., *Microcomputers and Physiological Simulation,* New York: Addison-Wesley; 1980.

SAGAWA, KIICHI, "Critique of a large-scale organ system model: the Guytonian cardiovascular model," *Annals BME,* Vol. 3, pp. 386–400; 1975.

SCHILS, G. F., F. J. SASSE AND V. C. RIDEOUT, "Automatic control of anesthesia using two feedback variables," *Ann. BME,* Vol. 15, pp. 19–34; 1987.

SHEINER, L. B. ET AL, "Simultaneous modeling of pharmacokinetics and pharmacodynamics: Application of d-tubocurarine," *Clin. Pharmacol.,* Vol. 25: pp. 358–71; 1979.

SHEPPARD, L. C., "Computer control of the infusion of vasoactive drugs," *Ann. BME,* Vol. 8, pp. 431–44; 1980.

SLATE, J. B. ET AL, "A model for design of a blood pressure controller for hypertensive patients," *Proc. Intl. Fed. of Auto. Control,* 5th Symposium on Identification and System Parameter Estimation, Darmstadt; 1979.

STOLWIJK, J. E. J. AND J. D. HARDY, "Regulation and control in physiology," Chap. 57 in *Medical Physiology,* (13th Ed.); Mountcastle, V. B. (Ed.); St. Louis: C. V. Mosby Co.; 1974.

TUCKER, G. T., "Pharmacokinetic models—different approaches," pp. 54–64 in *Quantitation Modelling and Control in Anesthesia;* H. Stoeckel (Ed.); New York: Thieme Inc.: 1985.

VOSS, G. I. ET AL, "Adaptive multivariable drug delivery: control of arterial pressure and cardiac output in anesthetized dogs," *IEEE-TBME,* Vol. BME-34, No. 8, pp. 617–23; 1987.

ZELANO, J. A. ET AL, "A closed-loop control scheme for intra-aortic balloon pumping," *IEEE-TBME,* Vol. BME-37, No. 2, pp. 182–92; 1990.

9
Parameter Estimation

9.0 MODEL-BASED PARAMETER ESTIMATION

Matching a model to a real system usually requires that a structural or topological correspondence between model and system be determined; this is sometimes called *structural* (or system) *identification*. After this has been done so that we can draw a model block diagram or write the equations needed to describe the system model, it is still necessary to find the numerical values of all unknown parameters. Various *parameter estimation* schemes may be used to determine these parameter values (Marquart-63, Fletcher-63, Lyung-87).

It is also possible to set up a "black box" model and use the same input signals for the system and this model. By matching the output signals as the black box transfer function is varied, we can make this function correspond to the unknown system. Something in between these two methods (often called "gray box" estimation), making some use of any structural knowledge of the system, may be preferred.

In parameter estimation relating to pharmacokinetics, use is often made of black box (or dark gray box!) models with one, two, or three compartments, but recently there has been an effort to use physically based or physiological models where possible (Himmelstein-79). In such model-based parameter estimation, we typically develop a model with definite structural resemblance to the system of interest and then subject the system and model to the same input drives and initial conditions. The output signals available from the system are then compared with corresponding outputs from the model (see Fig. 9.0.1), and unknown param-

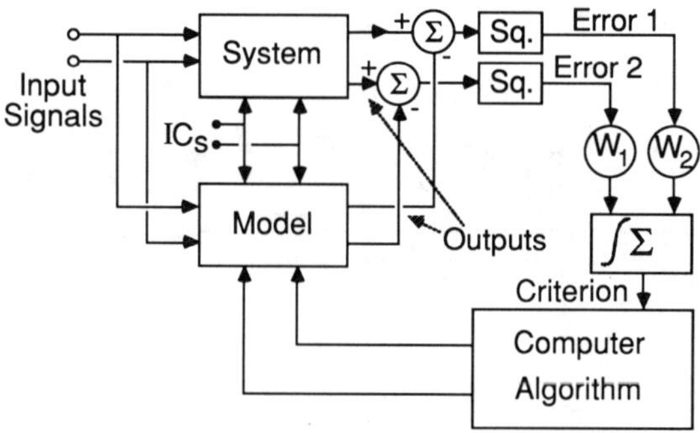

Figure 9.0.1. Block diagram of model-based parameter estimation.

eters in the model are adjusted with the aid of some algorithm until the model outputs correspond with the system outputs as closely as possible.

As shown in Fig. 9.0.1, corresponding outputs are subtracted and squared, and a weighted sum of these squared errors then gives a time-varying criterion function. This may be integrated to give a *criterion,* which is to be minimized by adjustment of model parameters, and thus yield a set of model parameter values that are close to the corresponding parameters in the real system.

9.1 LINEAR REGRESSION

A single compartment with linear outflow or decay of a solute will, in the linear case, have a concentration c that decays exponentially:

$$c = C_0 * \epsilon^{-t/T} \tag{9.1.1}$$

where C_0 is initial concentration, and T is the system time constant. Taking the natural log of both sides gives

$$\mathrm{Ln}(c) = -t/T + \mathrm{Ln}(C_0) \tag{9.1.2}$$

This is a straight-line equation that may be expressed as

$$Y = A*X + B \tag{9.1.3}$$

where the variables are $Y = \mathrm{Ln}(c)$ and $X = t$, and the constant parameters are $A = -1/T$ and $B = \mathrm{Ln}(C_0)$.

A typical *inverse problem* is, given a set of N observed points, X_i, Y_i, to find a straight line giving a least squared error fit to these points (see Fig. 9.1.1a). We can begin by finding the means, or averages, over the N points

$$\overline{Y} = (\sum_N Y_i)/N, \qquad \overline{X} = (\sum_N X_i)/N \tag{9.1.4}$$

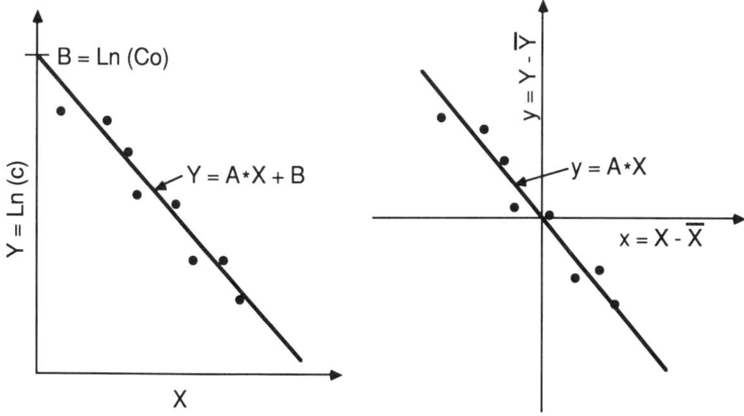

Figure 9.1.1. (a) Observation points, and linear regression line to be estimated.
(b) The same points and line after moving the axis center by the amount of the mean of X and of Y.

and moving the axes by these amounts (see Fig. 9.1.1b). It is now necessary to find a line $y = A*x$ that best fits the experimental points, which are at $x_i = X_i - \overline{X}$, $y_i = Y_i - \overline{Y}$; (B can be found later using $B = \overline{Y} - A*\overline{X}$). The mean square error is

$$E = \sum_N \frac{(y - y_i)^2}{N} = \sum_N \frac{(A*x_i - y_i)^2}{N} \tag{9.1.5}$$

For a minimum, $\delta E/\delta A$ must equal zero, whence

$$\sum_N \frac{2*(A*x_i - y_i)*x_i}{N} = 0 \tag{9.1.6}$$

$$\therefore \sum_N A*x_i^2 = \sum_N x_i*y_i$$

From this and the expression for B given above,

$$A = \sum_N N*x_i*y_i \Big/ \sum_N x_i, \qquad B = \overline{Y} - A*\overline{X} \tag{9.1.7}$$

Returning to the exponential concentration expression in (9.1.1), the estimates of the parameters are $C_0 = \epsilon^B$, $T = -1/A$. Note that the logarithm to base 10 is often used, in which case (9.1.2) will be replaced by

$$\log c = -t/(2.303*T) + \log C_0 \tag{9.1.8}$$

and $\epsilon = 2.7183$ will be replaced by 10.

The least squares regression method is widely used, but is only mathematically correct for this simple kind of parameter estimation if the errors have a normal distribution. Also, the simple model, a single compartment in this case, must adequately represent the system being studied (Deming-43).

The regression scheme may be extended to the inverse problem in polyexponential cases, where, for example

$$c = C_0(\epsilon^{-t/T_1} + \epsilon^{-t/T_2}) \tag{9.1.9}$$

Some numerical polyexponential cases are discussed by Gibaldi and Perrier (Appendix C in Gibaldi-82). Also note that Fortran programs have been developed for "peeling" in polyexponential regression (Sedman-76).

9.2 PARAMETER ESTIMATION BY GLOBAL SEARCH

Rather than making parameter estimation studies of a real system, it is instructive at this point to set up a fairly detailed system in model form with most of the important structural details included and a simpler model that is to be matched to this "system" (Chang-73). Here we begin our study of estimation techniques using a rather simple system described by two first-order differential equations. This system corresponds to a simple two-compartment diffusion-coupled system in which one compartment corresponds to all the extracellular fluid and the other corresponds to intracellular fluids. It is assumed that the system equations are

$$\begin{aligned} dX_n/dt &= -K_{11}*X_n + K_{12}*Y_n + L*X_n^2 + F \\ dY_n/dt &= K_{21}*X_n - K_{22}*Y_n \end{aligned} \tag{9.2.1}$$

where $F = 5.0*\exp(0.5*t)$, ICs are $X_n(0) = 0$, $Y_n(0) = 0$, and $K_{11} = 3.15$, $K_{22} = 1.07$, and $K_{12} = K_{21} = 0.5$, and $L = 0$.

We will begin by setting up a scheme for global search, and will assume as indicated above that L, the coefficient of the only nonlinear term, is zero, and that K_{12} and K_{21} are known. We will then have a model in which there are just two unknown parameters, K_{11} and K_{22}:

$$\begin{aligned} dX_m/dt &= -K_{11}*X_m + 0.5*Y_m + F \\ dY_m/dt &= 0.5*X_m - K_{22}*Y_m \\ F &= 5*\text{Exp}(0.5*\text{t}), \text{ and } X_n(0) = 0.0,\ Y_m(0) = 0.0 \end{aligned} \tag{9.2.2}$$

If the error signals are $X_n - X_m$ and $Y_n - Y_m$ and weighting functions are W_x and W_y, then an error integral criterion is

$$I_e = \int_0^{TF} W_x*(X_n - X_m)^2 + W_y*(Y_n - Y_m)^2 dt \tag{9.2.3}$$

where the integral is taken over a range TF that is large compared to the time constants expected in the system or in its driving function. To keep things simple, we shall assume initially that the weighting functions are each of value unity; 20 sec may be shown to be adequate for the upper limit of the error integral by some experimentation with the system.

An ACSL program, PAREST1, for a global search is shown below. Here the arrays for K11 and K22 are declared, and an initial guess of the ranges 1 < K11 < 5 and 0.5 < K22 < 2.5 and of suitable step-sizes is made, giving 25 pairs of points to be examined. (Note that we will now use ASCL terminology for X11 and the like.) The scheme used is to set up the "system" differential equations (Eq. (9.2.1) with XN, YN as variables) and those for the model (Eq. (9.2.2) with XM, YM) in the derivative section, together with the driving function F and the error integral from (9.2.3). The program is set up first to find the error integral IE for K11 = 5.0 and K22 = 0.5 and then to iterate through all 25 pairs of values of these parameters. Fortran statements in the TERMINAL section enable the grid or array of IE = I(P) to be printed.

```
PROGRAM PAREST1 $'Parameter Est. by Global Search'
   Constant  TF=20., L=0.0, WX=1.0, WY=1.0
   INTEGER P, PMAX
   ARRAY K11(25),K22(25),I(25)
   Constant K11 = 5.,5.,5.,5.,5., ...
                  4.,4.,4.,4.,4., ...
                  3.,3.,3.,3.,3., ...
                  2.,2.,2.,2.,2., ...
                  1.,1.,1.,1.,1.
   Constant K22 = 0.5,1.0,1.5,2.0,2.5, ...
                  0.5,1.0,1.5,2.0,2.5, ...
                  0.5,1.0,1.5,2.0,2.5, ...
                  0.5,1.0,1.5,2.0,2.5, ...
                  0.5,1.0,1.5,2.0,2.5


  INITIAL
   Constant P=1, PMAX=25    $'PMAX=25 because there'
   L1..CONTINUE             $'are 25 pairs of points to try'
  END $ 'Of Initial'

  DYNAMIC
   Cinterval CINT= 0.2
```

```
    DERIVATIVE
     Algorithm IALG = 4  $ 'Runge Kutta 2'
     Maxterval MAXT = 0.1
     Nsteps NSTP = 1

      'Differential Equations'
     XN =INTEG (-3.15*XN = 0.5*YN + L*XN**2 + F, 0.0)
     YN =INTEG (0.5*XN - 1.07*YN, 0.0)       $'System Eqns.'
     XM =INTEG (-K11(P)*XM + 0.5*YM + F, 0.0)
     YM =INTEG (0.5*XM - K22(P)*YM, 0.0)     $'Model Eqns.'
     IE =INTEG WX*(XN - XM)**2 + WY*(YN - YM)**2, 0.0)
                                              'Error Integral'
     F = 5.0*EXP(-0.5*T)
    END $ 'of Deriv.'

     TERMT (T .GE. TF)
   END  $ 'Of Dynamic'


   TERMINAL
     CALL LOGD(.TRUE.)         $'Here these four statements'
     I(P)=IE                   $'form a do-loop to iterate through'
     P = P + 1                 $'the error of integration PMAX times.'
     IF (P .LE. PMAX) GO TO L1
     WRITE(6,FMT)I             $'These two Fortran statements are'
     FMT..FORMAT(5F10.3)       $'needed to print the IE output array.'
   END $'Of Terminal'
  END  $'Of Program'
```

If we run this program with simply a START command, followed by STOP to end run time, then the command TYPE PAREST1.OUT will yield the global search error integral matrix shown in Table 9.2.1. It can be seen in the table that the minimum (which should be close to zero) is just a little above K11 = 3 and slightly more than K22 = 1, and a more restricted search in this region would yield better estimates. Since we know the system values in this case (K11 = 3.15, K22 = 1.07), we can check any algorithms we set up and also look for the error introduced by the nonlinear term in the "real system," which was not included in the model.

It can be seen that even a rough global search gives a painfully slow approach to estimation of parameters, and it becomes quite awkward as we go beyond two parameters (for four parameters we would need to examine six arrays like the one above, for example). Its chief value is as a way of discerning whether the error integral surface has more than a single minimum, and whether or not the contours are of a desirable near-

TABLE 9.2.1 Results of a Global Search of an Error Integral, Using Program PAREST1

	5	0.365	0.389	0.480	0.544	0.588
	4	0.252	0.123	0.203	0.270	0.318
K_{11}	3	0.606	0.0136	0.0292	0.082	0.128
	2	3.675	1.084	0.755	0.693	0.689
	1	42.987	15.443	11.262	9.787	9.076
		0.5	1.0	1.5	2.0	2.5
			K_{22}			

circular shape, so that methods of parameter estimation such as pattern search will work well.

9.3 PARAMETER ESTIMATION BY PATTERN SEARCH

Rather than using the tedious global search method for parameter estimation, much more efficient schemes may be employed. One of the simplest methods, but still rather crude, is *direct search*. Our version of this scheme (Fig. 9.3.1) may be easily converted to more efficient pattern search schemes (Hooke-61), or to a steepest descent scheme (Bekey-78).

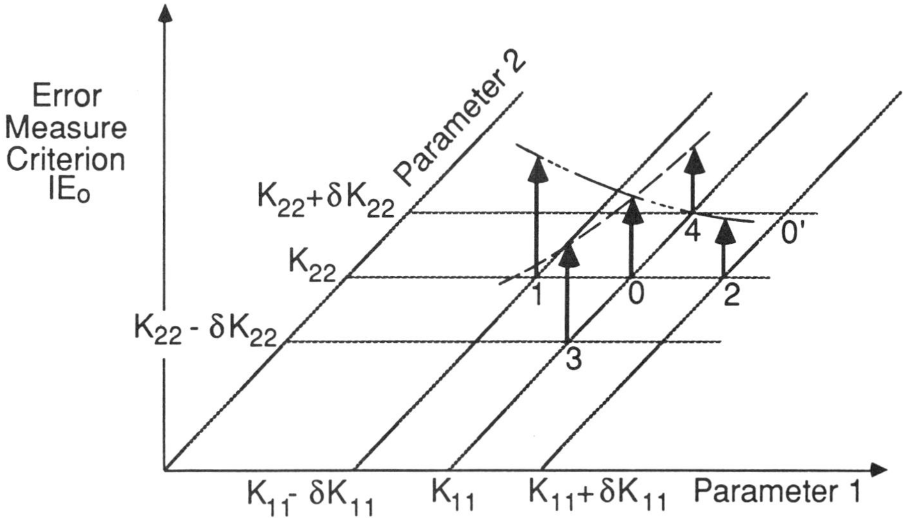

Figure 9.3.1. Five-point pattern for determining sequential parameter adjustment. Here the new center point will be at 0′. Note that if both IE1 and IE2 were larger than IE0, no step would be taken in K11, DK11 would be halved, and the new iteration center would be at point 4.

In our pattern search scheme, using an integral error criterion as in program PAREST1, we shall choose the same system and model, but during each run determine not only the integral error at the current values of K11 and K22 (point 0 in Fig. 9.2.1), but also at four surrounding points 1, 2, 3, and 4 at K11-DK11, K22 + DK22, and so on. This requires that model commands be repeated five times in the program. The arbitrary choice for the initial increment DK11 or DK22 is approximately one-tenth of the corresponding initial K. Note that in this program, DK11 is reduced by half each time that a step is *not* called for in the K11 direction, and similarly for DK22 (this feature of the algorithm was chosen to give smoother progress down "valleys" in criterion-parameter space).

Program PAREST2 is an ACSL program illustrating the implementation of this pattern search applied to our simple case (with the nonlinear term in the system initially at zero). Here a parameter sweep is used to iterate the search for a minimum value of the error criterion.

```
PROGRAM PAREST2
   Constant K11=2.1,DK11=.2,K22=4.2,DK22=.4
   Constant L=0., WX=1., WY=1.
   Integer A,AM
   Constant A=0,TF=20.,AM=20,AT=0.0
 INITIAL
   L1..CONTINUE
 END $ 'Of Initial'

 DYNAMIC
   Cinterval CINT= 0.2

  DERIVATIVE
   Algorithm IALG = 4  $ 'Runge Kutta 2'
   Maxterval MAXT =.1
   Nsteps NSTP = 1
 'Differential Equations'
   XN =INTEG (-3.15*XN + 0.5*YN + L*XN**2 + F, 0.0)
   YN =INTEG (0.5*XN - 1.07*YN, 0.0)        $'System Eqns.'
   F = 5.0*EXP(-0.5*T)                       $'Driving Function'

   X0 = INTEG(-K11*X0 + 0.5*Y0 + F, 0.0) $'Model Eqns. at'
   Y0 = INTEG( 0.5*X0 - K22*Y0, 0.0)      $'pattern center'
   IE0= INTEG(WX*(X-X0)**2 + WY*(YN-Y0)**2,0.0)

   X1 = INTEG(-(K11-DK11)*X1 + 0.5*Y1 + F, 0.0)
   Y1 = INTEG( 0.5*X1 - K22*Y1, 0.0)
   IE1= INTEG(WX*(XN-X1)**2 + WY*(YN-Y1)**2,0.0)

   X2 = INTEG(-(K11+DK11)*X2 + 0.5*Y2 + F, 0.0)
```

```
      Y2 = INTEG( 0.5*X2 - K22*Y2, 0.0)
      IE2= INTEG(WX*(XN-X2)**2 + WY*(YN-Y2)**2,0.0)

      X3 = INTEG(-K11*X3 + 0.5*Y3 + F, 0.0)
      Y3 = INTEG( 0.5*X3 - (K22-DK22)*Y3, 0.0)
      IE3= INTEG(WX*(XN-X3)**2 + WY*(YN-Y3)**2,0.0)

      X4 = INTEG(-K11*X4 + 0.5*Y4 + F, 0.0)
      Y4 = INTEG( 0.5*X4 - (K22+DK22)*Y4, 0.0)
      IE4= INTEG(WX*(XN-X4)**2 + WY*(YN-Y4)**2,0.0)
     END   $'Of Deriv.'

      TERMT (T .GE. TF)
      TT = T + A*TF                        $'TT is total time'
    END    $'Of Dynamic'

    TERMINAL
     CALL LOGD(.TRUE.)
     A =A+1
     IF ((IE1 .GT. IE2) .AND. (IE0 .GT. IE2)) K11=K11+DK11
     IF ((IE2 .GT. IE1) .AND. (IE0 .GT. IE1)) K11=K11-DK11
     IF ((IE3 .GT. IE4) .AND. (IE0 .GT. IE4)) K22=K22+DK22
     IF ((IE4 .GT. IE3) .AND. (IE0 .GT. IE3)) K22=K22-DK22

     IF ((IE0 .LE. IE1) .AND. (IE0 .LE. IE2)) DK11=DK11/2.
     IF ((IE0 .LE. IE3) .AND. (IE0 .LE. IE4)) DK22=DK22/2.

     IF (A .LT. AM) GO TO L1
    END        $'of Terminal'
   END         $'of Program'
```

In the Terminal portion of this program, logic statements are used to change K11 and K22 as needed at each iteration and also to decrease the size of DK11 and/or DK22 when a valley in criterion space has been reached.

In Fig. 9.3.2a plots of the input drive F(t) and of the system responses XN and YN are shown, and the error integral (Fig. 9.3.2b) may be seen to be steadily decreasing in value as the system iterates (and A increases). In Fig. 9.3.3 the abscissa has been changed to total time TT, and the paths followed by K11 and K22 are shown as iterations proceed. Note that in Fig. 9.3.3b, the values of the increments DK11 and DK22 decrease rather rapidly as K11 and K22 approach their correct values. A DISPLY command at the end of the run showed final estimated values of K11 = 3.15000, K22 = 1.06875 after 20 iterations as compared to the true values of 3.15 and 1.07.

Model-to-model studies of the combination of the parameter estima-

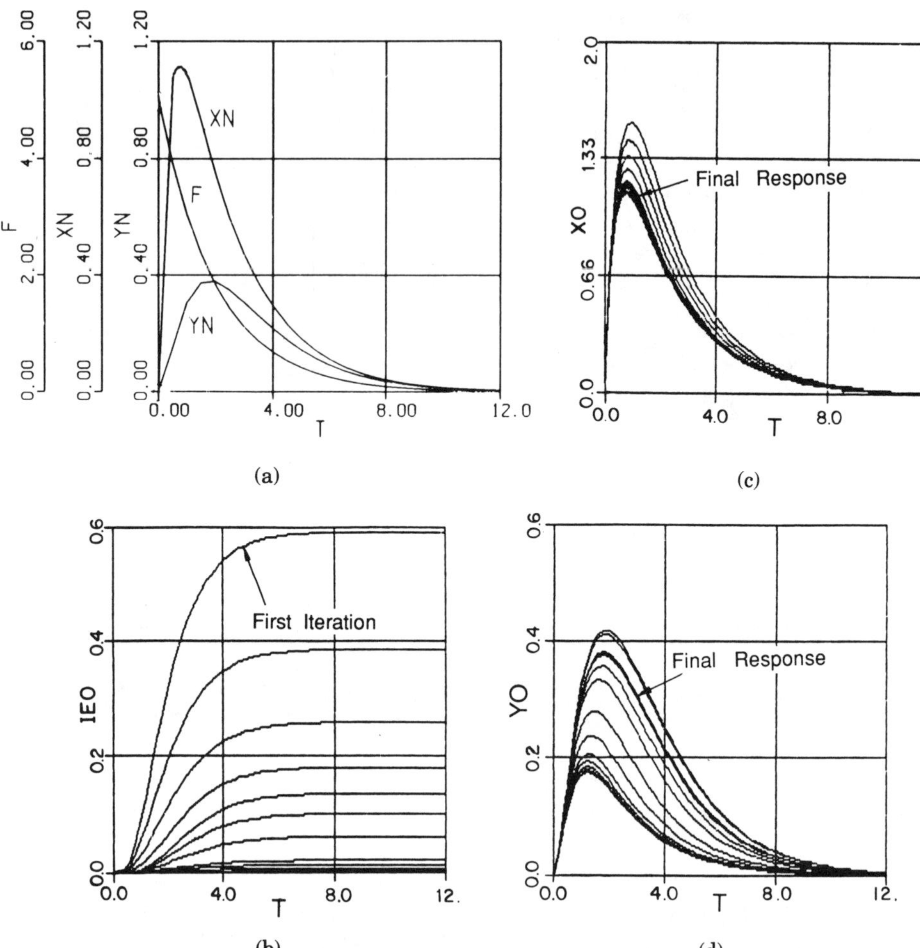

Figure 9.3.2. (a) System input F and responses XN and YN.
(b) Plots of error IE0 as iteration proceeds.
(c),(d) Sequence of responses X0, Y0.

tion algorithm and a rather good model approximation of the system to be studied are often helpful as work begins on a particular problem. Thus, as described in the work of Chang (see Section 9.4), it was found that model-to-model exercises permitted the model to be adjusted to the needs of parameter estimation in this case, and the minimization algorithm improved, so that animal-to-model studies could proceed more smoothly and rapidly.

The algorithm used here may be changed to one that converges with

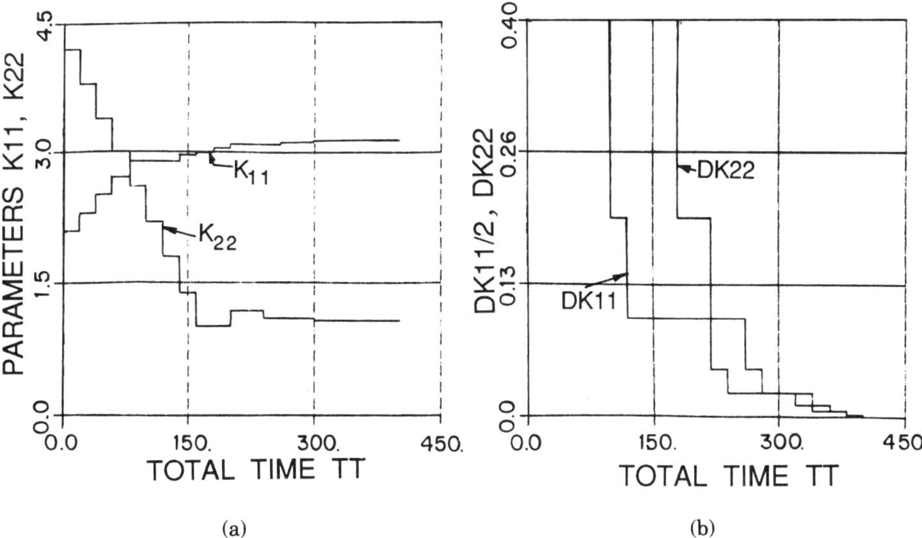

Figure 9.3.3. (a) Parameters K11 and K22 plotted against total time, TT = T + A∗TF, as iteration proceeds.
(b) Correction increments DK11 and DK22, also plotted against total time.

fewer iterations, if a successful step is followed by a similar step whenever a check of IEO shows that error was reduced (Hooke-61). This adds to program length and may not give much if any reduction in computer time, however. See other general references listed at the end of this chapter (Bekey-70, 78, Rideout-75, Hill-78, Grove-80, Möller-90).

9.4 PARAMETER ESTIMATION OF THE CANINE ARTERIAL SYSTEM

In a study of model-based parameter estimation of the canine arterial system, Pao-Ping Chang dealt with a number of problems preliminary to the actual estimation procedure, including the choice of model size and amount of detail, variables to be measured, parameters to be estimated, as well as criterion functions and minimization algorithms to be used (Chang-73, 74). His studies began with model-to-model studies of the estimation model to be adjusted to match a known model with much detail, resembling that of Snyder's shown in the frontispiece of this book (Snyder-68). It was soon found that if detail was reduced by combining too many sections the criterion began to show false minima, and wave shapes became hard to manage. The lumped circuit model finally chosen is shown in Fig. 9.4.1, with a main aorta terminating in the femorals (combined) and with two branches, one for the upper body and the other for the internal organs.

This model has 25 resistances, 9 inertances, and 12 compliances, a total of 46 elements. Such a large number would be very difficult to deal with, and since it was felt that there must be much resemblance between adjoining sections, a search was made for more basic parameters that might be easier to use. Ultimately, this led to a set of only 8 parameters to be estimated, but from which the 46 parameters in Fig. 9.4.1 could be determined. These 8 parameters included 3 upper-end vessel radii, a single vessel taper ratio, total peripheral resistance, characteristic impedance near the aortic valve, total main branch length, and the ratio of total head to total internal organ branch resistance. From these 8 parameters all R, L, and C parameters could be determined, with help from some assumptions (including linear tapering and uniform wall damping).

Six variables were measured; they included two flows widely separated in the aorta and three pressures also widely separated, together with a pressure in the carotid artery. Earlier studies had shown that it was important to have both pressure and flow measurements widely separated in order to have criterion surfaces of favorable shape.

The criterion that was selected weighed pressures most heavily and the characteristic and peripheral impedance the least. A hybrid computer was chosen because it had the best combination of speed and power for the many runs that had to be made. Finally, a Hooke and Jeeves type of

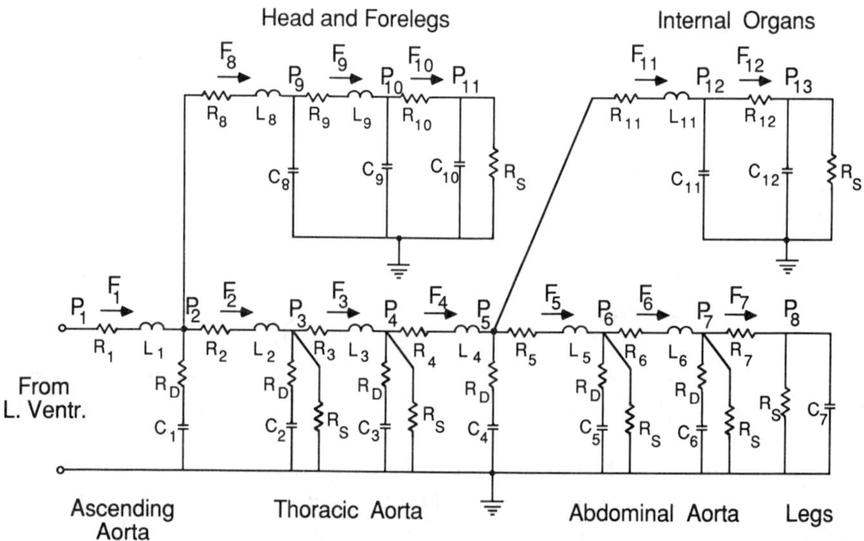

Figure 9.4.1. Model of the canine arterial system with detail reduced to a minimum that permits parameter estimation with good waveforms in the main arterial vessels (from Chang-73, with permission).

pattern search algorithm (Hooke-61) was used to help reduce total computer time needed.

After many model-to-model studies to help determine the choices listed above, studies were made using recordings obtained with a dog under normal anesthesia (with sodium pentathol), then with added norepinephrine, and then with isoproterenol. Checking the results was difficult because direct measurements of cardiovascular parameters can seldom be made without disturbing the whole system. An indirect check was done by examining all measured waveforms and comparing them with computer model waveforms after the estimation (requiring 50 iterations) was complete. Results are shown in Fig. 9.4.2 for the initial case (anesthesia only) and the second case, with added norepinephrine. Here it can be seen that the final model waveforms have a close resemblance to those measured in the dog, after initial guesses that were quite different. Measured error was under 15 percent, compared with 5 percent for the model-to-model study.

The entire parameter estimation method briefly described in this section is rather complex, despite the simplicity of the criterion minimization algorithm. It may be considered to be made up of seven steps (Chang-73), as follows:

1. *Determination of model form and approximate parameter values, based on physical principles.* The detail needed in the model may need to be increased to prevent the appearance of false minima of the criterion in parameter space. Nevertheless, it is possible in some cases to develop rather simple black-box models for use in adaptive control systems (Hynson-80).
2. *Choice of parameters to be estimated.* The number of parameters should be kept to a minimum, as determined by experience with the kind of system and parameter estimation method being used. It may be helpful that some parameters do not have to be estimated because they can be determined by direct measurement (this is often true for peripheral resistances in CV systems, for example).
3. *Choice of variables to be measured.* The difficulties of measurement of each variable must be balanced against the importance of using that variable in the criterion. Thus, in the CV system it may be important to have pressure and flow measurements at well-separated points in the system.
4. *Selection of a criterion whose minimum satisfactorily agrees with a correspondence between system and model.* A typical criterion has the form:

$$I = \int_0^T \sum_i W_i * |E_i|^Y dt$$

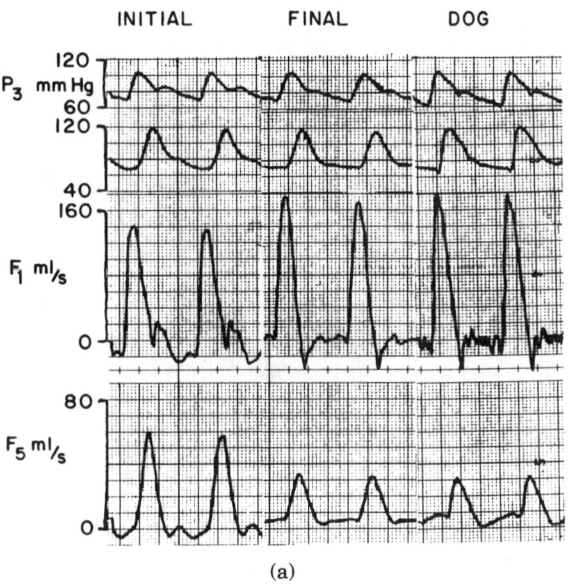

(a)

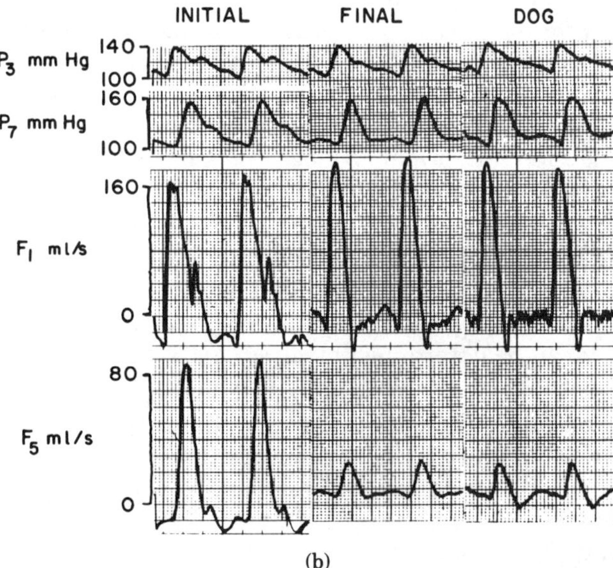

(b)

Figure 9.4.2. (a) Initial and final (after parameter estimation) model waveforms, and corresponding waveforms measured in the dog under normal anesthesia.
(b) Waveforms as in part (a), with norepinephrine injected.

where I is the criterion, E_i is the error between the ith model variable and the ith system variable, W_i is the weighting given to the ith error, and Y is the power to which the absolute value of the error is raised to make it a suitable measure. In the canine CV system parameter estimation example described in this section, it was found most satisfactory to use $Y = 1$. The time T of integration is determined by the time taken for variables to repeat; thus in the cardiovascular system about four heartbeats may be satisfactory.

5. *Choice of a minimization algorithm.* Often much attention is given to the design of complex minimization algorithms that converge rapidly despite undesirable contour shapes of criteria in parameter space. However, initial model-to-model studies may enable investigators to find more usable contours (near spherical in multispace), that permit fast approaches to the minimum with simpler algorithms.
6. *Choice of a computer.* The best computer for parameter estimation was once the hybrid computer, combining the speed of the parallel analog (for running the model) with the logic capability of an interconnected digital computer. Although the powerful digital machines of today are ordinarily used in parameter estimation, large problems with repetitive simulations of the modeled system may require the use of a fast parallel digital computer.
7. *Verification.* Model-to-model studies may be helpful in verifying the speed and accuracy of the parameter estimation scheme that has been developed. Animal-to-model or clinical studies are more difficult. One scheme is to exercise the model (as in the example described in this section), by changing the CV system by use of suitable drugs, and comparing system variables with those of the parameter-estimated model.

Although the steps listed above must be followed in most parameter estimation studies, some of them may be hidden. Also, the estimation methods used in various physiological systems may show almost as much variability as do the systems themselves. Many examples may be found in the literature (Bellville-88, Beneken-73, Campello-78, Clark-80, DiStefano-75, Katz-70, Loeve-72, Möller-90, and Sims-72). Many other problems may arise, such as the variation of some parameters of a system with time; it may be desirable to follow such changes with the estimation scheme used (Lyung-87).

PROBLEMS

9.1. **(a)** Run the global search program PAREST1 with a finer matrix of parameter trial values. For example, vary K_{11} from 1.5 to 5.0 in steps of 0.5 and

K_{22} from 0.25 to 2.0 in steps of 0.25 or less. Then try to draw contours (by hand) of the integral error criteria.

(b) Repeat part (a) for an included nonlinearity of L = 0.1 or 0.2; note any changes in the shape of the contours.

9.2. Run the pattern search model PAREST2 with L = 0.1 in the system equations, but do not include it in the model. Search for K_{11} and K_{22} as before and explain the results.

9.3. Indicate the changes needed in the pattern search program PAREST2 if L = 0.2 in the system and L is also included in the model. Set up the program to search for K_{11}, K_{22}, and L and discuss your results.

9.4. Change PAREST2 to a steepest-descent routine by adding commands in the TERMINAL program to move in the direction of greatest decrease in the criterion. Compare with the results obtained in your text.

REFERENCES

BEKEY, GEORGE A., "System identification—an introduction and a survey", *Simulation;* pp. 151–65; Oct. 1970.

BEKEY, G. A. AND J. E. W. BENEKEN, "Identification of biological and medical systems", *Identification and System Parameter Estimation,* Rajbman, (Ed.); North-Holland Pub. Co.; 1978.

BELLVILLE, J. W., D. S. WARD AND D. WIBERG, "Respiratory System: Modelling & Identification," *Systems and Control Encyclopaedia; Theory, Technology, Applications,* M. G. Singh, (Ed.); Oxford: Pergamon Press; 1988.

BENEKEN, J. E. W., "Estimation of heart function parameters by hybrid optimization techniques," Eykhoff, P. (Ed.) *Identification and System Parameter Estimation,* Proc. 3rd IFAC Symp.; Amsterdam: North Holland Pub. Co.; 1973.

CAMPELLO, L. AND C. COBELLI, "Parameter estimation of biological stochastic computational models—an application," *IEEE Trans. BME,* Vol. BME-25, No. 2, pp. 139–46; Mar. 1978.

CHANG, PAO PING, "Model-based Parameter Estimation of the Canine Systemic Circulation System," (Ph.D. thesis, Univ. of Wisconsin); 1973.

CHANG, P. P., G. L. MATSON, J. E. KENDRICK, AND V. C. RIDEOUT, "Parameter Estimation in the Canine Cardiovascular System," *IEEE Trans. Aut. Control;* Vol. AC-19, No. 6, pp. 927–31; 1974.

CLARK, J. W. JR., ET AL., "A two-stage identification scheme for the determination of the parameters of a model of left heart and systemic circulation", *IEEE Trans. Biomed. Engg.,* Vol. BME-27, No. 1; 1980.

DEMING, W. E. "Statistical Adjustment of Data," New York; John Wiley & Sons; 1943.

DISTEFANO, J. J., ET AL., "Identification of the dynamics of thyroid hormone metabolism," *Automatica,* Vol. 11, pp. 149–59; 1975.

FLETCHER, R. AND M. J. D. POWELL, "A rapidly convergent descent method for minimization," *Comput Jl.,* Vol. 6; pp. 163–68; 1963.

GIBALDI, M. AND D. PERRIER, "Pharmacokinetics," 2nd Ed.; New York: Marcel Dekker, Inc.; 1982.

GROVE, T. M., G. A. BEKEY AND L. J. HAYWOOD, "Analysis of errors in parameter estimation with application to physiological systems," *Am. Jl. Physiol.* 239 (Reg. Integ. Comp. Physiol. 8) pp. R390–R400; 1980.

HILL, W. S. ET AL., "Identification of complex biological systems through mathematical pattern recognition," *Identification and System Parameter Estimation,* Rajbman, (Ed.); North-Holland Pub. Co.; 1978.

HIMMELSTEIN, K. J. AND R. J. LUTZ, "A review of the applications of physiologically-based pharmacokinetic modeling," *Jl. Pharmacokin. and Biopharmaceutics,* Vol. 2, pp. 127–45, 1979.

HOOKE, R. AND J. A. JEEVES, "'Direct Search' solution of numerical and statistical problems," *Jl. ACM,* Vol. 8, pp. 212–29; Apr. 1961.

HYNSON, J. M., "Model studies for the Design of a Servoanesthesia System" (M.S. thesis, Univ. of Wisconsin-Madison), 1980.

KATZ, A. I. ET AL., "Parameter optimization for a model of the cardiovascular system," *Proc. 1970 Summer Computer Simul. Conf.* ACM, Denver CO, pp. 889–98; 1970.

LOEVE, J. "Estimation of hemodynamic parameters in the human leg arteries," (M.S. thesis, Tech. Univ., Eindhoven, Nds). 1972.

LYUNG, L., *System Identification; Theory for the User,* Englewood Cliffs, NJ; Prentice Hall; 1987.

MARQUART, D. W. "An algorithm for least-squares estimation of nonlinear parameters," *Jl. SIAM,* Vol. 11, pp. 431–41; 1963.

MÖLLER, D. P. F., "Parameter estimation: an advanced simulation tool in biomedicine," pp. 74–82 in *Advanced Simulation in Biomedicine,* D. P. F. Moller (Ed.), New York: Springer-Verlag; 1990.

RIDEOUT, V. C., AND J. E. W. BENEKEN, "Parameter estimation applied to physiological systems," *Proc. AICA,* Vol. 17, pp. 23–36; Jan. 1975.

SEDMAN, A. J. AND J. G. WAGNER, "CSTRIP, a Fortran IV computer program for obtaining initial polyexponential parameter estimations," *Jl. Pharm. Sci.,* Vol. 65, No. 7, pp. 1006–10; 1976.

SIMS, J. B., "Estimation of arterial system parameters from dynamic records," *Comput. Biomed.,* Vol. 5, pp. 131–47; 1972.

SNYDER, M. F., V. C. RIDEOUT AND R. J. HILLESTAD, "Computer modeling of the human systemic arterial tree," *Jl. Biomech.,* Vol. 2, No. 4, pp. 325–34; 1968.

Appendix A
Continuous System Simulation Programming

The sets of ordinary differential equations used to describe physiological (and other) dynamic systems may be set up for computer solution and solved using high-level languages such as Fortran, Pascal, or Basic (Randall-87). More convenient and efficient languages of still higher level (which we will refer to as third-level languages) are available that permit the use of very simple programming, then translate the original program into some powerful second-order language such as Fortran, after which follow compilation and running of the compiled program.

In 1967 standards were set up for such third-level languages, called CSSL or Continuous System Simulation Languages (Strauss-67). This appendix briefly describes the principles and programming techniques for one of these languages, ACSL (Advanced Continuous Simulation Language, pronounced "axle"), which is used in the examples given in this book (Mitchell-76). Other languages have appeared that conform to the CSSL standards, and so closely resemble ACSL that this appendix and the program examples elsewhere in this book should be quite useful to those who are learning and using other CSSL-type languages. These languages have been reviewed in several publications (Nilsen-74, Korn-78, Spriet-82, Cellier-86), and include IBM's CSMP (Speckhart-76) and the more recent IBM Simulation Programs, as well as ESL (Crosbie-85), DESIRE (Korn-86) and CSSL-IV (Nilsen-74); recent additions to this list of languages are SCOP (Kootsey-89), and ADAPT (D'Argenio-90), both designed for biomodeling. Note, however, that discrete system simulation languages, briefly discussed in Section 1.3 of this book, are aimed at the solution of problems involving queues, scheduling and the like.

There are other third-level languages that were developed for the solution of electric and electronic network problems. These languages, which include ECAP, SPICE (Nagel-75; Tuinengra-76), and SCEPTRE (Bowers-71), have sometimes been used in physiology (Mikulecky-77), but have the disadvantages that the set of equations describing the physiological system to be analyzed must first be expressed in network form.

Setting up equations to describe a physiological system is discussed in Chapter 3 and elsewhere in the examples in this book. Note that the set of differential equations corresponding to the system state variables will result in the need for one integration for each state variable in the program, but that algebraic equations may be separated out of these differential equations and appear as additional equations. Limiting and other nonlinear operations may conveniently be included, and delays, and logic operations are possible.

Once equations for a system are available, they must be written in ACSL form, as explained below, using a text editor or word processor. Detailed descriptions of ACSL commands and ACSL programming may be found in the *ACSL Manual* (Mitchell-86, Kloss-90), but the introduction given here and elsewhere in this book will enable the new user to begin to effectively use this powerful language. It is important to note that the main body of equations need not be arranged in any particular order, because ACSL is a nonprocedural language (unlike Fortran, in which the commands must be arranged in the order required for solution). This programming simplification is accomplished by a *sorting* algorithm included in ACSL and related languages.

Within ACSL a *translation* program is used to translate the equation into Fortran; coding for the particular integration algorithm selected by the user is included in ACSL, together with diagnostics. The chosen algorithm may be a self-starting program, such as Euler or one of the Runge-Kutta routines, or a predictor-corrector algorithm may be used with possibly a modification that enables more rapid solution of "stiff" systems—that is, systems with a wide range of time-constant values (Gear-71). The detailed structure of these integration algorithms is provided for the user in ACSL and similar languages. In ACSL, the default algorithm, if none is specified, is fourth-order Runge-Kutta, and the user need only make a reasonably good choice of integration step size, MAXT, which in this case remains fixed in length.

An ACSL program has the structure shown below, in which commands to begin (and end) the various portions of the program are shown in capitals and descriptions of what should be included in each part of the program are shown in lowercase, enclosed by square brackets:

```
PROGRAM [title]
  Constant [list numerical values of system constants,
            in the form K=.35, separated by commas.
            Note that constants may be included at any
            appropriate place in any of the sections of
            the program]
  INITIAL  [this section contains equations which must be
            solved once, before running the program proper]
  END      [of Initial commands]


DYNAMIC
           [commands which must be followed every com-
            munication cycle: an example is a test of a
            command, TERM, to stop the computation]
           [the value of the communication interval, th\
            CINTERVAL, with its name (usually CINT) is
            ordinarily given here.]

    DERIVATIVE
           [this most important section includes the system
            equations, in integral form. It should also
            include the maximum value, MAXT, of the integration
            interval, MAXTERVAL, the number of integration
            steps, NSTPS, per communication interval,
            (usually set equal to 1 if MAXTERVAL is given,
            and the chosen integration algorithm, IALG=N,
            where N is often 4 (for second-order Runge-
            Kutta integration) or 5 (for fourth-order)].
    END [of Derivative]

           [more DYNAMIC commands may be included here].
END   [of Dynamic]

  TERMINAL
           [final calculations may be made in this section
            at the end of the run; it is also used when the
            equivalent of a do-loop is set up to sweep para-
            meters through a range of values]

  END   [of Terminal]

END     [of Program]
```

Note that commands in the INITIAL and TERMINAL sections must be procedural, and that a PROCEDURAL section may be included in the DERIVATIVE section when needed. Remarks may be included, set off by single quotes, and two or more commands may be given in one line, separated by dollar signs.

A few of the more important ACSL commands will now be listed to enable the reader to follow some simple introductory programs and try some others.

1. Arithmetic expressions and assignment statements may be used in any section of the program, in statements written as in Fortran.
2. Differential equations are converted to integral form for solution. Thus the most important operation (used only in DERIVATIVE) is integration. Thus, if Y is the integral of Z, and Y has the initial condition value YIC, then this command is written

   ```
   Y = INTEG ( Z, YIC )                                   (A.1)
   ```

   Here the integrand might depend on other variables such as T and X that appear in the program and may be given by a separate command such as

   ```
   Z = X * T / (1 + A * X)**2                             (A.2)
   ```

   or the whole expression for Z may replace Z in (A.1).
3. The first order lag, or real-pole operator, is written as

   ```
   Y = REALPL (TAU, X, YIC)                               (A.3)
   ```

   where X is the input variable, TAU is the time constant, and YIC is the initial value of the output Y. This corresponds to the Laplace formulation, Y = X / (1 + TAU*s), (see Appendix B). Note that it is also possible to determine Y by using an integrator

   ```
   Y = INTEG((X - Y)/TAU, YIC)
   ```
4. A limiter or bound function is used to limit a function X to be greater than a lower limit L and less than an upper limit U, and is written as

   ```
   Y = BOUND ( L, U, X)                                   (A.4)
   ```

   Here L and U may be algebraic functions or numerical constants.

Other ACSL commands will be given later in this appendix; for a full description of all ACSL commands, refer to the *ACSL Manual* (Mitchell-86) or the *Beginner's Guide to ACSL* (Kloss-90). However, we now have enough commands to illustrate the use of ACSL in the simple motor position-control system example (see also Appendix C) shown in

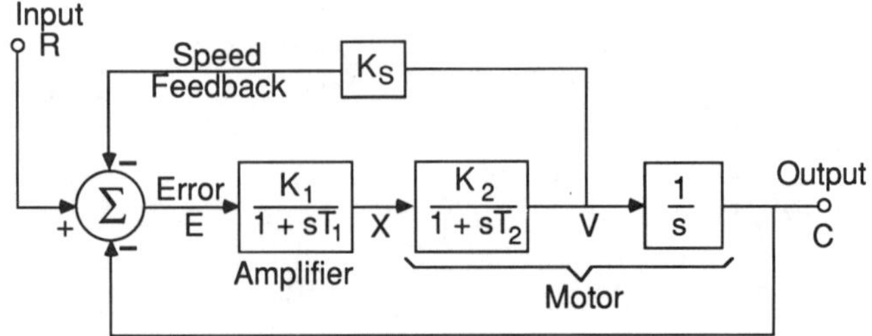

Figure A-1. A simple type-1 position control system with derivative (or speed) feedback stabilization.

block form in Fig. A.1. The equations for this system in Laplace notation are

$$\begin{array}{ll} \text{Error} & E = R - C - K_s*V \\ \text{Amplifier Output} & X = K_1*E/(1 + sT_1) \\ \text{Motor Velocity} & V = K_2*X/(1 + sT_2) \\ \text{Output Position} & C = V / s \end{array} \tag{A.5}$$

Here the first equation is algebraic, and indicates the negative feedback of position, C, and the negative speed feedback that provides system stabilization, K_s *V. The next two equations in (A.5) are simple lags, (see Appendix B) while the fourth equation expresses the integration needed to find output position, C, from speed, V.

The ACSL program needed to find time-varying outputs (for E, X, V, and C) from the four equations of (A.5) and the constants (K1, K2, T1, T2, KS) is shown below. Note that a rough calculation of the length of run time needed must be made; here we will choose a final time TF equal to 10 times the sum of the two main system time constants, T_1 and T_2. The program termination command, TERMT (logic expression), also appears in the DYNAMIC section of the program, and is examined once each communication interval. When the logic expression, T .GE. TF is TRUE, the program leaves the DERIVATIVE section. Note again that two commands or statements may be placed in a single line if they are separated by a dollar sign ($). Comment or remark statements must be enclosed by quotes.

The communication interval in CONSYS is named CINT, and appears in the DYNAMIC section. It value has been estimated at 0.2, equal to the shorter time constant in the loop. The choice of an integration algorithm is IALG = 5, which means fourth-order Runge-Kutta. This is the default algorithm, so this command could be omitted. The value of the maximum integration step size is the Maxterval, called MAXT here, and set equal to 0.04, or one-fifth of the smaller time constant in the feedback loop. Since Maxterval is given in this case, Nsteps (NSTP) must be set to unity. Note that the INITIAL and TERMINAL sections are omitted because no commands are required for these sections.

```
PROGRAM  CONSYS

DYNAMIC
   Cinterval CINT= 0.2
  Constant TF=10.0
   TERMT(T.GE.TF)

 DERIVATIVE
    Algorithm IALG = 5   $ 'Runge Kutta 4'
    Maxterval MAXT = .04 $ 'Integration Step'
    Nsteps NSTP = 1
    'Differential Equations'
   Constant R=10., K1=1., K2=1.5, T1=0.2, T2=0.8
   Constant KS=0.0       $ 'No speed feedback used initially'
    E = R - C - KS*V
    X = REALPL(T1, K1*E, 0.0)
    V = REALPL(T2, K2*X, 0.0)
   Constant CIC=0.0      $'Zero initial value for C'
    C = INTEG(V, CIC)
  END $ 'Of Deriv.'

 END  $ 'Of Dynamic'

END   $ 'Of Program'
```

When we call for this program to be translated and compiled into Fortran (following instructions for the computer configuration being used), completion is signaled by an ACSL> prompt appearing, and the following run-time commands may then be given:

```
OUTPUT T,V,C,'NCIOUT'=5
```

(This will call for tabular output of T and the output variables V and C every 5 communication intervals, or every 0.2 sec of problem time)

```
PREPAR T,V,C,E
```

(This will store values of T and the three dependent variables shown, at each communication period, for later plotting)

```
START
```

(This causes the compiled program to run) After the START command and a carriage return, tabular output will appear on the display. At the end of the run the prompt reappears and plots versus time T of variables in the PREPAR list may be requested with commands such as

```
PLOT 'XHI'= 9.0
```

This puts a limit of 9.0 on the x-axis for all plots in the run, until it is changed, as in

```
PLOT C
```

Another plot may be requested with the same x-axis scale

```
PLOT E, V
```

The results of these commands are shown in Figs. A.2a and A.2b. No graph size was indicated, and thus the original size of these graphs was the default size 4″ × 4″.

Here y-axis commands were used to override and slightly change the automatic scaling.

If the added run-time command SET KS = 1.0 is used, it will add some speed feedback, which will result in outputs for C and V that are less oscillatory by merely commanding START. The tabular results for the entire run may be obtained by stopping the run (command STOP) and calling for a printout of CONSYS.OUT, giving:

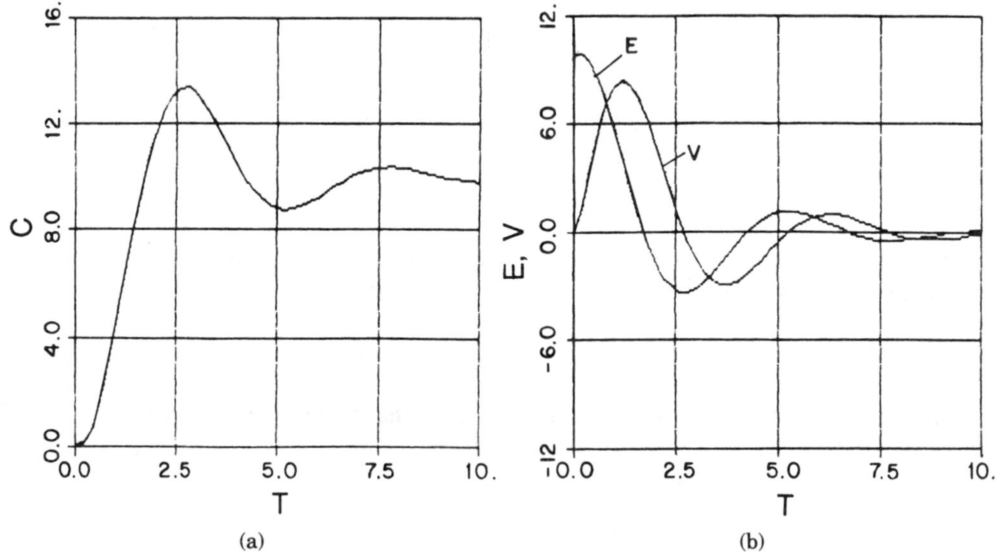

Figure A-2. Outputs for the simple control system CONSYS with KS = 0.0 for a step function input,
(a) Position output, C
(b) Velocity, V and Error E.

```
OUTPUT T,V,C,'NCIOUT'=5
PREPAR T,V,C,E
START
  T 0.                 V 0.                 C  0.
  T 1.00000000         V 8.11770000         C  4.32073000
  T 2.00000000         V 4.92217000         C 11.6840000
  T 3.00000000         V-1.45863000         C 13.1686000
  T 4.00000000         V-2.74687000         C 10.5942000
  T 5.00000000         V-0.51564500         C  8.87296000
  T 6.00000000         V 0.97681900         C  9.27067000
  T 7.00000000         V 0.63240500         C 10.1842000
  T 8.00000000         V-0.15956000         C 10.3937000
  T 9.00000000         V-0.34127800         C 10.0847000
  T 10.0000000         V-0.07346970         C  9.86451000
  T 10.2000000         V-0.01720490         C  9.85555000
 PLOT 'XHI'=9.0
 PLOT C, 'HI'=15.0
 DRAWING PLOT NUMBER    1
 PLOT E,'LO'=-12.,'HI'=12.0, V,'SAME'
 DRAWING PLOT NUMBER    2
 SET KS=1.0
 START
  T 0.                 V 0.                 C 0.
  T 1.00000000         V 5.11908000         C 3.33684000
  T 2.00000000         V 2.47260000         C 7.16441000
  T 3.00000000         V 1.02085000         C 8.79731000
  T 4.00000000         V 0.43709400         C 9.48506000
  T 5.00000000         V 0.18708700         C 9.77974000
  T 6.00000000         V 0.08000780         C 9.90580000
  T 7.00000000         V 0.03421900         C 9.95971000
  T 8.00000000         V 0.01463550         C 9.98277000
  T 9.00000000         V 0.00625956         C 9.99263000
  T 10.0000000         V 0.00267720         C 9.99685000
  T 10.2000000         V 0.00225897         C 9.99734000
```

Plots for this case (KS = 1.0) and for other values of speed feedback may be made as an exercise. However, it may be desirable to sweep through a range of values of KS and show the responses for all these values on the same set of axes. This parameter-sweep output may be obtained by adding an INITIAL section to the CONSYS program with the following commands:

```
INITIAL
 Constant KSIN = 0.0, DKS = 0.4, MKS = 2.1
  KS = KSIN
  L1..CONTINUE
END   $ 'Of Initial'
```

(Note that the command KS = 0.0 should be removed from the Derivative section in the original program CONSYS.)

It is also necessary to include a TERMINAL section with the following commands:

```
TERMINAL
  CALL LOGD(.TRUE.)
  KS = KS + DKS
  IF (KS .LE. MKS) GO TO L1
END  $ 'Of Terminal'
```

These changes will result in a complete run of the program for KS = 0.0, 0.4, 0.8, 1.2, 1.6, and 2.0, or from the original KS = 0.0 in steps of 0.4 to the largest KS below the MKS = 2.1 maximum. Note that it is necessary to include in the run-time expressions the LOGIC command SET FTSPLT = .TRUE., in order to kill the "flyback" trace. The result of this parameter sweep of the CONSYS program is shown in Fig. A.3.

Examples of other commands are to be found in the programs in this book, beginning with COMPART1 and COMPART2 in Section 3.2, where a FCNSW (function switch) is first used. A first use of an INITIAL section in a program appears in FLOTRAN1 in Section 3.3. In Chapter 4 the use of ZOH (zero-order-hold) and RSW (real switch) first appear in program LH-PF-1, and the LIMINT (limited integrator) first appears in program PF-1. Single-valued nonlinearities may be included in ACSL models: an example is the use of a TABLE function in program RESP-OX in Section 3.

It is sometimes convenient to set up a program of run-time com-

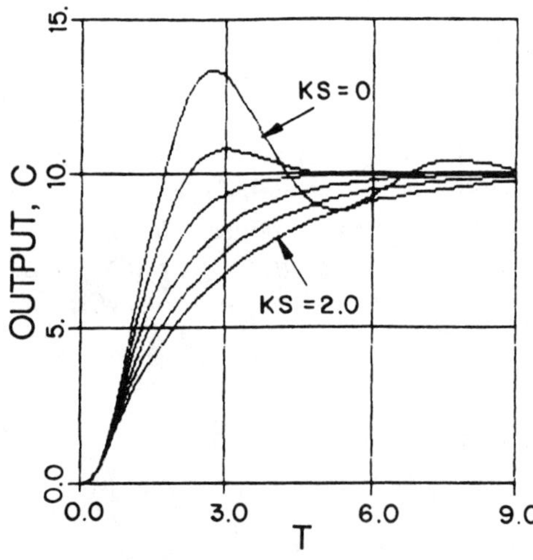

Figure A-3. Output C for the CONSYS program with sweep of parameter KS from 0.0 to 2.0. Here the run-time command SET XINCPL = 3.0, YINCPL = 3.0 gave 3″ × 3″ plots.

mands which are to be used several times. Such a command (CMD) program for the CONSYS system should be named CONSYS.CMD, and may be used, for example, to include all of the CONSYS run-time commands given above, except for the parameter sweep. In this program, as shown below, PAUSE commands are included so that output may be observed on the monitor, and hard copy made if so desired.

```
'CONSYS.CMD, Run-time Commands for Position-Control F-B System'
 OUTPUT T,V,C, 'NCIOUT' = 5
 PREPAR T,V,C,E,
 START
 PAUSE     $'Holds a view of the OUTPUT'
 SET TITLE = 'POSITION-CONTROL FEEDBACK SYSTEM'
PLOT 'XLO' = 0.0, 'XHI' = 10.0, C, 'LO' = 0.0, 'HI' = 16.0
 PAUSE     $'Holds a view of the plot C vs. T'
PLOT E, 'LO' = -12.0, 'HI' = 12.0, V, 'SAME'
 PAUSE     $'Note: X-Axis scaling is the same'
 SET KS = 1.0
 SET TITLE = 'POSITION-CONTROL SYSTEM, SPEED F-B'
 START
PLOT C,'LO' = 0.0, 'HI' = 16.0
 PAUSE
STOP
```

To use CONSYS.CMD, the CONSYS program must be translated and compiled, ready to run, with the ACSL prompt displayed. Then the command

```
SET CMD = 10
```

is made, followed by

```
CONSYS.CMD
```

in answer to a request for name. The run-time commands in this CMD program will then be executed, and a set of plots made. Note that both CONSYS.CSL and CONSYS.CMD appear in the program disk which is available for use with this book, to provide initial practice for any reader who is not familiar with ACSL. Also included in the disk are 26 other ACSL programs; 10 of these are accompanied by run-time command (.CMD) programs.

Some more advanced examples appear in the ACSL manual (Mitchell-86), including the following models related to biomodeling:

Example 8—PHYSBE
(A pressure-flow cardiovascular system simulation illustrating the

use of a MACRO to build up a new command which can be called up simply when needed.)

Example 11—Discrete Sampling Compensator
(Modeling of computer control of a continuous system)

Example 12—Aspirin Dosage Evaluation
(Introduction to variable-dose variable-time discrete drug infusion modeling)

PROBLEM

A.1. Set up and run the CONSYS program with the commands given for a sweep of parameter KS.

REFERENCES

ADI, "Preview of ADSIM on the AD100," *Applied Dynamics International:* Ann Arbor MI; 1971.

BOWERS, J. C. AND S. R. SEDORE, *SCEPTRE, a Computer Program for Circuit and Systems Analysis,* Englewood Cliffs, NJ: Prentice Hall; 1971.

CELLIER, F. D. (ED.), "Languages for Continuous System Simulation," *Proc. of a Conf. on Continuous System Simulation Languages;* San Diego, CA: Society for Computer Simulation; 1986.

CROSBIE, R. E., ET AL, "ESL—A new continuous system simulation language," *Simulation,* Vol. 44, pp. 242–46; May, 1985.

D'ARGENIO, D. Z. AND A. SCHUMITSKY, "ADAPT II User's Guide," *Biomed. Simulations Resource:* Univ. South. Calif., CA; 1990.

GEAR, C. W., *Numerical Initial Value Problems in Ordinary Differential Equations,* Englewood Cliffs, NJ: Prentice Hall; 1971.

HAY, J. L. AND R. E. CROSBIE, "ISIM–a simulation language for microprocessors," *Simulation,* pp. 133–36; Sept. 1984.

KARPLUS, W. J., "Support Languages for Model Simulation," *Computer-aided modelling and simulation* J. A. Spriet and G. C. Vansteenkiste (Eds.), New York: Academic Press, pp. 337–87; 1982.

KHEIR, N. A. (ED.), *Systems Modeling and Computer Simulation,* New York: Marcel Dekker; 1988.

KLOSS, MARILYN B., "Beginner's Guide to the Advanced Continuous Simulation Language," Concord, MA: Mitchell & Gauthier Assoc.; 1990.

KOOTSEY, J. N., *"Introduction to Computer Simulation,"* Durham NC: Duke University Medical Center; Sept. 1989.

KORN, G. A. AND J. V. WAIT, *Digital Continuous-system Simulation,* Englewood Cliffs, NJ: Prentice Hall; 1978.

KORN, G. A., "One hundred differential equations on the IBM PC," *Simulation,* Vol. 45, No. 3; Sept. 1986.

MIKULECKY, D. C., ET AL, "A simple network thermodynamic method for modeling series-parallel coupled flows," Parts I & II; *Jl. Theor. Biol.,* Vol. 69, pp. 72–78; 1977.

MITCHELL, E. E. L., AND J. S. GAUTHIER, *Advanced Continuous Simulation Language (ACSL) Reference Manual,* Concord MA: Mitchell and Gauthier Associates; 1986.

MITCHELL, E. E. L., AND J. S. GAUTHIER, "Advanced continuous simulation language (ACSL)," *Simulation,* pp. 72–78; March, 1976.

NAGEL, L. W., "SPICE2—A computer program to simulate semiconductor circuits, Electronics Research Lab.;" *Memo. ERL-M520;* May 1975.

NILSEN, R. N., AND W. J. KARPLUS, "Continuous-system simulation languages: a state-of-the-art survey," *Proc. Intl. Assoc. for Analog Comp., (AICA),* Vol. 16, No. 1, pp. 17–25; January 1974.

RANDALL, J. E., *Microcomputers and Physiological Simulation,* (Second Edition), New York, Raven Press, 1987.

SIMULATION COUNCILS, INC., "Catalog of Simulation Software," *Simulation,* pp. 152–58; Oct. 1986.

SPECKHART, F. H. AND W. L. GREEN, *A Guide to using CSMP,* Englewood Cliffs, NJ: Prentice Hall; 1976.

SPRIET, J. C. AND G. C. VANSTEENKISTE, *Computer-Aided Modelling and Simulation,* (Chap. 6), New York: Academic Press; 1982.

STRAUSS, J. C. ET AL, "The SCI continuous system simulation language (CSSL)," *Simulation,* pp. 281–303; Dec. 1967.

TUINENGRA, P. W., *SPICE–A Guide to Circuit Simulation and Analysis using PSPICE,* Englewood Cliffs, NJ: Prentice Hall; 1976.

Appendix B
Laplace Transform Analysis

Among the mathematical transform methods that are useful in simulation studies are the use of Fourier transforms, Laplace transforms, Z-transforms, and Wiener kernels (Stremler-90, D'Azzo-81, Jury-64, Sakuranaga-86). These methods involve the integral transformation of variables in the equations describing a system. This transforms the system to a new domain in which the independent variable is replaced by another variable. Thus, in Fourier transformation, the variable time, in equations describing a linear system with sinusoidal inputs, is replaced by $j\omega$, where ω is frequency. This is convenient in many studies involving filtering, in communication engineering, for example (Stremler-90). Laplace transformation is related to Fourier transformation but is somewhat more powerful. Here the new variable, s, has a real part, σ, such that $s = \sigma + j\omega$, and Laplace transformation of the linear equations describing a system may be used to determine transient as well as steady-state response. Wiener kernel methods may be used to deal with certain nonlinear systems (Marmarelis-72).

The objective in all transform methods is to put the equations into a form that is more convenient to solve or is in some way more revealing of important aspects of the system. Some examples of simple applications are provided in this appendix.

The Laplace transform of a function $f(t)$ is defined as

$$L\{f(t)\} \equiv F(s) = \int_{0-}^{\infty} f(t)e^{-st}dt \tag{B.1}$$

where s is the complex variable $\sigma + j\omega$; its imaginary part is j times frequency, and its real part is large enough that the integral converges for most functions of practical interest. Note the use of 0− (zero minus) for the lower limit of the definite integral; this is important where $f(t)$ is an impulse centered at zero and for other such functions.

The power of the Laplace transform method in the solution of dynamic linear systems is dependent on the fact that it is easy to find the transforms of derivatives. Thus the Laplace transform of the first derivative of $f(t)$, df/dt, is

$$\begin{aligned} L\{df/dt\} &\equiv \int_{0-}^{\infty} (df/dt)e^{-st}dt \\ &= e^{-st}f(t) \Big|_{0-}^{\infty} + s\int_{0-}^{\infty} f(t)e^{-st}dt \\ &= sF(s) - f(0-) \end{aligned} \tag{B.2}$$

where $F(s)$ is the Laplace transform of $f(t)$, from (B.1), and $f(0-)$ is the initial value of $f(t)$. (Note that $f(t)$ cannot be some quantity raised to a power of t^2, or any other function that will increase faster than the real part of e^{-st}.)

The second derivative of $f(t)$ can be transformed in similar fashion, giving

$$L\{d^2f/dt^2\} = s^2F(s) - sf(0-) - df/dt(0-) \tag{B.3}$$

The transforms of several commonly occurring waveforms are also needed in order to solve for the response of system to various inputs. Note that we are using one-sided Laplace transforms, and are only concerned with waveforms (and solutions) that begin at, or after, $t = 0$. A simple example is the step function of amplitude A, starting at $t = 0$, $f(t) = Au(t)$, where $u(t)$ is the unit step function. Here

$$\begin{aligned} F(s) &= \int_{0-}^{\infty} Au(t)e^{-st}dt \\ &= -Ae^{-st}/s \Big|_{0-}^{\infty} = A/s \end{aligned} \tag{B.4}$$

The inverse transform of a unit impulse at $t = 0$, $\delta(t)$, is

$$L\{\delta(t)\} \equiv \int_{0-}^{\infty} \delta(t)e^{-st}dt = \int_{0-}^{0+} \delta(t)dt = 1 \tag{B.5}$$

Note that if the impulse is $A\delta(t)$, it has area A and will have a Laplace transform $L\{s\} = A$.

If a step function begins at time t_1, then $f(t) = Au(t - t_1)$, and it may be shown that

$$F(s) = Ae^{-st_1}/s \tag{B.6}$$

In general, a "dead-time" delay of τ appears as a multiplicative term $e^{-s\tau}$ in the transform and the transform of a delayed unit impulse $\delta(t - \delta)$ is $e^{-s\tau}$ and that of a delayed input step is $e^{-s\tau}/s$.

Rather than employing the method shown, based on the integral in (B.1) to find transform pairs (or the inverse transform, which is still more difficult to use), the transform pairs that are most needed may be found in tables that have been worked out (McCollum-65). A short table of this type is included at the end of this appendix.

Some of the expressions obtained above may be used to study the response of a simple system to various inputs. Suppose that we have a linear system that responds to a time domain input $f(t)$ with an output $g(t)$ according to the simple first-order differential equation

$$dg/dt = f - k*g \tag{B.7}$$

where k is a constant of the system. If we now take the Laplace transform of both sides of (B.7), then, for the case of zero initial conditions on g, we will obtain

$$sG = F - k*G, \qquad \text{or}$$

$$G = F/(s + k) \tag{B.8}$$

where F and G are the Laplace transforms of the time functions f and g.

The transfer function of this system in Laplace form is the output/input ratio

$$H(s) = G(s)/F(s) = 1/(s + k) \tag{B.9}$$

Here $H(s)$ is the impulse response of the system (in Laplace form); that is, it is the output G(s) for an input $F(s) = 1$, the transform of a unit impulse.

Input signal	System Impulse Response	Output signal
$f(t) = A\delta(t)$	$h(t) = e^{-kt}$	$g(t) = Ae^{-kt}$
Input transform	Transform of Impulse Response	Output transform
$F(s) = A$	$H = 1/(s + k)$	$G(s) = HA = A/(s + k)$

For another input that has a Laplace transform, the unit step $u(t)$, with transform $1/s$ the output transform will be $1/s(s + k)$. The inverse transform, from Table B.1, is $(1 - e^{-kt})/k$. The step response of a simple lag such as H is discussed is Section 3.2.

In the example given here the initial condition on $g(t)$ was assumed to be zero. To call attention to the inclusion of an initial condition, which is one of the strong points of the Laplace approach, consider Eq. (B.7). If the initial value of the output is $g(0)$, then the transformation will give

$$sG - g(0) = F - kG, \qquad \text{or}$$

$$G = (F + g(0))/(s + k) \tag{B.10}$$

If F is a unit step, then

$$G = \frac{1}{s(s + k)} + \frac{g(0)}{(s + k)} \tag{B.11}$$

TABLE B.1 A Short Table of Laplace Transform Pairs

	F(s)	$f(t)$, $t \geqq 0-$
1.	1	$\delta(t)$, unit impulse, at $t = 0$
2.	$1/s$	$u(t)$, unit step, at $t = 0$
3.	$1/s^2$	$tu(t)$, ramp function
4.	$e^{-s\tau}/s$	$u(t - \tau)$, unit step at τ
5.	$(1 - e^{-s\tau})/s$	$u(t) - u(t - \tau)$, rectangular pulse
6.	$1/(s + a)$	e^{-at}, exponential decay
7.	$1/s(s + a)$	$(1 - e^{-at})/a$
8.	$1/(s + a)(s + b)$	$(e^{-at}-e^{-bt})/(b - a)$
9.	$s/(s + a)(s + b)$	$(be^{-bt}-ae^{-at})/(b - a)$
10.	$1/s(s + a)(s + b)$	$\frac{1}{ab} + \frac{be^{-bt} - ae^{-bt}}{ab(a - b)}$
11.	$1/(s + a)(s + b)(s + c)$	$e^{-at}/(b - a)(c - a) + e^{-bt}/(c - b)(a - b) + e^{-ct}/(a - c)(b - c)$
12.	$1/\{(s + \alpha)^2 + \beta^2\}$	$(e^{-\alpha t}/\beta)\sin \beta t$
13.	$\frac{s}{(s + \alpha)^2 + \beta^2}$	$\frac{1}{\beta}(-\alpha \sin \beta t + \beta \cos \beta t)e^{-\alpha t}$
14.	$\frac{1}{s\{(s + \alpha)^2 + \beta^2\}}$	$\frac{1}{\alpha^2 + \beta^2} - \frac{e^{-\alpha t}}{\beta(\alpha^2 + \beta^2)}\{\alpha \sin \beta t + \beta \cos \beta t\}$

and the expression for $g(t)$ may be obtained by using two of the transform pairs (No. 7 and No. 6) in a table such as B.1 (McCollum-65, D'Azzo-81, Stremler-90).

Thus the procedure involved in the Laplace transform solution of problems involving linear ordinary differential equations often consists of algebraic manipulation and the use of a table of transforms, as shown for the simple cases above. Obtaining the solution in numerical or graphical form may be most conveniently done with a computer program. Since this may be done using numerical analysis applied directly to the original differential equations, a question may be asked as to the need for Laplace transform solutions. The answer is that the Laplace methods yield "closed-form" solutions in algebraic form, that may be meaningful and helpful to the investigator using them. Of course the vast majority of systems in physiological systems are nonlinear, and Laplace methods cannot be used; however, it is sometimes possible to linearize problems, under certain conditions, and to use transform methods to get approximate but useful general solutions in algebraic form (see Section 8.1).

REFERENCES

D'Azzo, J. J., and C. H. Houpis, *Linear Control System Analysis and Design*, Second Ed., Chapter 4; New York: McGraw-Hill; 1981.

JURY, ELIAHU I. *Theory and Application of the Z-transform Method,* New York: Wiley; 1964.

MARMARELIS, P. Z., AND K.-I. NAKA, "White-noise analysis of a neuron chain: an application of the Wiener Theory," *New England Jl. of Medicine,* Vol. 175, pp. 1276–78; 1972.

MCCOLLUM, P. A. AND B. F. BROWN, *Laplace Transform Tables and Theorems,* New York: Holt Rinehart & Winston; 1965.

SAKURANAGA, M. ET AL., "Nonlinear analysis: mathematical theory and biological applications," *Critical Reviews in Biomed. Eng.,* Vol. 14, Issue 2: pp. 127–84; 1986.

STREMLER, F. G. *Introduction to Communication Systems,* Chapter 3; Reading, Mass: Addison-Wesley; 1990.

Appendix C
Negative Feedback Control Systems

C.0 INTRODUCTION

Feedback control systems are briefly discussed in Section 2.3, with some references to books and papers dealing with both engineering and a biological systems of this type. Biological control systems are much more complex than the systems designed by engineers, but the basic notions, invented ages ago by nature but only recently by man, are much the same. This introduction to feedback control is necessarily brief, and the reader who has not had an introductory course in control may wish to refer to some standard text (Kuo-88, or D'Azzo-81). As discussed in Section 2.3, mathematical methods alone are of limited application in physiological system analysis, and much use of numerical methods and computer simulation is in general necessary in the study and modeling of physiological control systems (Bassingthwaighte-85). The synthesis and design of prosthetic control systems for a purpose such as the control of drug infusion are rather different and require that the designer be familiar with more advanced control theory (Jones-69, Katona-82, Harris-85, Nalecz-87, and Bar-Kana-87), and descriptions of advanced applications of control (Hardy-78, Steer-75, Jaklitsch-87 and Houk-88).

Closed-loop feedback control has many advantages over simple feedforward open-loop control. This is illustrated in Fig. C.0.1 by the comparison of simple open- and closed-loop control of a system of gain G_s, in which the output C should be caused to follow an input signal, R (in a

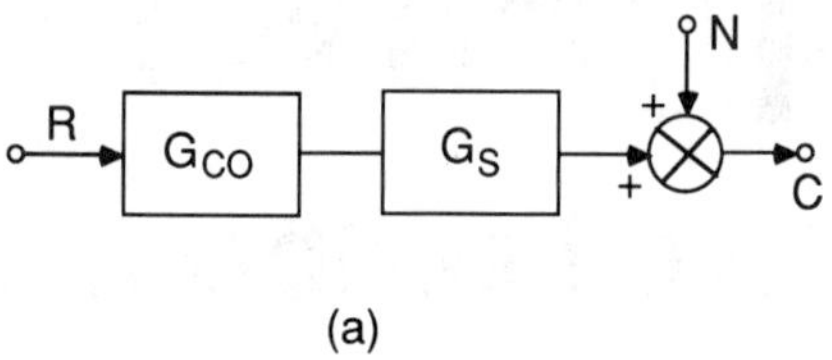

(a)

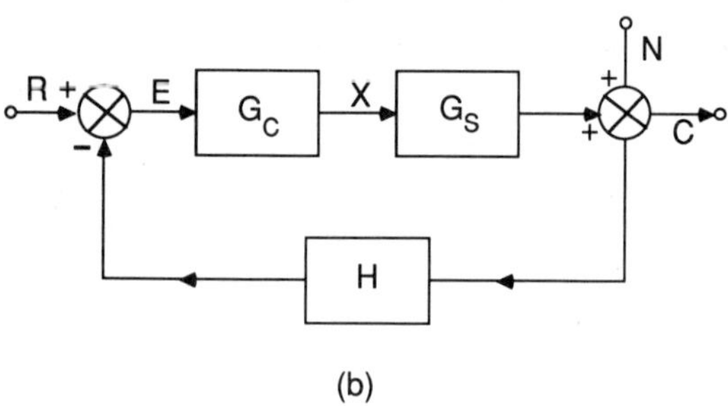

(b)

Figure C.0.1. (a) Feed-forward or open-loop control of a system of gain G_S. (b) Negative feedback control of a system of gain G_S.

follow-up system), or settle to a value equal to a constant, R (in a regulator), despite noise or other problems in the system being controlled.

In the open-loop case, if a controller G_{co} is added as shown in Fig. C.0.1a, the output will be

$$C = G_{co}{*}G_s{*}R + N \tag{C.0.1}$$

where we consider only the frequencies in R for which G_{co} and G_p are at a maximum constant value, and N is any noise or disturbance, effectively added in at the output.

In the closed-loop or negative feedback case shown in Fig. C.0.1b, if the noise N is zero and if it is assumed that the system, controller, and feedback blocks have constant gains, the error E is

$$E = R - H{*}C \tag{C.0.2}$$

But $C = G_c{*}G_s{*}E$, and if this is used in (C.0.2) to eliminate E,

$$C = \frac{G_c{*}G_s{*}R}{1 + G_c{*}G_s{*}H} \tag{C.0.3}$$

Here it is interesting to examine the case for which the "loop gain" or gain around the closed loop, $G_c{*}G_s{*}H$, is much greater than unity, so that

$$C \approx G_c{*}G_s{*}R/(G_c{*}G_s{*}H) = R/H \tag{C.0.4}$$

Thus, for large loop gains, the output depends only on the input R, and the feedback H, which may be a passive constant (and is often simply unity, if $C \approx R$ is desired).

The noise output N_o due to the disturbance N in the closed-loop case may be solved for independently, since we have assumed a linear system in which superposition holds. Here the output noise only (with $R = 0$) will be

$$N_o = G_c*G_s*E + N \quad \text{(C.0.5)}$$

Since $E = -H*N_o$, substitution in (C.0.5) and elimination of E give

$$N_o = N/(1 + G_c*G_s*H) \quad \text{(C.0.6)}$$

Here it may be seen that the effect of the negative feedback is to reduce the output noise, particularly if the loop gain is large.

It is interesting to examine the effect of negative feedback as given by the important equation (C.0.3) for a numerical case. If we choose $H =$ 1 (so that $C \approx R$), and if $G_c*G_s = 100$, then

$$C = 100*R/(1 + 100) = 0.99009*R \quad \text{(C.0.7)}$$

which shows that C follows R within 1 percent. (Note, however, that this result only holds for steady-state or very low frequency inputs; transient response is discussed in the next section.)

If the controlled system changes gain by 5 percent, then

$$C = 105*R/(1 + 105) = 0.99056*R \quad \text{(C.0.8)}$$

Thus the effect of a 5 percent change in the gain of G_s, is less than 0.05 percent, whereas it would be 5 percent in the nonfeedback case. Furthermore, N_o will be equal to $N/101$, and thus reduced to less than 1 percent of its value without feedback.

C.1 TRANSIENT RESPONSE OF LINEAR CONTROL SYSTEMS

The simple analysis of the preceding section provides no information on the time-domain response of control systems. Here we shall examine linear system response and, in a later section, some of the problems of stability.

If the controller and the system in Fig. C.0.1b are simple low-pass (or first-order lag) devices, their transfer functions may be expressed in Laplace notation as

$$G_c = C_{co}/(1 + sT_c) \quad \text{(C.1.1)}$$

$$G_s = G_{co}/(1 + sT_s) \quad \text{(C.1.2)}$$

The loop gain of the system will be

$$G_{\text{loop}} = G_{co}*G_{so}*H/\{(1 + sT_c)*(1 + sT_s)\} \quad \text{(C.1.3)}$$

Substitution of (C.1.1) and (C.1.2) in the basic control system equation (C.0.1) gives, after some reduction

$$C(s) = \frac{G_{co}*G_{so}*R(s)}{(1 + G_{co}*G_{so}) + s(T_c + T_s) + s^2 T_c*T_s} \quad \text{(C.1.4)}$$

where $H = 1$, and $R(s)$ is the Laplace transform of the input $r(t)$.

If $G_{co} = 10.0$, $G_{so} = 1.0$, $T_c = 2.0$, and $T_s = 5.0$, then the control system transfer function (C.1.4) gives

$$C(s) = 10.0*R(s)/(21.0 + 7.0s + 10.0s^2)$$
$$= \frac{1.0*R(s)}{(s + 0.35)^2 + 0.9887^2} \quad \text{(C.1.5)}$$

Using transform pair 12 in Appendix B, for the case where the input is a unit impulse, $R(s) = 1$, (C.1.5) gives a time-domain response c_i, where

$$c_i = 1.011*\epsilon^{-.35t}* \sin(0.9887t) \quad \text{(C.1.6)}$$

Similarly, for a unit step function input, $R_s = 1/s$, transform pair 14 in Appendix B gives

$$c_s = 0.9091 + e^{-0.35t}*[0.3218*\sin(0.9887*t)$$
$$+ 0.9091 * \cos(0.9887*t)] \quad \text{(C.1.7)}$$

The system discussed above has response to an impulse, from (C.1.6), and to a step input, from (C.1.7), as shown in Figs. C.1.1a and C.1.1b. These results can be determined either by use of FORTRAN, BASIC, or PASCAL from (C.1.6) and (C.1.7), or they can be obtained more directly from the original equations using an ACSL or similar time-domain program; for the impulse case, using ACSL, a program may easily be written using the methods discussed in Appendix A. This has been done in the program CTL below; the step response may be found in the same way, except that the constant RS = 1.0 is substituted for the approximation to an impulse, RI, and the solution for the output to a unit input step, CS is obtained in the same program with CI, the impulse response.

```
PROGRAM CTL
 DYNAMIC
   Cinterval CINT=.05
   Constant TF=15.
   TERMT (T .GE. TF)
  DERIVATIVE
   Maxterval MAXT=.001
   Nsteps NSTEP=1
```

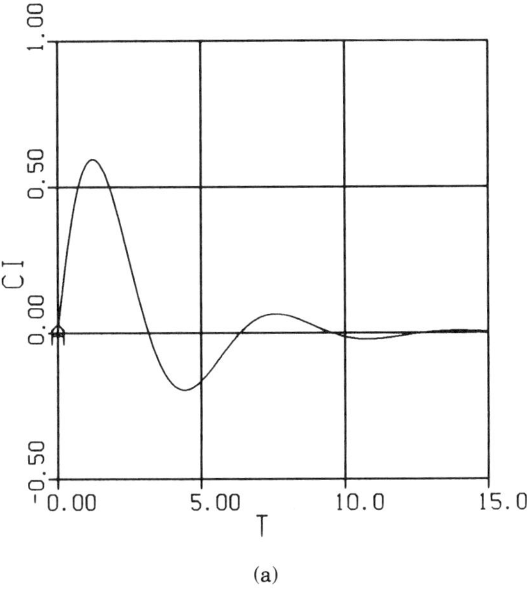

(a)

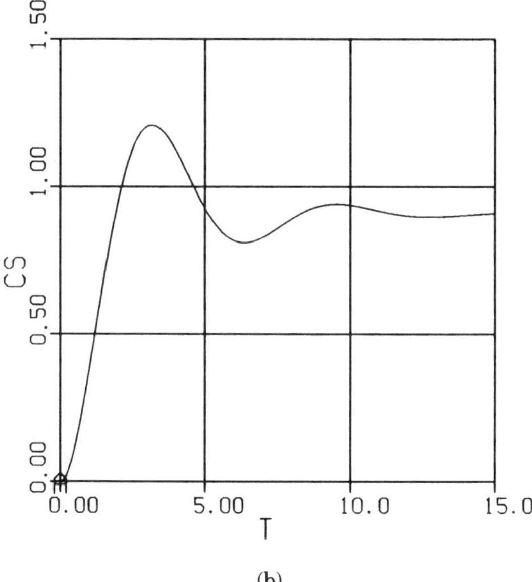

(b)

Figure C.1.1. (a) Response CI of the system of program CTL to an input unit impulse.
(b) Response CS of the system to an input unit step.

```
'Response,CI, to unit impulse input, RI'
   Constant GC=10.                    $'GC = Gco*Gso'
   RI = 200.*PULSE(0.0,1.E10,.005)    $'Impulse Approx.'
   XI = GC*REALPL(2.0, RI-CI, 0.0)
   CI = REALPL(5.0, XI, 0.0)          $'Impulse Response'
'Response,CS, to unit step input, RS'
   RS = 1.
   XS = GC*REALPL(2.0, RS-CS, 0.0)
   CS = REALPL(5.0, XS, 0.0)          $'Step Response'
  END   $'Of Derivative'
 END    $'Of Dynamic'
END     $'Of Program'
```

Note that in the case of a unit step input the output of this system settles at CS = 0.9091 (or 10/11). This system, called a type 0 system because it has no integrators in the loop, will always have a final error of this kind, although it will be reduced if the maximum loop gain is increased.

Another common kind of control system (called a type 1 system) includes a single integration in the loop, as in the case of the example in Fig. A.1. In theory, such a system will settle to zero error for a step input, although minor nonlinearities may result in small final error.

C.2 STABILITY OF CONTROL SYSTEMS

If the components of a linear feedback system are set up to give positive feedback, and if the loop gain is greater than unity, oscillations will appear and increase exponentially in amplitude until some limiting due to overload is reached. Thus, if the feedback is made positive in the program CONTROL of Sec. C.1 (by changing RI − CI in the XI command to RI + CI), growing oscillations will appear unless GC is reduced from its present value of 10.0 to a value less than unity.

Simple negative feedback control systems may also become unstable and oscillate if the gain around the loop exceeds unity at a frequency for which the phase shift is 180°. This amount of phase shift amounts to sign reversal, converting negative feedback to positive.

Program CONTROL as presented in Section C.1 is quite stable, because the maximum phase shift possible is only 90° in each simple lag, and the total phase shift only reaches 180° at infinite frequency, where gain will be reduced to zero. But, if some additional element with a negative phase shift is placed in the loop, instability may occur. It will be interesting to add a transport delay to this system and to examine its effect on stability.

To deal conveniently with linear transfer functions in stability studies, it is helpful to use the Fourier transform in place of the Laplace transform (Stremler-90). This may be readily accomplished if we substitute $j\omega$ for s in expressions where it appears. Thus, for a simple first-order lag, $1/(1 + sT_a)$, the Fourier transform or frequency domain expression is

$$\frac{1}{1 + j\omega T_a} = \frac{1}{1 + j\omega/\omega_a} * \frac{1 - j\omega/\omega_a}{1 - j\omega/\omega_a} = \frac{\underline{/-\tan^{-1}\omega/\omega_a}}{\sqrt{1 + (\omega/\omega_a)^2}} \tag{C.1.2}$$

where $\omega = 1/T_a$ is the characteristic (or "corner") frequency (in radians/s), and electrical engineering notation is used for the phase angle, a lagging phase shift of $\tan^{-1}\omega/\omega_a$.

Similarly, a transport lag of T_1 with input $x(t)$ has a time-domain output

$$y = x(t - T_1) \tag{C.2.2}$$

In the s-domain of Laplace transforms

$$Y(s) = X(s)\epsilon^{-sT_1} \tag{C.2.3}$$

whence, in the frequency domain

$$Y(jw) = X(j\omega)\epsilon^{-\omega T_1} \tag{C.2.4}$$

Transport delays are common in the systems of the human body, in nerves, and in fluids carrying substances. Such delays are often troublesome in the body's control systems because they can cause instability in control loops. Let us now examine a linear control system loop of program CTL with its two simple lags and an added transport delay of 0.5 unit of time, as shown in Fig. C.2.1.

In this system the loop gain and phase is

$$G_{\text{loop}}(j\omega) = \frac{10 \underline{/-\tan^{-1}2\omega - \tan^{-1}5\omega - 0.5\omega}}{\sqrt{1 + 4\omega^2} * \sqrt{1 + 25\omega^2}} \tag{C.2.5}$$

There are graphical methods for finding the gain and phase shift versus frequency curves and determining stability, and these graphs may also be determined by use of an ACSL program (see the *ACSL Manual* referred to in Appendix A). In this simple case we do not need to use the more formal Nyquist criteria (Kuo-88; D'Azzo-81), and can determine stability by setting

$$\sqrt{1 + 4\omega^2} * \sqrt{1 + 25\omega^2} = 10.0 \tag{C.2.6}$$

and using the marginal value of ω (for unity loop gain) so determined in the expression for phase shift appearing in (C.2.5). If the calculated nega-

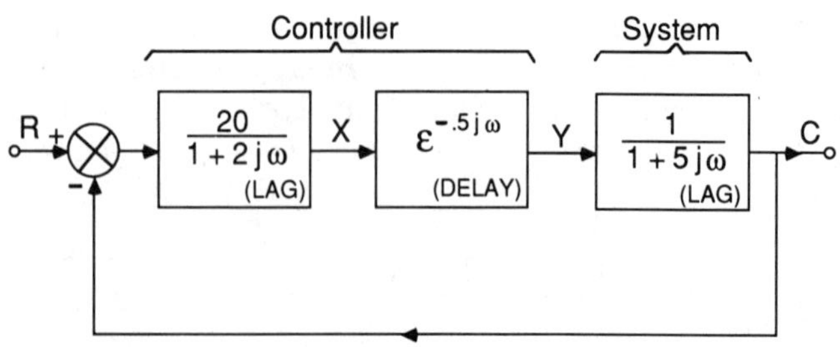

Figure C.2.1. A simple negative feedback control system with two first-order lags and a transport delay in the loop. Here GC = 20.0 (gain at W = 0.0).

tive phase shift is equal to or greater than 180°, then growing oscillations may be expected.

It is helpful to study stability in a system using a time-domain program such as ACSL, and this may be done for the system of program CTL by adding the command for transport delay

$$\begin{aligned} &Y = \text{DELAY}(XI, 0.0, TD, 5000) \\ &\text{Constant } TD = 2.0 \end{aligned} \tag{C.2.7}$$

and changing the command for CI to

$$C = \text{REALPL}(5.0, Y, 0.0) \tag{C.2.8}$$

This change, which can also be made in the step response commands, will be found to add considerably to the oscillatory nature of the responses. This can best be studied with a parameter sweep program, which will be called CTL-SWP, giving delays ranging from TD = 0.2 to 1.6 in steps of 0.2. The program for CTL-SWP (for step input only and with GC = 5.0) follows:

```
PROGRAM CTL-SWP
  INITIAL
     Constant TDIN=0.2, DTD=0.20, TDM=1.6
     TD = TDIN
     L1..CONTINUE
  END $ 'Of Initial'
  DYNAMIC
     Cinterval CINT=0.1
     Constant TF = 15.0
     TERMT (T .GE. TF)
   DERIVATIVE
     Maxterval MAXT=.01 $ Nsteps NSTP = 1
     R = 1.0
     Constant GC=5.0
```

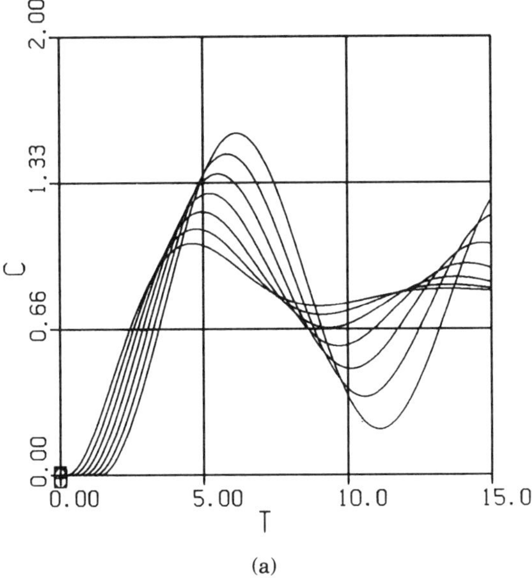

(a)

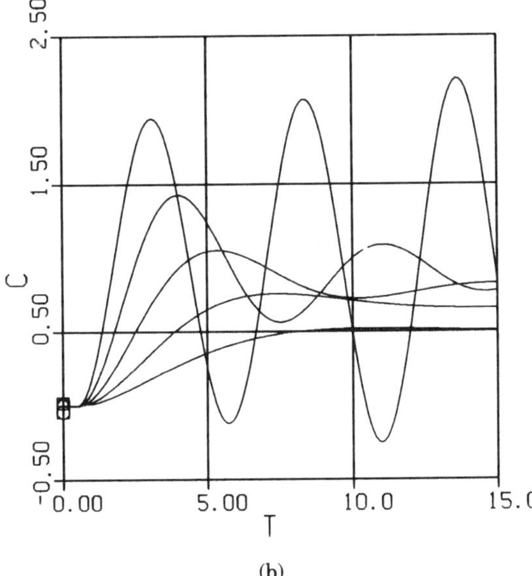

(b)

Figure C.2.2. (a) Step response C of the system of program CTL-SWP for a sweep of delay through values TD = 0.2.,0.4.,0.6.,0.8,1.0,1.2,1.4, with controller gain fixed at GC = 5.0.
(b) Step response of the same system to a sweep of controller gain through values GC = 1.0,2.0,4.0,8.0, and 16.0, with TD = 0.0, using program CTL-GAIN, (see Problem C.1).

```
          X = GC * REALPL(2.0,R - C, 0.0)
          Y = DELAY (X, 0.0, TD, 5000)
          C  = REALPL(5.0, Y, 0.0)     $ 'Step response'
        END $'Of Deriv.'
      END  $'Of Dynamic'
      TERMINAL
        CALL LOGD(.TRUE.)
        TD = TD + DTD
        IF (TD .LE. TDM) GO TO L1
      END  $'Of Terminal'
    END    $'Of Program'
```

The response of this system as given by the program CTL-SWP is shown in Fig. C.2.2a. It can be seen that the response for the largest delay (TD = 1.4) is close to being a continuing oscillation. A similar program may be used to study effects of controller gain increase as shown in Fig. C.2.2b.

PROBLEMS

C.1. Re-run CTL with GC = 5.0 and with GC = 20.0 and compare with Fig. C.1.1.

C.2. Write a program CTL-GAIN as a modification of program CTL-SWP with TD = 0.0, using a sweep of GC from 1.0 to 16.0; check your results against the output C shown in Fig. C.2.2b.

C.3. Repeat Problem C.2 with TD = 0.4.

C.4. Repeat Problem C.3 with some derivative feedback.

REFERENCES

BAR-KANA, I., "Adaptive control—a simplified approach," in *Advances in Control and Dynamic Systems,* C. T. Leondes (Ed.), Vol. 25; Reading, MA: Addison-Wesley; 1987.

BASSINGTHWAIGHTE, J. B. "Using computer models to understand complex systems," *The Physiologist,* Vol. 28, No. 5, pp. 439–42; 1985.

D'AZZO, J. J. AND C. H. HOUPIS, *Linear Control System Analysis and Design,* 2nd Ed., New York: McGraw-Hill; 1981.

HARDY, J. G., A. P. GAGGE AND J. A. J. STOLWIJK, (EDS.), *Physiological and behavioral temperature regulation,* Springfield IL: Chas. C. Thomas; 1978.

HARRIS, C. J. AND S. A. BILLINGS, (EDS.), *Self-Tuning and Adaptive Control: Theory and Applications,* (2nd Ed.); New York: Peregrinus; 1985.

HOUK, JAMES C., "Control strategies in physiological systems," *FASEB* Vol. 2, pp. 97–107; 1988.

JAKLITSCH, R. R. AND D. R. WESTENSKOW, "A model-based self-adjusting 2-phase controller for vecuronium-induced muscle relaxation during anesthesia," *IEEE-TBME,* Vol. BME-34, No. 8, pp. 583–94; Aug. 1987.

JONES, RICHARD W., "Biological control mechanisms," Chap. 2 in *Biological Engineering,* H. P. Schwan (Ed.); New York: McGraw-Hill; 1969.

KATONA, P. G., "On-line control of physiological variables and clinical therapy," *CRC Rev. Bio. Engg.,* Vol. 8, Issue 4, pp. 281–310; 1982.

KUO, B. C., *Automatic Control Systems,* Englewood Cliffs, NJ: Prentice-Hall; 1988.

NALECZ, M., (ED.), *Control Aspects of Biomedical Engineering,* Oxford: Pergamon Press; 1987.

STEER, E. B., "Application of control theory to endocrine regulation and control," *Annals Biomed. Engg.,* Vol. 3, pp. 439–55; 1975.

STREMLER, F. G., *Introduction to communication systems,* Reading MA: Addison-Wesley; 1990.

Appendix D

Model Programs

A computer disk containing a copy of each ACSL model program developed and discussed in the book may be ordered (see order form in the back of this book). This was done to make it more easily possible for anyone using the book to enter these ACSL programs into any computer equipped with the requisite software.

ACSL is presently available for use in about 20 different machines, ranging from PCs, such as the IBM/AT and its clones, to the Cray-XMP. The programs provided on disk are in the form used in machines (such as PCs) using the DOS operating system, and have the extension .CSL with the 3-symbol limit of DOS. In larger machines using the UNIX operating system the end-of-line indicators are different, and some program such as the netware program DOS2UNIX must be used to strip off DOS and add UNIX end-of-line indicators. Also, the extension .ACSL may be used with UNIX.

Because some of the programs (such as PF−0, PF−1, PF−1−REG and PF−1−BP) require 18 or more integrators, it is not convenient to use the ACSL Classroom Kit (limited to 12 integrators) or other differential-equation-solving programs if they are limited to less than 30 integrators. Also, a convenient plotting capability such as that provided with ACSL is essential.

A list of the model programs in this text, (and provided on the disk) follows, with a descriptive addition to each title included, together with the section in which each program appears. Command (CMD) programs to make it more easily possible to duplicate results shown in this text are included for several of the ACSL programs (see Appendix A).

Program	Section	Description
CONSYS.CSL	App.A	Control system—a first ACSL exercise
CONSYS.CMD	App.A	Output command program for CONSYS
COMPART1.CSL	3.2	Single compartment with diffusion
COMPART1.CMD	3.2	Output command program for COMPART1
COMPART2.CSL	3.2	Parameter sweep in a compartment model
COMPART2.CMD	3.2	Output command program for COMPART2
FLOTRAN1.CSL	3.3	Flow transport in an open-loop system
FLOTRAN1.CMD	3.3	Output command program for FLOTRAN1
IND-DIL1.CSL	3.4	Indicator tranport in a CV loop
IND-DIL2.CSL	3.4	Effects of a VSD in a CV loop
IND-DIL3.CSL	3.4	Parameter sweep in a CV loop with VSD
IND-DIL3.CMD	3.4	Output command program for IND-DIL3
IND-DIL4.CSL	3.4	Indicators used to find CO and Volume
ENZ-MM1.CSL	3.6	Enzyme (Michaelis-Menten) studies
LH-PF-1.CSL	4.2	Model of left heart and systemic flow
LH-PF-2.CSL	4.2	LH-PF-1 with improved heart simulation
LH-PF-3.CSL	4.2	LH-PF-2 with improved valve modeling
LH-PF-3.CMD	4.2	Output command program for LH-PF-3
PF-0.CSL	4.3	Pressure-flow model of simple CV loop
PF-1.CSL	4.3	Improved model of the CV loop
PF-1.CMD	4.3	Output command program for PF-1
PF-1-REG.CSL	4.5	Baroreceptor control added to PF-1
PF-NP.CSL	4.6	Non-pulsatile model of the CV loop
RESP-PF.CSL	5.2	Respiratory system PF model
RESP-OX.CSL	5.3	Oxygen transport added to RESP-PF
RESP.CMD	5.2,5.3	Output command program for RESP-PF or RESP-OX
MULMOD3.CSL	6.1	Multiple model using LH-PF-3
THERMO.CSL	7.3	Thermal diffusion and regulation
B-FLUID.CSL	8.1	Fluid balance and hypertension
B-FLUID.CMD	8.1	Output command program for B-FLUID
PF-1-BP.CSL	8.2	Balloon pumping in the human aorta
GLUC-TOL.CSL	8.3	Glucose tolerance testing
PAREST1.CSL	9.2	Global parameter estimation
PAREST2.CSL	9.3	Pattern methods of parameter estimation
PAREST2.CMD	9.3	Output command program for PAREST2
CTL.CSL	App.C	Control system
CTL-SWP.CSL	App.C	Sweep study of a control system

Index

Thank you for purchasing this book.

The publisher would like to offer you the opportunity to obtain the applications and examples in this book on diskette.

To save keyboard input time, all of the applications and examples in this book are available on the disk. Each application has the original template(s), named ranges, program(s), etc., Described in the book.

To send for the *Mathematical and Computer Modeling of Physiological Systems* disk, just photo copy this page, fill out the information completely and return to the address listed below. Thank you.

Date Purchased: ____________

Name: ____
Title: ____
School/Company: ____
Department: ____
Street Address: ____
City: ________________ State: ________________ Zip: ________________
Telephone: ( )____

Ben R. Colt
College Marketing
Prentice Hall
Englewood Cliffs, NJ 07632